PEDIATRIC

NEUROLOGY

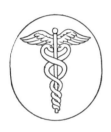

PEDIATRIC

NEUROLOGY

STANLEY S. LAMM, M.D.

Clinical Professor of Pediatrics, State University of New York,
College of Medicine at New York City

Neurological Consultant, Pediatric Dept., Kings County Hospital,
(State Univ. Div.) Brooklyn, N. Y.

Formerly Instructor in Neurology, Long Island College of Medicine,
Brooklyn, N. Y.

Director, Cerebral Palsy Clinic, Long Island College Hospital,
Brooklyn, N. Y.

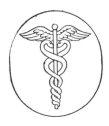

LANDSBERGER MEDICAL BOOKS · INC·

New York

TO MY WIFE AND MY SON

PREFACE

The specialty of pediatrics has been influenced by various branches of medicine in the past thirty-five years, the period of the author's experience. In the twenties, emphasis was placed on the changing patterns of infant feeding and the application of biochemistry. During the thirties, the scope of pediatric care was further enlarged by the utilization of psychiatric principles in the raising of children. In recent years the nervous system has received intensive study.

The author believes that the relationship between pediatrics and neurology is constantly growing closer, and he has endeavored to point out the influence upon each other of recent advances in both fields. Examples of allied disorders in which much has been learned in the past decade include cerebral palsy, epilepsy, and those related to inborn errors of metabolism. In like manner both specialties have benefited by the increased knowledge of the effects on brain development of such prenatal factors as anoxia, infection, radiation, and Rh incompatibility.

Detailed anatomy of the nervous system has not been included since many excellent texts of neuroanatomy are available. However, the anatomy and physiology required for understanding certain specific diseases are described. For similar reasons a separate section on the neurologic examination of the child has likewise been omitted. The method of performing a specific neurological test and its significance are described as indicated in the discussion of the individual diseases. Included also are descriptions of reflexes, both normal and pathological, and an outline of normal motor development. As Crothers has pointed out, however, the approach toward the examination of the infant and child should be one of observation of physiologic and spontaneous behavior rather than a compilation of the conventional neurologic signs to fit a classic syndrome. In the chapter on cerebral palsy there is a detailed description of history taking, which may be suitably applied to any neurological condition. Comment on electroencephalography is made in the presentation of epilepsy, and the meaning and value of electrodiagnosis and electromyography are covered in the chapter on diseases of muscle.

In disorders in which therapy is of great value, specific treatment and daily management have been outlined in detail. Some of the diseases in this group are the meningitides and encephalitides, cerebral palsy, epilepsy, intracranial birth injury, lead encephalopathy, and certain brain tumors.

While a classification of diseases is necessary, it is never wholly satisfactory since some disorders cannot at present be properly categorized. In fact, it is often more effective to group together those conditions which require differentiation, even though they may be of different origin. Diseases which are brought in only as a part of differential diagnosis are not listed in the table of contents; their location may be found in the index.

I should like to express my appreciation to the members of my department and others of the faculty of the State University Medical School who read some of the chapters and offered valuable advice. I also wish to thank Dr. S. Aaronson, Professor of Neuropathology, State University Medical School and Dr. T. Morrione, Director of Pathology, Long Island College Hospital, for their permission to use some of their pictures. I am indebted to Dr. R. Pinck and Dr. D. Rosenblum for the use of X-ray films taken from their department at the Long Island College Hospital. I am also grateful to my publisher Mr. E. K. Georg Landsberger, for his cooperation.

CONTENTS

Thallium
Diphtheria
Diabetes
Reaction of the Nervous System following Injections of Sera, Vaccines,
    Drugs, and Antibiotics
Neuropathy of the Facial Nerve (Bell's Palsy)

Cranial
Spinal Column (Cord)
Peripheral Nerves
Tetanus

Gaucher's (Infantile)
Familial Amauroses

Electrodiagnosis and Electromyography
Amyotonia Congenita
Infantile Progressive Muscular Atrophy (Werdnig-Hoffman)
Arthrogryposis Multiplex Congenita
Muscular Dystrophy
Chronic Progressive External Ophthalmoplegia
Myotonia Atrophica
Myotonia Congenita (Thomsen)

Intracranial Aneurysms
Venous Angiomas
Telangiectases
Vascular Malformations of the Spinal Cord
Cerebral Embolism and Thrombosis
Hypertension

                 BLOOD DISORDERS

PEDIATRIC

NEUROLOGY

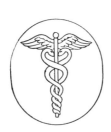

CHAPTER 1

MENTAL GROWTH AND DEVELOPMENT

The transmission of mental and physical qualities is based on inheritance. However, the development of the embryo and fetus depends not only on genetic forces, but also upon the influence of the prenatal and natal environment. The latter is expressed in good part through the health of the mother during her pregnancy.

MEDICAL GENETICS

The fertilized ovum or zygote contains 48 chromosomes within its nucleus, 24 from each parent. Variations in total number have been reported. The chromosomes differ somewhat in size and shape. However, 46 of them are arranged into pairs, forming 23 similar or homologous pairs, lying opposite each other in the nucleus. These are referred to as autosomal chromosomes. The 24th pair contains the sex chromosomes. In the female there is a pair of like sex chromosomes (X-chromosomes), one from each parent, whereas the male contains a pair of unlike sex chromosomes, an X from the mother and a smaller Y-chromosome from the father. Experimental evidence suggests that desoxyribonucleic acid (DNA) present within the chromatin of the nucleus is the genetic transmitter.

Within the chromosomes are located the genes. Just as the chromosomes are arranged in homologous pairs, so too the genes, which carry the inherited characters or traits, occupy definite places or loci within the chromosome. They similarly are arranged as partners, each member of the pair of genes being referred to as an allele. When the alleles of a pair are different, the individual is heterozygous for the gene; a person is homozygous when the alleles of a pair are similar. Many traits or characters may be due to the interplay of multiple genes, or a single gene may affect more than one trait. There are also modifying genes; hence, multiple ab-

3

normalities in a child may be due to single gene effects, or to other genes which modify the single gene effect, or to multiple genes. Also, in rare instances, a gene may become pathologic through mutation. In these cases the results are liable to be severe.

The external appearance of the individual is referred to as his phenotype. It is the result of the interaction of his genetic constitution (genotype) fixed at the time of fertilization and his environment in the course of embryonic development. It follows that the phenotype is not necessarily an indication of the genotype.

We have referred to the genotypic interplay of genes which may affect the appearance or phenotype. The environmental factors include nutrition, infection, hormones, and the characteristics of the various organs in man. There thus may be a variety of gene effects appearing in different organs based on the genotype and environment.

Forms of Inheritance

Dominant Inheritance. In this form, the effect of one allele of a pair of genes prevails over the other. The dominant gene, therefore, expresses the trait or character in a heterozygous individual. In dominant inheritance either one of the parents always exhibits the trait or disease. This parent will transmit the disease to 50 per cent of the children. The offspring who are free of the trait will produce normal children, if they marry a person free of the trait. This, of course, presupposes all other conditions are satisfactory.

Dominant Transmission (Heterozygous) 1:1 Ratio

Dd × dd   D-dominant
d-recessive

Offspring Dd (50%) show the trait D
dd (50%) normal phenotype and genotype

In the general population D usually occurs in a heterozygous individual. It is likely to be a rare abnormality if pathological, and therefore occurs in only one parent, the other allele transmitted to the child being recessive. If, however, it is frequent, then it may be both heterozygous Dd and homozygous DD (the last might be lethal as in Ichthyosis congenita).

Recessive Inheritance. The recessive gene does not express itself in the presence of the dominant allele, so that its effect or phenotype can only be evident when there are two recessive alleles; in other words, the person is homozygous for the pair. In this type the parents appear normal and do not show the trait, each one carrying a recessive allele. They are carriers.

Recessive transmission (Heterozygous) 3:1 Ratio

Dd × Dd   D-dominant
d-recessive

Offspring: DD   Dd   Dd   dd-homozygous recessive.

In this case, the heterozygous parents, who are carriers, produce according to the Mendelian ratio of 3:1, that is, there is one chance in four of the same recessive abnormality (gene) appearing in any one sibling of the affected individuals. This is especially noted when there is parental consanguinity, for this increases the chances of a child's receiving the same gene from each parent.

In summary, recessive abnormalities appear only in the homozygous state. They are rare and because of the small size of families are likely to show up sporadically. When they occur, the abnormality is usually severe. Consanguinity, by bringing together heterozygous members of the same family, increases the potential for the more rare recessive abnormality to occur.

Sex-Linked Inheritance. The female has two X-chromosomes, one from each parent. The male pair contains one X-chromosome from the mother and a Y-chromosome from the father. The latter is relatively less active and does not inhibit its X allele. In sex-linked recessive inheritance it is the male who inherits the genetic trait. In a female the recessive X cannot be effective in the presence of its dominant allele, whereas in the male, even though X is recessive, it is unopposed by its allele, the less active Y-chromosome. The females are thus heterozygous carriers, who themselves are unaffected and appear normal. As a result, male siblings of the affected male may also show the trait (50:50 chance). It is also evident that fathers will not transmit the effect directly to their sons, but to their daughters—these in turn will transmit the trait to their sons, since they themselves are unaffected carriers. One-half of the sons will be affected and one-half of the daughters will be carriers.

Sex-linked dominant inheritance is characterized by the fact that daughters of affected males will show the trait, but not the sons, since the father gives his X-chromosome to his daughter only, whereas the son gets his X-chromosome from the mother.

Y-chromosome inheritance is rare. It occurs only in males, being passed from father to son.

Genetic Inheritance. The genetic type of inheritance is mentioned in the course of the discussion of the various diseases as they are taken up in this book. This brief description of terminology has been offered, not only to promote better understanding of the inheritance pattern of a particular condition such as muscular dystrophy, optic atrophy, Friedreich's ataxia, etc., but also to encourage that it be considered in taking a history of the family. The history should include the illnesses of the parents of the patient, and the condition of each of the siblings. There should also be a statement of any consanguinous marriages by the parents or relatives and any abnormalities among the latter.

In estimating the risk of another child's being affected similarly to the patient, the presence of small families must be considered. This factor alters the normal calculations. It must also be recognized that in the general population there are mixtures of dominant and recessive alleles. The latter if rare may not appear for generations. Sporadic cases also occur. At times, a dominant may mutate to a recessive gene. Another consideration is the factor of penetrance, which refers to the degree with which a dominant gene expresses itself. If the frequency with which a pathologic gene produces clinical abnormality is diminished, it is referred to as reduced penetrance, which may cause the disease state to be skipped for a generation in some families. Other genes may show irregular dominance in that they show variability of expression in different individuals and also reduced penetrance.

SUMMARY: A long pedigree is necessary before a decision is made whether an allele is dominant or recessive. If there is a definite hereditary disease, the ratio of 3:1 for a Dd × Dd Recessive or 1:1 for a Dd × dd Dominant marriage may be used to predict the disease in the offspring in terms of a 25 per cent or 50 per cent risk. This risk rate of one in four for recessive inheritance and one in two for dominant, repeats itself with each new pregnancy. Statistical risk rates may be referred to, which take into account the size of the family, correcting for the small sized ones. The other factors previously discussed should also be considered.

With this knowledge, some advice may be offered the parents as to the potential risk of another child's having the same defect, the seriousness of the latter, etc. Since the physician cannot tell the exact order or the exact character of the next offspring, but only what the general risks are, he should leave the decision as to what action to take to the parents.

Childs, B. and Sidbury, Jr., J. B.: A survey of Genetics as it applies to Problems in Medicine. Supplement to Pediatrics, No. I, Part II, 20:177, 1957.

Ford, C. E. and Hamerton, J. L.: The Chromosomes of Man. Nature 178:1020, 1956.

Fraser, F. C. J.: Medical Genetics in Pediatrics. Pediat. 44:85, 1954.

Halpern, S.: Human Heredity and Mental Deficiency. Am. J. Ment. Def. 51:153, 1946.

Neel, J. V.: The Clinical Detection of the Genetic Carriers of Inherited Disease. Medicine 26:115, 1947.

Reed. S. C.: Counseling in Medical Genetics. Philadelphia, W. B. Saunders Co. 1955.

Sorsby, A.: Clinical Genetics. St. Louis, C. V. Mosby Company, 1953.

Warkany, J. and Fraser, F. C.: The Role of Genetics and other Prenatal Factors in Disorders of Childhood. Summary of Round Table Discussion. Pediat. 18:314, 1956.

ENVIRONMENT

In addition to genetic inheritance, environmental factors acting prenatally also influence mental development and the occurrence of congenital malformations; hence a congenital disease may be inherited or acquired through environmental influences: an example is microcephaly. It should also be remembered that not all inherited conditions are congenital, some appearing in later life. Natal and postnatal factors may also exert an influence on mental development.

Prenatal. These are environmental influences operating during pregnancy, which may exert a profound effect upon the embryo and fetus. The period of gestation is of marked importance. An abnormal factor, such as anoxia or infection, if active in the first trimester of pregnancy, the period when there is organ differentiation, may produce congenital malformation in the brain or other organs of the body. If severe enough, it may produce death of the embryo. At a later period of pregnancy, when the various organs of the fetus are already formed, the same abnormal factor may produce only general lack of normal development with subsequent evidence of mental deficiency. Not only may different results ensue in the same organ by virtue of the period of gestation, but different organs may be involved in various degrees.

Ingalls has used a low pressure chamber to induce anomalies in the young of pregnant mice. The latter were left for five hours at low oxygen levels corresponding to altitudes of about 30,000 feet. This was done on the 1st, 9th, or 15th day (pregnancy in the mouse is about 20 days). Gross defects of the brain resulted in the young of the pregnant mice exposed on the 9th day. Anomalies of other systems were also present, for example, fused ribs. Exposure on the 15th day produced cleft palate. It has also been shown that different forms of stress may produce the same malformation in mice: for example, cleft palate is produced by radiation, vitamin deficiency, and anoxia.

Hicks has shown that irradiation of rats in their early stages of development when the organs are being differentiated produces massive effects on the brain and eyes. He points out, however, that the experimental animal is subjected to noxious agents to a degree to which the pregnant woman would not find herself exposed. The work of Apgar and her associates should be mentioned. They found no significant correlation between "level of blood oxygen content measured in the first three hours after birth and intelligence as gauged by Stanford-Binet testing in early childhood." They did concede, however, that anoxia prior to birth could conceivably injure cerebral cells and produce delayed intellectual development and yet the damage might be undetected by their experiment. Usdin and Weil compared children who were apneic following delivery for three or more minutes with a control group who breathed spontaneously at birth. The children were 13 to 14 years of age at the time of the study. Intelligence tests revealed no significant difference between the intelligence of the apneic and control groups. On the other hand, reference to the articles by Courville, Yant, Schreiber, and Lamm would seem to offer evidence for the role of anoxia in mental deficiency.

We have referred to irradiation prenatally in animals (Hicks) to indicate how deleterious the effects may be on the fetus. There are genetic sequelae of two types which may follow sublethal doses of ionizing radiation. These are gene mutations and chromosome aberrations which lead to somatic mutations and result in the abnormal development of one or more organ systems. The problem of gene mutations involves subsequent generations and is a subject too controversial to discuss at present. Genetic injury from radiation has thus far not been demonstrated in man, according to Robinow and Silverman, who, however, feel the question is still open and that it may be a matter of finding methods to prove the production of mutations. As to somatic mutations that lead to developmental defects, two factors are involved, the amount of dosage and the time during gestation when it is delivered. In the mouse, the critical period of gestation corresponds to the second to sixth week in man. In general, the larger the dose and the shorter the period over which radiation is given, the greater the damage.

The Atomic Bomb Casualty Commission has reported that of eleven Hiroshima children exposed in utero to amounts of gamma radiation that approximated the median lethal dose, seven had microcephaly plus mental retardation, two were mongolian idiots, and two were apparently normal. Most pregnant women miscarried soon after the exposure. In a follow-up ten years after the explosion at Hiroshima, 33 children (including the eleven previously mentioned) who were exposed in utero at the time had head circumferences 2 or more standard deviations below normal. Twenty-four of these were between the 7th and 15th weeks of gestational age at the time of detonation of the bomb. The incidence and severity of microcephaly increased as the distance from the hypocenter* decreased. Mental retardation occurred in 15 of the 33 patients. The incidence of this defect was also related to distance from the hypocenter and gestational age. No other embryonic effects of exposure to the atomic bomb have been detected to date. Births of microcephalic, mentally retarded children have resulted from the accidental overexposure of women during the first half of their pregnancy to radiation given as treatment for pelvic disease.

German measles and toxoplasmosis are cited as instances in which infection injures the developing nervous system during embryonic and fetal life. With respect to viral infections, Adams and associates have suggested a concept of a spectrum of involvement of the embryo. Severe viral infections result in death. On the other hand, mild infections may produce at birth abnormalities of the fetus or a normal appearing fetus. In some instances the latter might show abnormalities at a later age.

Warkany cites an experiment occurring in nature to show the

* The hypocenter is a point directly under the atomic bomb when it explodes.

effects of nutrition on the development of the nervous system. "Swayback" or "enzootic ataxia" is a disease occurring in sheep who are fed in pastures deficient in copper. The young of such ewes show spastic paralysis, lack of coordination, and anatomically a small brain with flattened convolutions. Feeding copper sulfate to pregnant ewes reduces the incidence of this anomaly in the young.

We have dwelt on the effects of anoxia, radiation, infection, and maternal nutrition upon the growing embryo. To these should be added endocrine factors, such as diabetes. A baby born of a diabetic mother is usually overly large and may show congenital abnormalities, including those of the brain and mental deficiency. There are also other possible environmental effects on the fetus due to position of the ovum (ectopic) or malposition in the uterus with the development of congenital anomalies, presumably due to pressure. The amount of amniotic fluid is invariably increased in anencephaly.

Natal influences on mental development include birth injury associated with either intracranial hemorrhage, asphyxia resulting in cerebral anoxia, or both.

Postnatal factors include meningitis, encephalitis, and trauma, which may alter mental development or behavior. In addition, nutrition, especially protein deficiency, may unfavorably affect the psychomotor development of the infant. With the addition of protein Gitlin has indicated that the process is reversible if the child survives.

In summarizing the effect of environment, it may be said that phenotypes which resemble a hereditary condition can be produced by abnormal environmental factors. For example, microcephaly in the offspring may be produced by irradiation of the pregnant mother, infection of the fetus (viral or toxoplasma), or as an inherited genetic recessive condition.

The degree of abnormal exposure and the period of gestation when the environmental stress is applied are highly significant. It has also been shown that specific agents will produce a particular picture irrespective of the time factor, for example, trypan blue produces in rats primarily hydrocephalus and other cerebral defects, whereas Vitamin A deficiency in rats is exemplified primarily by ocular defects such as post-lental fibroplasia and retinal coloboma.

While there are as yet no hereditary conditions in humans which can be altered by therapy during pregnancy, both Fraser and Warkany suggest that "the phenomena of variable penetrance and ex-

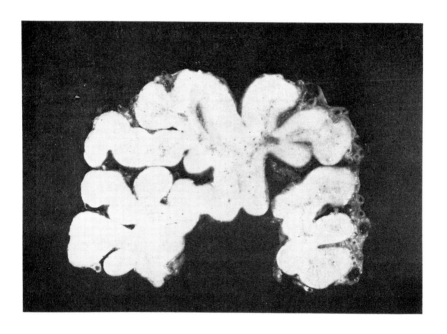

1. Frontal fusion of cerebral hemispheres. Note vascular anomalies and thickened leptomeninges on the right side.

pressivity offer hope that environmental features may be adjusted to modify the expression of the genes."

CONCLUSION: It is obvious from the previous discussion that an abnormality may be inherited, may be due to environmental agencies, or both. One must evaluate these factors and account for them in taking a history and in making a final decision whether a pathological condition is inherited or not. As Warkany has pointed out, the fact that the mother has appeared healthy during pregnancy does not guarantee a normal baby because agents which the mother may tolerate with safety may be noxious for the fetus. The age of the parents is important, as in mongolism, where there is a marked increase in incidence in mothers who are over thirty-five when pregnant. It is also noted that the greatest incidence of malformations occurs in women who conceive in the period just past puberty. The greatest number of lethal malformations occur in the central nervous system, especially anencephaly, according to Potter.

When the final decision is made, if the condition is acquired, another pregnancy can generally be advised with good assurance. If inherited, then the principles of genetics must be reviewed prior to counseling.

Adams, J. M., Heath, H. D., Imagawa, D. T., Jones, M. H. and Shear, H. H.: Viral Infections in the Embryo. A.M.A. J. Dis. Child. 92:109, 1956.

Apgar, V., Girdany, B. R., McIntosh, R., and Taylor Jr., H. C.: Neonatal Anoxia. A study of the Relation of Oxygenation at Birth to Intellectual Development. Pediat. 15:653, 1955.

Cohlan, S. Q.: Congenital Anomalies in the Rat Produced by the Excessive Intake of Vitamin A during Pregnancy. Pediat. 13:556, 1954.

Dekaban, A. S., and Magee, K. R.: Occurrence of Neurologic Abnormalities in Infants of Diabetic Mothers. Neurology 8:193, 1958.

Gitlin, D.: Protein Metabolism in Relation to Mental Retardation. Report of the Twenty-third Ross Pediatric Research Conference, M and R Laboratories, Columbus, Ohio, p. 89, 1957.

Hicks, S. P.: Injury of the Central Nervous System Incurred during Fetal Life. A. Res. Publ. Ass. Nerv. Ment. Dis. Proc. 34:86, 1954.

Ingalls, T. H.: Causes and Prevention of Developmental Defects. J.A.M.A. 161:1047, 1956.

Kugel, R. B.: Mental Deficiency. Pediat. 18:997, 1956.

Lamm, S. S.: Asphyxia as a Cause of Mental Deficiency—Suggestions as to Prevention. Am. J. Ment. Def. 43:131, 1943.

Miller, R. W.: Delayed Effects occurring within the First Decade after

Exposure of Young Individuals to the Hiroshima Atomic Bomb. Pediat. 18:1, 1956.

Murphy, D. P.: Maternal Pelvic Irradiation in Congenital Malformations, 2nd Edition. Philadelphia, Lippincott, p. 87-100, 1947.

Robinow, M., and Silverman, F. N.: Radiation Hazards in the Field of Pediatrics. Supplement to Pediatrics, 20:921, 1957.

Supplement to Pediatrics—19: No. 4, Part 2, April, 1957.

Usdin, G. L., and Weil, M. L.: Effect of Apnea Neonatorum on Intellectual Development. Pediat. 9:387, 1952.

Warkany, J., Kalter, H., and Geiger, J. F.: Experimental Teratology. Pediat. Clin. N.A. Philadelphia, W. B. Saunders Co., p. 995, Nov. 1957.

REFLEXES

Since the nervous system in the newborn infant is not fully developed, cortical inhibition is not as yet established. There is thus a great deal of reflex behavior expressed in the motor reactions of the infant. Development appears to be related to myelination, cephalad to caudad.

The reflex patterns which are generally elicited in an infant to establish the presence of normal development shall be described. Their significance will be commented upon both here and in the subsequent discussions where their presence or absence is of particular diagnostic import, as in mental deficiency or cerebral palsy.

Along with other symptoms and signs of value in neurological diagnosis, the importance of additional reflexes will be stressed in the sections dealing with the individual diseases. They are not of diagnostic value in the infantile period, since a Babinski, for example, may or may not be present. It may even disappear and reappear during this time. Between two and three years of age the presence of a Babinski may be interpreted as indicative of pyramidal tract pathology. A spontaneous Babinski seen in the newborn period is not suggestive of clinical pathology (Dietrich).

At birth the infant yawns and sneezes. Corneal reflex and pupillary reaction to light are present. These reflexes are permanent.

Rooting Reflex. Stroking the cheek of an infant with the finger causes the baby to turn his head towards the finger and at the same time to open his mouth. This reflex tends to disappear by the latter portion of the first year. It is related to the sucking reflex.

Sucking Reflex. The touch of the nipple to the lips of the infant will cause opening of the mouth and sucking movements. This also gradually weakens and disappears by the end of the first year.

Moro Reflex. The infant is placed on his back. A loud noise is made by slamming the hand of the examiner against the table or crib. The reflex which follows consists of symmetrical extension and abduction of the upper and lower limbs. This is immediately followed by a movement of the arms toward each other (adduction) resulting almost in a clasp. This reflex normally disappears after four months of age. Its persistence suggests brain damage, either mental retardation or cerebral palsy. Its absence following birth or a delay in its appearance may indicate birth injury. If absent on one side, it may point up a fractured clavicle or brachial plexus injury with an Erb's palsy.

Postural and Righting Reflexes. The postural reflexes maintain posture and equilibrium. The righting reflexes orient the individual in space. Stimuli received from the labyrinths, eyes, neck, and body (muscles and joints) are mediated by way of the medulla and brain stem to accomplish these ends.

Tonic Neck Reflex (*T.N.R.*). Place the infant flat on his back. Rotate the head to one side as far as it will go. This results in extension of the arm, leg, or both on the side towards which the face is turned and flexion of contralateral extremities (occipital side). This procedure should be done on both sides. The tonic neck reflex should disappear before the end of the first year. Its persistence means damage to the higher areas of the brain and may be indicative of retarded mental development or severe motor dysfunction due to destruction of brain tissue. In cerebral palsy its persistence is of bad import with respect to the ability of the child to benefit from therapy.

Postural Adjustment to Inverted Position (McGraw). The infant is suspended by the ankles in an inverted position.

A. Newborn or Flexor Phase—The infant flexes the knees and hips to maintain position of flexion against the pull of gravity.

B. Extensor Phase—The flexor position is now replaced by hyperextension of the vertebral column with arching of the back and extension of the arms. This is noted at four to six months of age.

Both of these phases are subcortical. There are later phases referred to by McGraw as the Righting phase and Mature or Relaxed phase. These are cortical.

In an infant over six months, in the presence of suspected motor retardation (cerebral palsy), a newborn or flexor position would suggest cortical injury.

Palmar Grasp Reflex. The newborn baby grasps and holds on to a finger or rod put into its palm. This reflex normally disappears by the third to sixth month, but may reappear if there is damage to the frontal areas.

Plantar Grasp Reflex. When a finger is placed firmly across the ball of the foot directly under the toes, the baby will immediately flex the toes as if intent on grasping the finger. This reflex is present shortly after birth and disappears between six and twelve months of age.

Landau Reflex. The normal infant between six months and three years, when supported under the abdomen and held freely in the air, will extend the head, spine and legs.

When the infant is lowered or momentarily dropped while held securely round the waist, there is extension of the arms upward. This test is useful in cerebral palsy, since an infant with the latter involvement does not have the protective extension of the normal infant, but draws the arms in flexion.

Bobath, K. and Bobath, B.: Diagnosis of Cerebral Palsy in Infancy. Arch. Dis. Child. 31:408, 1956.

Byers, R. K.: Tonic Neck Reflexes in Children Considered from a Prognostic Standpoint. Am. J. Dis. Child. 55:696, 1938.

Dietrich, H. F.: A Longitudinal Study of the Babinski and Plantar Grasp Reflexes in Infancy. A.M.A. J. Dis. Child. 94:265, 1957.

Gentry, E. F. and Aldrich, C. A.: Rooting Reflex in the Newborn Infant. Incidence and Effect on It of Sleep. Am. J. Dis. Child. 75:528, 1948.

Gesell, A.: The Tonic Neck Reflex in the Human Infant. J. Pediat. 13:455, 1938.

Magnus, R.: Korperstellung. Berlin, Julius Springer, 1924.

McGraw, M. B.: Neuromuscular Mechanism of the Infant. Development Reflected by Postural Adjustments to an Inverted Position. Am. J. Dis. Child. 60:1031, 1940.

Moro, E.: Das Erste Trimenon: München. Med. Wchnschr. 65:1147, 1918.

Silver, A. A.: Postural and Righting Responses in Children. J. Pediat. 41:493, 1952.

PSYCHODYNAMICS

The physician is of necessity as much concerned with mental as with physical development. He is frequently called upon to diagnose and make recommendations in cases where the main complaint is failure of the child to speak, or when there is evidence of impaired learning ability or generally retarded mental development. In older children there may be an inability to adjust or make progress in school. There may be extremes of hostile, aggressive, and destructive behavior. Any behavior which indicates significant deviation from normal expectancy in the areas of social, emotional, or intellectual functioning demands a full study to determine the etiology.

The differential diagnosis must involve consideration of several basic factors. These include mental retardation, either endogenous or exogenous, pseudo-retardation, and a personality disorder with neurotic conflicts or psychotic disorganization.

The developmental history is of great importance. The use of psychological tests may provide valuable aid in differential when there is retardation. They also offer an estimate of the degree or severity of involvement. The use of neurological and laboratory techniques in the diagnosis of specific kinds of retardation, and the behavioral sequelae of organic brain damage have been described elsewhere. Here will be presented a general discussion of psychodiagnostic testing and some of the tests in common use.

For the most part the physician who is called upon to make recommendations in cases of suspected mental deficiency or severe emotional disorder is advised to refer his patient to a qualified psychologist or to the psychodiagnostic clinic of the local community for an evaluation of the mental level. When a quick, gross estimate of mental development is desired, the Kent EGY Scale, the Goodenough Draw-A-Man test, and/or the Raven Progressive Matrices (1947 revision) may prove valuable. Some caution must be exercised in administering any of these tests, lest their validity be decreased as a function of the lack of standardized procedures. Normative data for any of these tests is valueless when administration does not follow standard techniques. The question of rapport is of great importance. We might say simply that quite a different relationship between examiner and patient is required to obtain a valid and reliable sample of behavior as compared to a sample of blood or urine.

In judging the test results one must take into account the presence of specific disabilities like cerebral palsy, hearing or visual deficit, cultural limitations such as lack of understanding of the language, and personality disorders. Keeping in mind these reservations one may use the results of testing to classify mental deficiency.

I.Q.

Normal	90-110
Dull Normal	80- 90
Borderline	70- 80
Moron	50- 70
Imbecile	25- 50
Idiot	Below 25

The significance of these levels will be interpreted in the discussion of mental deficiency.

GUIDE TO NORMAL DEVELOPMENT

Since the physician will rarely have either the time or the facilities for comprehensive psychological or psychomotor testing of infants, the following is offered as a guide to normal developmental expectancies from the first through the thirty-sixth month of life.

At Birth: Moro, rooting, palmar and plantar grasp reflexes present
yawns, sneezes
sucking and rooting reflexes present
pupillary and corneal reflexes present

One Month:
predominantly positive tonic neck reflex
hand brought to mouth
both fists clenched
head sags when infant is held in sitting position
some throaty noises

Two Months:
looks at examiner alertly
follows moving person or light
responds to sound
lifts head when held, keeps it erect and steady
can raise chest when in prone position
smiles
babbles or coos

Four Months:
reaches for objects
holds rattle and observes same in purposeful manner
sits with support, steadily, leaning forward

Six Months:
sits when supported with trunk erect
grasps toy
lifts cup to mouth
rolls to prone position

Nine Months:
sits with good control, no back support required
drops and reaches for cube
stands when held, full weight, legs extended
imitates sounds, says "dada," etc.
holds bottle
pulls self up
some respond to bowel training

Twelve Months:
walks if held by one hand
begins to talk—two words
comprehends words like "no," "name," "Bye-Bye,"
   "give"
co-operates in dressing activities
drinks from cup

Eighteen Months:
turns several pages in a book
looks selectively at pictures in a book; points to one
   picture correctly
spontaneous scribbling
walks fast—runs stiffly
walks up stairs if one hand is held
seats self in chair
speaks ten words
attempts to feed self
pulls toy; carries and hugs doll
daytime toilet regulated

Twenty-Four Months: attempts to fold paper
                      turns pages of book one at a time
                      names pictures and objects—cat, dog
                      imitates vertical and circular pencil strokes
                      kicks ball
                      runs fairly well
                      goes up and down stairs alone
                      speaks two to three word sentences
                      verbalizes toilet needs consistently
                      refers to self by name
                      bladder control

Thirty Months: definitely folds paper with a crease
                      builds tower of eight cubes
                      holds crayon in fingers
                      imitates horizontal stroke
                      tries to stand on one foot
                      jumps on both feet
                      speech repetitious
                      refers to self using pronoun
                      helps put things away
                      carries breakable object
                      gives full name

Thirty-Six Months: describes action in pictures
                      imitates building bridge with blocks
                      copies circle
                      names own drawings
                      repeats three digits
                      gives full name and sex
                      stands on one foot with momentary balance
                      rides tricycle
                      alternates feet going upstairs
                      begins to assume full responsibility for toilet needs
                      feeds self well—no spilling
                      pours from pitcher
                      puts shoes on
                      unbuttons accessible buttons
                      knows several rhymes
                      understands taking turns

Blum, L. H., and Fieldsteel, N. D.: Cumulative Record of Motor Behavior, New York, World Book Co., 1952.

Cattell, P.: The Measurement of Intelligence of Infants and Young Children. New York, The Psychological Corp., 1940.

Gesell, A., and Amatruda, G. S.: Developmental Diagnosis. Ed. 2. New York, Paul B. Hoeber, 1954.

Terman, L. M., and Merrill, M. A.: Measuring Intelligence. New York, Houghton Mifflin Co., 1937.

CHAPTER 2

MENTAL RETARDATION

Simply expressed, mental retardation refers to a lack of normal development so that the individual is unable to participate educationally. There is, in other words, subnormal intellectual behavior. Others have used the term in the sense of social inadequacy as well. In England the legal conception is that "mental defectiveness means a condition of arrested or incomplete development of mind, existing before the age of eighteen years, whether arising from inherent causes or induced by disease or injury." A variety of terms have been used more or less interchangeably including mental deficiency, feeblemindedness, amentia, and oligophrenia. The Committee of the American Association on Mental Deficiency has referred to mental retardation as being characterized by inadequate social adjustment, reduced learning capacity, and slow rate of maturation. Mental retardation may include one or more of these features and is due to subaverage intellectual functioning present usually from birth or early childhood. The committee considers mental retardation to be a generic term which has incorporated "all that has been meant in the past by such terms as mental deficiency, feeblemindedness, idiocy, imbecility, and moronity, etc."

There are no satisfactory data on the number of mental defectives. Estimates place the figure at one per cent of the total population in the United States. From two to three per cent of school children have been considered mentally deficient.

There have been a number of clinical classifications of mental deficiency based on medical factors, especially with respect to etiology (Tredgold, Yannet, Jervis). Tredgold originally used the terms endogenous or primary, indicating germ plasm or genetic relationship to the mental deficiency, and exogenous or secondary, implying adverse environmental factors as the cause. At the present time it is realized that it is often difficult to know in a given instance whether the defect is due to genetic or environmental influence or both, when the condition appears to be caused by prenatal factors.

Malamud has presented the neuropathologic findings in 543

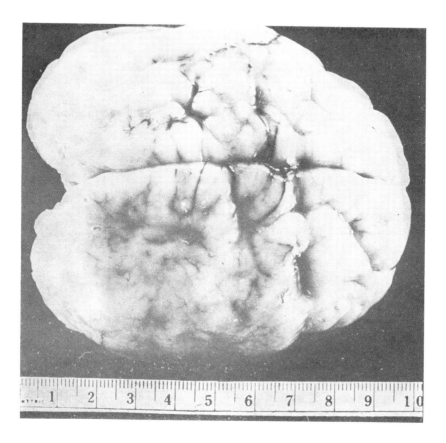

2. Hypogenesis with agyria. Dorsal view of cerebral hemispheres showing marked diminution and total absence of gyri.

autopsied cases of mental deficiency. He found that 400 showed malformations such as microgyria, porencephaly, microcephaly, etc., and 121 presented destructive processes (atrophy, cysts, scars, old hemorrhages) as the result of trauma, kernicterus, or postnatal infection. Together, the malformations and destructive processes comprised 96 per cent, leaving only 4 per cent for the metabolic disorders such as amaurotic idiocy, gargoylism, and phakomatoses, e.g., tuberous sclerosis and angiomatosis. He did not feel that the pathological data could be correlated with distinctive, clinical, etiological factors such as infection or trauma, and he therefore felt that an etiologic classification of mental deficiency was not warranted.

Some general observations may be made concerning the accumulated data on mental retardation. The vast majority of cases are due to prenatal etiology. This includes the subcultural group or familial amentia, due to multiple genes which are inadequate as to quality. The qualitative defect in the genes is passed along through generations. Another large prenatal group is associated with anomalies in other systems. These are produced by the exogenous or environmental factors previously discussed, such as infection, radiation, Rh incompatibility, hormones, and anoxia. (See Chapter 1.)

The congenital cerebral maldevelopment may be of a specific type, e.g., following German measles, or the clinical characteristics may be undifferentiated and the etiology unknown. At present, the latter comprise over 30 per cent of the total population in institutions for the mentally retarded.

There is a small group of genetic disorders classified as inborn errors of metabolism, such as gargoylism, phenylketonuria, and galactosemia. Birth trauma (hemorrhage and asphyxia) comprises only a small percentage, perhaps three per cent. Postnatal infection, including meningitis and the encephalitides, both viral and allergic, lead encephalopathy, and trauma are of greater significance.

In summary, it is recognized that in addition to the retardation which is due to inheritance, usually of poor multiple genes or rarely of a single pathologic gene, there are other factors operating both prenatally, natally, and postnatally to produce mental impairment. These prenatal factors are in some instances the same as those operating to produce cerebral palsy and congenital anomalies in general. We have made reference to a large group of cases of mental deficiency due to prenatal causes at present not clearly defined, who present malformations of various systems, including the brain. There are some who feel that these prenatal causes have been given undue influence and that the problem is mainly genetic. The stress on the influence of environment may sometimes be due to a desire to find causes which can be influenced by a prophylactic medical approach. Certainly this has been true of congenital neurosyphilis, which is rare today, and kernicterus due to Rh incompatibility, which is also becoming a negligible factor. Another observation is that mental deficiency, even when due to a genetic defect, e.g., phenylketonuria, may now be prevented or modified through dietary control.

In evaluating mental retardation, one should take account of the effect of factors other than the intelligence level (I.Q.) which influence intellectual progress. Emotional factors may retard the child. This is shown to an extreme degree in the autistic type of schizophrenia. Woodward and Siegel have reported a preliminary study on eight such retarded children. There was no organic pathology demonstrable, and the family was free of mental deficiency. They feel that psychiatric study will sort out a number of such children now classified as mental defectives, who will be found retarded on a psychological basis. Poor nutrition, lack of proper home environment (environmental retardation), or prolonged institutionalization (hospitalism, rejected children, maternal deprivation) may affect the child so that he appears to be retarded. Finally specific defects such as blindness, poor hearing or speech as in cerebral palsy, or seizures may affect the child's ability to demonstrate a satisfactory intellectual level. The term "pseudo-feeblemindedness" has been applied to these factors, just mentioned, which are outside the nervous system but affect the child so that he behaves as a mental deficient. It is suggested that the child with a high IQ may overcome these handicaps, whereas a borderline type may be affected by the extraneous factor so as to exhibit mental deficiency.

The clinical or etiological classification of mental retardation which follows is that suggested by a committee of the American Association on Mental Deficiency. It is referred to as Part 1, Etiological Classification, by the Committee on Nomenclature. For details as to code numbers, etc., reference may be made to the original manual.

Cerebral birth trauma
Cerebral infection, postnatal (specify)
Congenital cerebral maldevelopment due to prenatal infections (specify)
Congenital cerebral maldevelopment (non-specific)

Congenital cerebral maldevelopment—other forms (specify)
Congenital cerebral maldevelopment with cerebral palsy
Congenital cerebral maldevelopment with congenital ectodermoses (specify)
Congenital cerebral maldevelopment with cranial anomalies (specify)
Congenital cerebral maldevelopment with mongolism
Congenital cerebral maldevelopment with phenylketonuria
Due to convulsive disorder
Familial
Hypothyroidism
Kernicterus (iso-immunization, other)
Other postnatal forms (specify)
Progressive neuronal degeneration (specify)
Psychogenic
Unclassified
Unknown

Most of the conditions referred to in the classification will be discussed separately in their respective chapters. These include cerebral birth trauma; postnatal cerebral infections such as meningitis or encephalitis; congenital cerebral maldevelopment with cerebral palsy; congenital cerebral maldevelopment with congenital ectodermoses such as tuberous sclerosis, neurofibromatosis, and cerebral angiomatosis; congenital cerebral maldevelopment associated with cranial anomalies such as the craniostenoses, congenital hydrocephalus, or hypertelorism; mongolism; phenylketonuria; mental retardation due to convulsive disorder, hypothyroidism, kernicterus; other rare postnatal forms including lead encephalopathy; progressive neuronal degeneration such as Tay-Sachs, and demyelinating diseases such as Schilder's. Congenital cerebral maldevelopment due to prenatal infections includes German measles, congenital syphilis, and toxoplasmosis. The non-specific congenital cerebral maldevelopment group includes those cases of prenatal origin which are undifferentiated clinically and of unknown etiology. The classification of "congenital cerebral maldevelopment—other forms (specify)" refers to conditions which can be diagnosed and are of prenatal origin, but rare; included are fetal irradiation, hereditary mental retardation, and known maternal intoxication.

I will not attempt to follow any classification of mental deficiency in this book, since many of the specific entities cannot be adequately placed with our present knowledge.

FAMILIAL OR SUBCULTURAL AMENTIA

In the preceding discussions on genetic inheritance and mental deficiency reference has been made to inferior strain or stock.

Inheritance has been effected with transference of a poor grade of genes to the offspring. There is a familial defect in the quality of multiple genes, both sides adding to the general inferiority; there is no single pathological gene effect, or alteration of a gene. Subcultural standards are presumed to be at fault. If one were to plot a distribution curve of intelligence for the general population, it would be expected that the majority of people would be located in the IQ zone of normal, i.e., 80-120. It follows that the remainder would be in the very superior or retarded group. The latter would lie mostly in the 50-74 range, or moron level. As Jervis remarks, this is an "integral" part of the population. It is in this latter group that we find the subcultural population. The remainder or lowest range in the scale comprise the congenital idiocy population. The deficiency in the subcultural group may not be too apparent in infancy, but as these children go to school their mental limitations are soon noted. The siblings of such children are also likely to be in the same moron level. Yannet has stated that these make up the largest single group among mental defectives that can be classified and comprise one-third of institutional admissions. Pathological examination may not reveal anything distinctive; there may be a small brain, undifferentiated, with a paucity of nerve cells; or there may be developmental anomalies of the brain and cord (Benda, Malamud).

Examination of these children reveals no neurological abnormalities. Therefore, the diagnosis is made on psychological evaluation and tests of social adjustment. In summary, the significant features are the presence of a retarded child of borderline or moron level, normal history except for inferior intelligence of the parents, and an essentially normal physical and neurological examination. Siblings are of similar intellectual level. Their treatment is educational, within the limits of their mental ability. Given a simple society, these children can make a satisfactory adult adjustment.

At this point mention should be made of another theory of etiology. This would emphasize adverse environmental factors acting prenatally, or postnatal conditions such as protein deficiency, emotional deprivation, and poor educational opportunities. Jervis feels that there may be different etiologies accounting for the subcultural group. It is probably advisable to look at factors such as environmental inadequacy, and personality or behavior disorders with associated physical defects, as additions to the genetic mechanism.

CONGENITAL IDIOCY

These children make up the lowest end of the scale of a distribution of intelligence. The IQ is at the idiot or imbecile level. Their only manifestation or symptom is mental deficiency. There are no neurological or laboratory changes. However, they do have associated malformations of other systems. There may be peculiarly shaped ears, palatal defects, webbing of fingers or toes, abnormality of the iris or lens, or genitourinary or gastrointestinal anomalies. The parents of these children are of normal intelligence. If the retarded child is isolated, diagnosis is difficult; but when there is another defective sibling without any ascertainable cause, then the diagnosis is more readily made. Halpern places the chances of such a family producing another defective at 7 to 10 times greater than for the normal population.

MANAGEMENT: The parents should be told the truth as soon as the physician is sure of the diagnosis. This should include a statement as to whether the condition is inherited or acquired or whether the cause is unknown. The etiological classification of the American Association on Mental Deficiency, previously given, may be used.

In discussing the prognosis for the child, account should be taken of the level of mental development. This may be influenced by the presence of specific disabilities. The physician must be certain that the low IQ is not due solely to failure of hearing, vision, reading disability, aphasia, or personality disorder. If, however, there is retardation plus a specific disability, such as cerebral palsy or any of the above, the outlook is less hopeful. These facts will also influence the question of schooling and the possibilities for the child in later life (marriage and children).

There are no known drugs which are appreciably effective in raising the mental level, except for specific defects like cretinism where thyroid extract is of value. If seizures are present, these should be treated as indicated in the chapter on epilepsy. Attempts at revascularization of the brain to raise the IQ have largely been abandoned. The tranquilizing drugs like chlorpromazine may be of value to combat the hyperactivity, withdrawal, and restlessness seen in some of these children. Be careful of convulsive seizures following the use of phenothiazines.

The disposition of the patient depends on many factors. All infants should be cared for at home when possible. This permits the parents to feel they are doing all they can. It lessens guilt feelings about having rejected the baby. If there is a specific reason why this cannot be done, then a small residential plan should be utilized, such as a foster home. Later on, the parents can come to a decision as to placement in a special institution. When the community offers resources, many children in the borderline, and IQ groups above 50 may adjust satisfactorily at home. These children can be educated in special classes. In their teens they should get vocational training and be prepared for a job. As previously indicated, this IQ group represents about 75 per cent of the retarded population; therefore, the majority can be integrated at home. For children with a very low IQ, below 25 (about 5 per cent of the total retarded population), institutional care will be required, at about three to five years of age. The moderately retarded, IQ between 25 to 50, who represent about 20 per cent of the total population and of whom mongols form the majority, may need institutions if the home is inadequate. The reaction of the family itself is a consideration. There are situations in which the high intellectual level of the parents prevents them from accepting the fact that their child is slow, or the mother believes it is all her fault, or in which the parents look on the retarded child as a social disgrace. Coleman and Provence have reported two cases of infants reared in their own families who became retarded developmentally because of inadequate maternal care. Lack of maternal stimulation produced a picture similar to the environmental retardation of institutionalized infants. Treatment was effected through temporary transfer of the baby to a hospital setting where the staff provided proper attention and love and through modification of the parents' attitude by psychotherapy.

In addition to diagnosis, etiology, prognosis, treatment, and disposition, there should also be discussed the chances for recurrence in future pregnancies, the effect on the other children of the presence of the mentally deficient child, whether anything can happen to the normal children in the way of subsequent deterioration, and how to explain the deficient child to relatives and friends.

Bakwin, H.: Informing the Parents of the Mentally Retarded Child. Pediat. 49:486, 1956.

Benton, A. L.: The Concept of Pseudo-feeblemindedness. Arch. Neurol. & Psychiat. 75:379, 1956.

Coleman, R. W. and Provence, S.: Environmental Retardation (Hospitalism) in Infants Living in Families. Pediat. 19:285, 1957.

Doll, E. A.: The Essentials of an Inclusive Concept of Mental Deficiency. Am. J. Ment. Def. 46:214, 1941.

———: Counseling Parents of Severely Mentally Retarded Children. J. of Clin. Psychol., 9:114, 1953.

Etiological Classification. Statistical Manual of the American Association on Mental Deficiency, ed. 4, Willimantic, Conn., 1957.

Glaser, K. and Eisenberg, L.: Maternal Deprivation. Pediat. 18:626, 1956.

Jervis, G. A.: Etiologic Factors in Mental Deficiency. Am. J. Public Health, 47:63, 1957.

Kanner, Leo: Parent's Feelings about Retarded Children. Am. J. Ment. Def. 57:375, 1953.

Lewis, E. O.: Types of Mental Deficiency and Their Social Significaance. J. Ment. Sc. 79:298, 1933.

Malamud, N.: Recent Trends in Classification of Neuropathological Findings in Mental Deficiency. Am. J. Ment. Def. 58:438, 1954.

Masland, R. L.: The Prevention of Mental Retardation. A.M.A. J. Dis. Child. Part 2. 95:3, 1958.

———, R. L.: The Prevention of Mental Retardation. Am. J. Ment. Def. 62 (Part II): 991, 1958.

McQuarrie, I.: Idiopathic Spontaneously Occurring Hypoglycemia in Infants: Clinical Significance of Problem and Treatment. A.M.A. J. Dis. Child. 87:399, 1954.

Moncrieff, A. and Wilkinson, R. H.: Sucrosuria with Mental Defect and Hiatus Hernia. Acta Paediat. 43 (Supp. 100); 495, 1954.

Sarason, S. B.: Psychological Problems in Mental Deficiency. New York, Paul B. Hoeber, 1953.

———, and Gladwin, T.: Psychological and Cultural Problems in Mental Subnormality: A Review of Research. Am. J. Ment. Def. 62 (Part 2):1115, 1958.

Sjögren, T. and Larsson, T.: Oligophrenia in Combination with Congenital Ichthyosis and Spastic Disorders: Clinical and Genetic Study. Acta psychiat. et. neurol. scandinav. Vol. 32, supp. 113, 1957.

Spitz, R. A.: Hospitalism: An inquiry into the genesis of psychiatric conditions in early childhood: Psychoanalytic Study of the Child. Vol. 1, New York, Internat. University Press, 1945.

Tarjan, G., Lowery, V. E., Wright, S. W.: Use of Chlorpromazine in Two Hundred Seventy-Eight Mentally Deficient Patients. A.M.A. J. Dis. Child. 94:294, 1957.

Tredgold, A. F. and Bailliere, R. F.: Mental Deficiency, 8th ed., London, Tindall and Cox, 1952.

Watson, E. H.: Counseling Parents of Mentally Deficient Children. Report of a Round Table Discussion. Pediat. 22:401, 1958.

Wolf, S. and Lourie, R. J.: The Impact of the Mentally Defective Child in the Family Unit. J. Pediat. 42:521, 1953.

Woodward, K. F. and Siegel, M. G.: Psychiatric Study of Mentally Retarded Children of Pre-school Age. Pediat. 19:119, 1957.

Yannet, H.: The Community Responsibility for the Care of the Mentally Retarded. J. Pediat. 50:397, 1957.

———, H.: Classification and Etiological Factors in Mental Retardation. J. Pediat. 50:226, 1957.

CHAPTER 3

DEVELOPMENTAL DEFECTS

For a general discussion of prenatal factors, either genetic or environmental, in relation to congenital malformations, refer to Chapter 1.

ANENCEPHALY

Anencephaly, which is due to failure of closure of the neural tube, occurs approximately 1/1000 in the general population, with a ratio of two males to three females. It is probably due to a lethal genotypic factor. The baby is born dead or may live a few hours.

A subsequent pregnancy has a six times greater risk of producing a central nervous system congenital defect compared to the general population, and a twenty per cent chance of aborting.

According to Vogel, angiogenesis is an important causative factor in the production of anencephaly.

Böök, J. A. and Rayner, S.: A Clinical and Genetical Study of Anencephaly. Am. J. Human Genet. 2:61, 1950.

Penrose, L. S.: Familial Data on 144 Cases of Anencephaly, Spina Bifida, and Congenital Hydrocephaly. Ann. Eugen. 13:73, 1946.

———, L. S.: Genetics of Anencephaly. J. Ment. Def. Research. Vol. 1, Part 1, July 1957.

Record, R. G. and McKeown, T.: Congenital Malformations of the Central Nervous System; Risk of Malformation in Sibs of Malformed Individuals. Brit. J. Social Med. 4:217, 1950.

Vogel, F. S.: The Association of Vascular Anomalies with Anencephaly. Am. J. Path. 34:169, 1958.

SPINA BIFIDA

In spina bifida there is a failure of fusion of the vertebral column, leaving a cleft or defect due to the lack of closure of the posterior arches.

A number of types have been described.

29

1. *Spina Bifida Occulta*. This is the most common type. It is stated to be present in twenty-five per cent of the normal population. There is no protrusion of intraspinal tissues, hence no external sac; but there is defective closure of the vertebral column, which can be demonstrated roentgenographically. There may be a tuft of hair, or a subcutaneous fat pad overlying the area, which is almost always in the lumbosacral region. In other children, dimpling or a port wine stain of the skin may be noted.

The majority of children with this condition have no symptoms since the spinal cord is unaffected. The peculiar appearance of the skin in the lumbosacral region may be noted in the course of routine examination, but there are no other abnormal physical signs. These children require no therapy and should not be operated upon unless neurological symptoms develop.

2. *Myelodysplasia with Spina Bifida Occulta*. In some instances there may be a complaint of enuresis, failure of bladder and rectal control, or dribbling of urine. In others there may be difficulty in beginning to walk, bilateral talipes equinovarus or valgus, or deformities of the toes. Examination may reveal a relaxed rectal sphincter, dribbling of urine with pressure on the abdomen, loss of deep tendon reflexes, sensory defects in the extremities, or trophic changes. In these cases there is a myelodysplasia along with the spina bifida occulta.

PATHOLOGY: The lumbosacral area of the spinal canal is filled with a fatty mass to which is attached the lower end of the spinal cord, or there are numerous strands of connective tissue attached to the cord, which bind it to the spinal canal membrane which has replaced the bony defect; the cord is prevented from ascending cephalad as the spinal column grows.

There is a question whether this condition is a germ plasm defect or acquired in utero. It is established that the neural tube is fused by the third to fourth week of development of the embryo. The central nervous system is formed by the differentiation of the cells of the neural plate (ectoderm). The mesoderm, which forms the vascular, fat, and connective tissues, and also the meninges surrounding the neural tube, is presumed by some to be the instigating factor in producing malformation. At any rate, the disturbance is in these two layers. By the third month the bony canal is closed and the spinal cord which is attached to the brain stem appears more cephalad in relation to the vertebral column in the succeeding months. In the anomalies described, where the cord is fixed by adhesions or a fat pad, it remains at a lower level and is impaired. Instead of reaching the level of the second lumbar vertebra, the conus medullaris remains anchored at the level of the sacrum. It is therefore evident that with the traction of longitudinal growth, progression of neurological findings may be anticipated throughout infancy and childhood.

Myelography and spinal fluid pressure readings may be carried out, as indicated, to show the type of abnormality of the spine.

DIAGNOSIS: The problem of diagnosis arises only where there are complaints such as enuresis, failure of bowel control, etc. X-ray of the spine reveals the defect in the vertebral column. It then must be decided whether spina bifida occulta is a factor or an incidental finding. In enuresis which is only nocturnal the cause is likely to be psychological. If it persists, then a complete genitourinary survey is indicated and the associated spina bifida is evaluated accordingly.

When there are associated weakness and paralysis of the lower extremities, other causes such as Werdnig-Hoffman, spinal cord paralysis due to breech extraction, poliomyelitis, and amyotonia congenita should be ruled out.

TREATMENT: Surgery may be attempted to relieve some of the pathological conditions with which spina bifida occulta may be associated, especially if there is progression of symptoms. These include lipomas of the spinal cord, fibrous bands which tie down the cord to the bony canal, tight filum terminale, or a bony spicule (diastematomyelia) which also fixes the cord.

3. *Meningocele.* A protrusion of spinal cord membranes only, into a sac, with overlying normal skin. There are no neurological symptoms.

4. *Myelomeningocele.* A protrusion of spinal cord or nerve roots along with membrane into a sac covered with skin or epithelial membrane. The cord itself is usually imperfectly formed with distension of the central canal. Adhesions to the sac are present.

The differences between these last two groups are essentially theoretical since it is clinically difficult to separate them. Myelomeningocele occurs much more often.

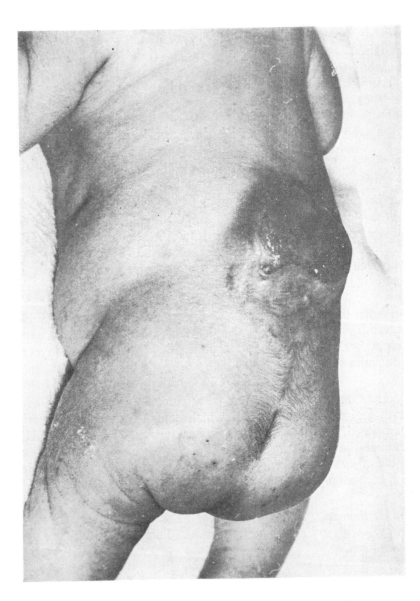

3. Myelomeningocele—lumbar area—hemorrhagic and ulcerated.

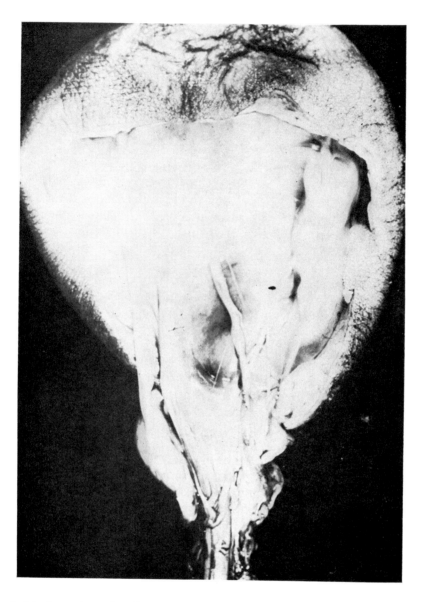

4. Myelomeningocele—large sac composed of dural membrane. Spinal cord is flattened and loses its identity in wall of sac.

CLINICAL PICTURE: The clinical picture is usually apparent after birth. The sac most often occurs in the lumbosacral area, occasionally cervical, and rarely thoracic. It is covered by normal skin or a thin translucent membrane (meninges) or the spinal cord is completely exposed (complete rachischisis or myeloschisis). This latter type often ulcerates, is easily infected, and is associated with complete paralysis of the legs and loss of sphincter control; it ends in death in a few months. The sac may be transilluminated in a darkened room to see whether nerve tissue is present. The legs will show flaccid paralysis and absence of deep tendon reflexes. To test for paralysis lift up the legs, then allow them to drop to the bed. If no attempt is made by the infant to break the fall, or if the legs drop lifelessly with no subsequent attempt at movement, they are paralyzed. There is also loss of sphincter control. If the sac is a pure meningocele there may be no paralysis, but this is not common. If the sac is cervical, there are spasticity and increased deep tendon reflexes in the lower extremities. Hydrocephalus due to an associated Arnold-Chiari syndrome is often present.

The incidence of meningomyelocele, meningocele, and encephalocele is given as 1:1000 births. There is a greater number of females, 1:6 to 1. A marked increase is seen in the frequency of these anomalies in families where it has once occurred, a 56 times greater chance than in the general population. This preponderance in females and the greater recurrence rate in families where it once occurred suggest to some authors a familial incidence. However, others do not find this experience. The question is as yet still open.

DIAGNOSIS: The presence at birth of a mass over the lumbosacral spine, or rarely cervical or thoracic, should suggest the diagnosis of spina bifida with meningomyelocele. Other congenital anomalies should be looked for, including club feet, dislocated hips, and hydrocephalus. The mass is soft and transilluminates. Sacrococcygeal teratoma does not have these characteristics. X-ray may be of aid in the differential.

PROGNOSIS: In infancy, the major risk is the associated hydrocephalus, which raises the question of the status of the mental development. The sac itself, if not covered by good skin, is likely to become infected or punctured in some areas with leakage of spinal fluid which subsequently becomes infected. This in the past meant meningitis and death, but is more controllable today because of antibiotics and chemotherapy.

TREATMENT: Surgery is questionable when there are complete paralysis of the legs and loss of sphincter action. Therefore, it should be delayed until a good neurological evaluation is made. The addition of hydrocephalus and mental retardation lessens the indications for repair of the sac. This is perhaps the general view. There are contrary ideas by others who advise early removal of the sac and immediate habilation. They feel this improves the morale of the patient and family. On the other hand, in meningocele the sac should be removed surgically as soon as possible. The outlook in this type is good.

As we have stated, one of the major problems in connection with spina bifida with meningomyelocele is the presence of associated hydrocephaly, which is due to the presence of the Arnold-Chiari malformation. (See chapter on hydrocephalus.) Hydrocephalus may also become evident after repair of the sac.

LIPOMAS OF THE CONUS MEDULLARIS AND CAUDA EQUINA

A lipoma is a soft, nonfluctuant mass covered by normal skin. It may be located over the sacral area in or near the midline and be present from birth. It is not associated with meningocele. It penetrates the dura and is attached to the conus. As a result it produces traction on the conus and the cauda equina as the spinal cord migrates cephalad in the course of the development of the infant. This traction accounts for the clinical picture.

Incontinence of urine or nocturnal enuresis is present. There is peripheral neuropathy with pain in the limbs, flaccid weakness, disturbed bowel and bladder function, and skeletal and trophic changes. X-ray shows a spina bifida of the sacrum.

DIAGNOSIS: This is based on the presence of a tumor at or near the midline with normal overlying skin associated with bowel and bladder disturbances, neurological deficit, and x-ray evidence of lumbosacral spina bifida.

PROGNOSIS: This is good if surgery is done early.

TREATMENT: Since the lipoma is not an integral part of the nerve roots as in the meningomyelocele, it can be readily removed without neurological deficit. Surgical removal should be performed in the first three or four months of life to avoid the effects of traction.

CRANIUM BIFIDUM

This is a defect in the skull, usually midline, due to lack of fusion of the cranial bones. The protruding sac is referred to as an encephalocele and occurs most often in the occipital area. In Ingraham and Matson's series of 187 cases, 139 were occipital. As in the spina bifida group, there may be just meninges (meningocele) or meninges with brain tissue (encephalomeningocele). The incidence of cranial encephalocele in relation to spina bifida is about 1 to 7.

The mass is detected most often in the occipital region; other areas include the parietal, frontal, nasal, and nasopharyngeal. The sac is covered by normal skin or a thin translucent membrane. Its shape and size are variable; it may be sessile or pedunculated.

The important factors are the contents of the sac and the presence of other anomalies of the brain. There may be some dura containing fluid within the sac, which may be reducible by pressure causing bulging of the fontanel. In other cases there may be brain contents connected with the remaining neural tissue by way of the ventricular system, the latter contained within the contents of the sac. The brain itself may show hydrocephalus, microgyria, or deformities of the brain stem including the cerebellum. There may be a hemangioma causing enlargement of the head, either by blocking the flow of cerebrospinal fluid or through increase in its own size.

DIAGNOSIS: There is usually little difficulty in diagnosis. In the newborn, cephalhematoma must be ruled out. This is parietooccipital in location, does not pulsate, and decreases in size after several weeks. In every case X-ray of the skull and perhaps ventriculography should be performed. This will settle the problem of the amount of brain tissue and ventricular system involved in the sac.

One of the problems in connection with encephaloceles is the presence of ectopic brain tissue in other areas, such as the nose and throat.

Brain tissue may be present in tumors of the nose, or at times may be found intranasally in a mass which is producing obstruction. The neural tissue consists of glial elements within a connective tissue meshwork. Two problems in diagnosis arise; one, that the nasal tumor may be connected with the brain or meninges with the risk of subsequent meningitis if the mass is operated upon unknowingly; the other is that the presence of neural or brain tissue extra or intranasally or in the pharynx raises the question of possible encephalocele.

PROGNOSIS: This depends on the location of the encephalocele, the contents of the sac, and associated anomalies. Since most encephaloceles are occipital and the latter is particularly associated with cerebral anomalies, the general picture is not bright. However in Ingraham and Swan's series, 21 of 59 patients (34 per cent) were normal after surgery.

TREATMENT: The therapy is surgical. Operation should be done early, within a few weeks of birth.

Bassett, R. C.: The Neurological Deficit Associated with Lipoma of the Cauda Equina. Am. Surg. 131:109, 1950.
Bluestone, S. S. and Deaver, G. G.: Habilitation of the Child with Spina Bifida and Myelomeningocele. J.A.M.A. 161:1248, 1956.
Chambers, W. R.: Hydrocephalus Consequent to Cranium Bifidum. A.M.A. J. Dis. Child. 88:466, 1954.
Ingraham, F. D.: Spina Bifida and Cranium Bifidum. Cambridge, Mass., Harvard University Press, 1944.
————, F. D. and Matson, D. D.: Neurosurgery of Infancy and Childhood. Springfield, Ill., Chas. C. Thomas, 1954.
Jones, P. H. and Love, J. G.: Tight Filum Terminale. A.M.A. Arch. Surg. 73:556, 1956.
Kahn, E. A.: Developmental Defects of the Skull and Spine Associated with Lesions of the Central Nervous System. A. Res. Publ. Ass. Nerv. Ment. Dis. Proc. 34:68, 1954.
Low, N. L., Scheinberg, L. and Anderson, D. H.: Brain Tissue in the Nose and Throat. Pediat. 18:254, 1956.
Schwidde, J. T.: Spina Bifida, A.M.A. J. Dis. Child. 84:35, 1952.

KLIPPEL-FEIL SYNDROME (BREVICOLLIS)

In this condition there is fusion of the vertebrae. There may be a reduction in the number of cervical vertebrae, which are fused into one bony mass. There may be a variety of anomalies in which the upper thoracic vertebrae are fused with the cervical mass. There may also be defective fusion of the occipital bone or thoracic spine with the development of spina bifida, either occulta or with meningocele.

The significance of brevicollis lies in its association with other congenital deformities, such as spina bifida, Sprengel's deformity, or syringomyelia, with consequent neurological disturbances. Torticollis and defects of the trapezius and pectoral muscles may also be present.

ETIOLOGY: This is a congenital, developmental defect, probably inherited in some families as a dominant with reduced penetrance.

CLINICAL PICTURE: There are a short neck and lowering of the hair line on the back of the neck. Motion of the head is limited. The neurological symptoms, if present, depend on the associated pathology. Cerebellar signs have been noted. Other neurological features include spastic hemiplegia, mental defect, convulsions, and defective hearing.

DIAGNOSIS: This is based on the essential clinical features with X-ray evidence of fusion of the cervical vertebrae. Pterygium colli should be ruled out.

TREATMENT: There is no specific therapy.

Bauman, G. I.: Absence of the Cervical Spine, Klippel-Feil Syndrome. J.A.M.A. 98:129, 1932.
Mosberg, Jr., W. H.: The Klippel-Feil Syndrome. Etiology and Treatment of Neurologic Signs. J. Nerv. and Ment. Dis. 117:479, 1953.

CONGENITAL DERMAL SINUS

This term is applied to a tract which leads from the skin in the midline of the back towards the meninges and is lined with stratified squamous epithelium.

Normally the cutaneous and neural ectoderm separate at about the fourth week of embryonic life. When this is incomplete, the sinus or skin aperture occurs at that point. The skin and connective tissue are then connected to the meninges of the spinal cord or brain. The most frequent area is the lumbosacral region. The ends of these sinus tracts may form epidermoid or dermoid cysts, with secondary cord pathology.

CLINICAL PICTURE: The child is usually seen with meningitis, which may often be recurrent. In the absence of a meningeal focus, the midline should be searched for evidence of a dermal sinus. These are present especially in the lumbosacral and occipital regions and are about 1-2 mm. in diameter. The lumbosacral sinuses are usually associated with spina bifida, which can be demonstrated by X-ray.

In the lumbosacral type, the organism is usually b. coli. The occipital type is often associated with s. aureus. In the occipital type there is often a dermoid cyst extending into the posterior fossa, which may be infected with an abscess.

DIAGNOSIS: In the presence of recurring meningitis, especially s. aureus or b. coli, or with signs of increased intracranial pressure in the posterior fossa, dermal sinus should be considered. One looks for midline dimpling of the skin.

TREATMENT: If there is meningitis or a local abscess in the area of the sinus, these should first be cured. Then the tract should be excised. The same procedure should be followed if there are spinal cord symptoms and an associated dermal sinus. In this case a dermoid cyst may be found. From a prophylactic point of view, when there are local signs of infection, a dermal sinus is removed immediately after the infection has been cleared with antibiotics, to avoid development of meningitis.

Matson, D. D. and Ingraham, F. D.: Intracranial Complications of Congenital Dermal Sinuses. Pediat. 8:463, 1951.
Walker, A. E. and Bucy, P. C.: Congenital Dermal Sinuses; Source of Spinal Meningeal Infection and Subdural Abscesses. Brain, 57:401, 1934.

DIASTEMATOMYELIA

In diastematomyelia the spinal cord is divided into two portions, each surrounded by its own dura. Accompanying this is the presence of a spicule of bone arising from the posterior surface of the body of a vertebra and passing through the middle of the spinal canal to transfix the spinal cord or cauda equina. Spina bifida is present in these cases. Traction on the cord results from growth of the vertebral column.

CLINICAL PICTURE: These children are brought for examination because of inability to walk or because their gait and balance are poor. There is also a lack of sphincter control of the bowel and bladder.

Examination of the skin over the back reveals unusual tufts of hair, dimpling of the skin, or a lipoma. The lower extremities show weakness of the muscles with diminished tendon reflexes, or there is spastic paralysis and increased reflexes with lesions higher in the cord. Deformities of the feet may be seen.

X-ray shows spina bifida in the same area where the skin manifestations are noted. In this same location there is a line of increased density in the middle of the spinal canal. Myelography reveals the separation around the spicule and the level of the lesion.

DIFFERENTIAL DIAGNOSIS: This condition is not to be confused with diplomyelia which refers to a doubling or reduplication of the spinal cord. In the latter there may be no symptoms; if however, spina bifida or other cord anomalies are present, clinical evidence of the associated abnormality may be observed. Diastematomyelia should be considered in any child who is not walking properly, or when a diagnosis of cerebral palsy is being entertained.

PROGNOSIS: Patients surgically treated improve or the progression of their symptoms is halted.

TREATMENT: Surgical removal of the bony spicule should be performed. This eliminates traction on the spinal cord.

Matson, D. D., Woods, R. P., Campbell, J. B. and Ingraham, F. D.: Diastematomyelia (congenital clefts of spinal cord); Diagnosis and Surgical Treatment. Pediat. 6:98, 1950.
Neuhauser, E. B. D., Wittenberg, M. H., Dehlinger, K.: Diastematomyelia. Transfixion of Cord or Cauda Equina, with Congenital Anomalies of Spine. Radiology. 54:659, 1950.

BASILAR IMPRESSION

(PLATYBASIA)

Basilar impression or basilar invagination involves a deformity of the base of the skull (occipital bone). Portions of the occipital bone are softened and flattened, allowing them to be pushed upward into the posterior fossa by the more rigid cervical spine. Along with this abnormality, there are associated anomalies, including narrowing and upward displacement of the foramen magnum, fusion of the atlas with the occipital bone, or fusion of atlas and axis. The odontoid process is displaced forward and upward.

As a result of these abnormalities, the medulla, pons, and cerebellum may be compressed or their structural relationships distorted. Aqueduct obstruction with hydrocephalus may result. The cranial nerves and cervical cord may also be involved.

ETIOLOGY: This is primarily a congenital anomaly. There is a familial tendency, and many of the patients have concomitant malformations of the brain, cord, or skeleton. Rarely basilar impression may develop in association with Paget's disease or rickets.

CLINICAL PICTURE: While the anomalies are present since birth, the neurological effects are usually not markedly evident until adolescence and adult life. There is a short neck with limited mobility, often held at an odd angle and hyperextended. Weakness of the extremities of a spastic type may be seen due to pressure on the pyramidal tracts. Headache and visual disturbances (papilledema) may occur due to subarachnoid block or hydrocephalus, with resultant increased intracranial pressure. Cranial nerve palsies, nystagmus, ataxia, and sensory disturbances may be present.

LABORATORY: X-ray confirms the diagnosis. In the lateral view, when a line is drawn from the posterior margin of the foramen magnum to the posterior margin of the hard palate (Chamberlain's line), it is seen that the odontoid process is displaced above the line (normally is below).

There are also cephalic bulging of the clivis, and upward and forward displacement of the atlas and axis. There are narrowing and invagination of the posterior rim of the foramen magnum. Instead of using the posterior margin of the foramen magnum, the line may also be drawn from the posterior margin of the hard palate to the lowermost point of the occipital bone (McGregor).

While basilar impression and platybasia are used interchangeably by many authors, others use each term more specifically. Basilar impression is confined to the posterior fossa including the area of the foramen magnum. Platybasia refers to abnormalities in the region of the anterior and middle fossae and involves the posterior fossa from the dorsum sellae only to the anterior margin of the foramen magnum. If one draws a line from the root of the nose to the center of the sella turcica, and another from the center of the sella to the anterior border of the foramen magnum, the inferior angle formed at the point of junction is referred to as the basal angle, and normally it is about 135 degrees. In platybasia the lines straighten, forming an angle closer to 180 degrees.

DIAGNOSIS: Basilar impression should be considered in infancy when there is weakness of the extremities with hyperactive reflexes. An X-ray of the skull and spine should be taken which will reveal the associated abnormalities. The clinical neurological picture may simulate multiple sclerosis. It may also be associated with a picture of hydrocephalus or syringomyelia.

PROGNOSIS: The outlook is poor.

TREATMENT: Surgical decompression of the occipital and upper cervical region should be performed.

Chamberlain, W. E.: Basilar Impression (Platybasia). Bizarre Developmental Anomaly of Occipital Bone and Upper Cervical Spine, with Striking and Misleading Neurologic Manifestations. Yale J. Biol. Med. 11:487, 1939.

McGregor, M.: The Significance of Certain Measurements of the Skull in the Diagnosis of Basilar Impression. Brit. J. Radiol. 21:171, 1948.

Poppel, M. H., Jacobson, H. G., Duff, B. K. and Gottlieb, C.: Basilar Impression and Platybasia in Paget's Disease. Radiology 61:639, 1953.

Spillane, J. D., Pallis, C. and Jones, A. M.: Developmental Abnormalities in the Region of the Foramen Magnum. Brain 80:11, 1957.

AGENESIS OF THE CORPUS CALLOSUM

Agenesis or failure of development of the corpus callosum is a congenital anomaly of the brain, which may occur alone or often in conjunction with other malformations. The corpus callosum is formed between the third and fifth months of fetal life, so that interference with development will result in complete or partial absence, depending on the time when the arrest took place.

Since the corpus callosum develops from the lamina terminalis, other structures similarly derived are also involved. There is therefore absence of the hippocampal and anterior commissures and septum pellucidum. Alteration in the convolutions is noted, with microgyria or agyria. Heterotopic masses are observed. Hydrocephalus, meningoencephalitis, porencephaly, or cortical atrophy may be present.

ETIOLOGY: Intrauterine infection producing meningitis or ependymitis, congenital syphilis, and viral inflammation (maternal rubella) have been noted in some reports. In others, vascular lesions

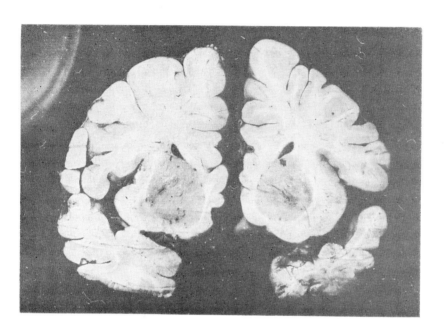

5. Agenesis of the Corpus Callosum.

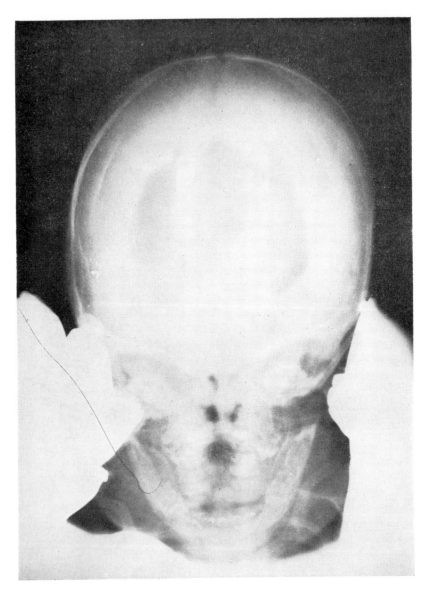

6. Agenesis of the Corpus Callosum. Lateral ventricles are dilated. Third ventricle is displaced dorsally and dilated.

and developmental failures of unknown cause have been considered because of the presence of other midline closure defects such as harelip, cleft palate, and spinal anomalies.

CLINICAL PICTURE: If the corpus callosum alone is absent, there may be no symptoms. With the presence of other cerebral anomalies, the presenting picture is one of mental deficiency and seizures. The head is usually enlarged. Cerebral palsies, with spasticity or athetosis, may be present. Associated anomalies may be observed such as hypertelorism, cleft palate, and optic atrophy. The electroencephalogram shows diffuse cortical dysrhythmia.

Pneumoencephalography (Davidoff and Dyke) reveals:
1. Marked separation of the lateral ventricles.
2. Dilation of the 3rd ventricle, which is extended dorsally beyond the normal.
3. Radial arrangement of the medial cerebral sulci around the roof of the 3rd ventricle and their extension into the zone usually occupied by the corpus callosum.

DIAGNOSIS: This is usually made in childhood by pneumoencephalography. Agenesis of the corpus callosum should be suspected in any child with a low I.Q., seizures, large head, cerebral palsy, and other associated anomalies.

TREATMENT: There is no corrective therapy.

Bell, W. E. and Summers, T. B.: Agenesis of the Septum Pellucidum. Neurology 8:234, 1958.
Davidoff, L. M. and Dyke, C. G.: Agenesis of the Corpus Callosum: Its Diagnosis by Encephalography. Am. J. Roentgenol. and Rad. Therapy 32:1, 1934.
Koch, F. P. and Doyle, P. J.: Agenesis of the Corpus Callosum, Report of Eight Cases in Infancy. J. Pediat. 50:345, 1957.
Savitsky, E. and Spinella, V. A.: Agenesis of Corpus Callosum in Infancy: Clinical and Roentgenologic Aspects. Am. J. Dis. Child. 76:109, 1948.
Van Epps, E. F.: Agenesis of the Corpus Callosum with Concomitant Malformations, Including Atresia of the Foramens of Luschka and Magendie. Am. J. Roentgenol. 70:47, 1953.

HYDROCEPHALUS

This is a condition in which there is distension of the ventricular system of the brain, caused by accumulation of cerebrospinal fluid, which is under increased pressure.

The cerebrospinal fluid is contained and flows within a closed system, originating primarily in the lateral ventricles, continuing into the foramina of Monro, the 3rd ventricle, aqueduct, and 4th ventricle; there are exits from the roof of the 4th ventricle by way of the lateral foramina of Luschka and the central foramen of Magendie. This allows for communication dorsally with the cisterna magna cerebellomedullaris. From the latter, the fluid flows caudally into the subarachnoid space surrounding the spinal cord and anteriorly or ventrally around the bulb into the cisterna basalis and a series of cisternae under the pons and midbrain. The cerebrospinal fluid reaches the subarachnoid spaces over the convexity by way of the lateral surfaces of the cortical hemispheres. It is finally absorbed into the dural venous sinuses, especially the superior longitudinal, by way of the arachnoid villi. The formation of the cerebrospinal fluid occurs primarily in the ventricles, especially the lateral, but also the 3rd and 4th. The fluid itself is essentially a secretion of the choroid plexuses located in these ventricles. But there is some quantity of fluid which enters by way of the ependyma and walls of the subarachnoid space. This occurs as an ultra-filtrate. The amount is determined by the hydrostatic and osmotic pressures of the blood in the cortical blood vessels and cerebrospinal fluid, as well as by the permeability of the perivascular space between them. The absorption takes place in various ways. Primarily the cerebrospinal fluid is absorbed by way of the arachnoidal villi which protrude into the large dural sinuses. The venous blood has a lower pressure and is hypertonic relative to the fluid in the villi. There is also some absorption into the blood by way of the subarachnoid space, both cortical around the cranial nerves and spinal around the peripheral nerves, and in the ventricles by way of the choroid plexus.

ETIOLOGY AND PATHOLOGY: How is hydrocephalus caused? Primarily by obstruction somewhere along the pathway of the circulating cerebrospinal fluid, from the lateral ventricles to the subarachnoid spaces over the cortex. There are two other mechanisms of minor importance, namely oversecretion or excessive production of cerebrospinal fluid, and secondly, defective absorption. Let us consider the latter two first. There is definite evidence that hypersecretion is a factor in the production of hydrocephalus. Removal of a papilloma of the choroid plexus in the lateral ventricle, when hydrocephalus had occurred without any evidence of obstruction to the flow of fluid or defective absorption, has been followed by relief of the signs of increased intracranial pressure and diminution of the hydrocephalus. This tumor occurs primarily in early infancy, and Matson stresses that apart from this age group hypersecretion is a rarity and extremely unusual.

The question of defective absorption of the cerebrospinal fluid has been raised with respect to longitudinal sinus thrombosis. As we have previously indicated, the dural sinus is the main absorbing area by way of the arachnoidal villi, so that a pathological process involving the sinus might theoretically produce non-absorptive hydrocephalus. Russel has provided illustrations of sinus thrombosis associated with increased intracranial pressure in which there were normal ventricles and other instances with dilated ventricles. In some cases there is no increased intracranial pressure. The condition has never been produced experimentally. If therefore this type of defective absorptive hydrocephalus does occur, it is extremely rare. This leads us to a discussion of the major type, that is, obstructive hydrocephalus. In infants and children there are several major etiological factors, namely, maldevelopments, inflammations, and neoplasms.

I. Maldevelopments. These are of various types:

    A. Spina bifida, myelomeningocele + Arnold-Chiari syndrome.

    B. Cranium bifidum.

    C. Aqueduct. Pathology here is the most common cause of non-communicating hydrocephalus.

Spina bifida with myelomeningocele is often associated with the Arnold-Chiari complex. In the latter, the tonsillar tissue or inferior portions of both cerebellar hemispheres are pushed through the foramen magnum. There is also elongation of the medulla and displacement of the fourth ventricle into the spinal canal with resultant compression of the cervical cord. There is some obliteration of the ventricle, and part of the choroid projects into the spinal canal. The end result is a block in the flow of cerebrospinal fluid resulting in hydrocephalus, usually of the communicating type; that is, the ventricular system is patent and the fluid flows from the 4th ventricle to the spinal canal but does not reach the anterior surfaces for eventual absorption in the venous sinuses. If there is associated stenosis of the aqueduct or a block at the foramina of Luschka and Magendie, there is then a non-communicating type of hydrocephalus (no communication between the ventricular system and the outside subarachnoid spaces). In cranium bifidum where there is encephalomeningocele present, hydrocephalus also occurs. This is attributed to the associated abnormalities such as congenital atresia of the aqueduct, failure of formation of the foramina of Luschka and Magendie, or obliteration of the cisterna magna. Benign tumors may be present with cranium bifidum, which also produce hydrocephalus by blocking the flow of cerebrospinal fluid. These are removable surgically.

a) Stenosis—the aqueduct is abnormally small, but histologically normal. There is no increase in subependymal glia. This form may be genetic.

b) Forking—This is more common than simple stenosis; the aqueduct is divided into several components, with small tubules or channels, but the intervening neural tissue is normal. Also probably genetic. Russel feels that stenosis and forking are not uncommon as factors in hydrocephalus in the cases of spina bifida associated with Arnold-Chiari syndrome.

c) Gliosis of the aqueduct causes gradual obliteration of the lumen due to the overgrowth of fibrillary subependymal neuroglia. There may be subdivisions into various channels. The present weight of evidence seems to favor the inflammatory hypothesis as a cause for this condition. Since hydrocephalus gradually develops during childhood due to closure of the aqueduct, surgical relief must be carried out.

d) Atresia of the foramina of Luschka and Magendie results in a large cyst with a bulging 4th ventricle and compression of the vermis and cerebellar hemispheres. Clinically it may produce prominence of the occipital area, whereas usually hydrocephalus causes enlargement of the frontal and parietal regions. If dye is injected in the lateral ventricle, it may come through to the spinal canal; this means the obstruction is not complete. The ventriculogram shows symmetrical dilatation of the lateral and 3rd ventricles and of the aqueduct. The cyst is seen projecting into the cervical canal.

II. Hemorrhage and Inflammations. Hydrocephalus may be produced by either hemorrhage or inflammation. Intracranial hemorrhage, associated with prenatal anoxia or birth injury, may result in organization of the clot with fibrosis of the meninges, causing block of the basilar cisterns with secondary hydrocephalus. Intrauterine encephalitis or meningitis may produce aqueduct obliteration (ependymitis). Most often, however, this form of hydrocephalus is due to postnatal meningitis with subarachnoid block around the brain stem, chiasm, and cortex.

III. Neoplasms. These may obstruct the flow of cerebrospinal fluid. They are usually gliomas. One of our cases was a dermoid filling the 3rd ventricle and obstructing the flow of cerebrospinal fluid from both lateral ventricles.

CLINICAL PICTURE: The clinical picture is based upon the development of increased intracranial pressure secondary to block of the flow of cerebrospinal fluid. Since the sutures of the newborn infant are not united and the fontanels are open, there is room for expansion of the head, which enlarges and thus accommodates the increased pressure. If we use a mean circumference of 13.5" or 35 cm. as standard for the skull at birth, we may allow an increase of about ½" or 1¼ cm. a month as maximal. In progressive hydrocephalus this rate of increase will be much greater, as will the relationship of the head to chest measurements. The face also appears to be much smaller by comparison with the head. Another feature is the presence of distension of the veins of the forehead. The cranial sutures are separated beyond normal, and the anterior fontanel may be large, tense or bulging. Percussion of the skull may give a hollow "cracked pot" tone. The eyeballs may be displaced downward, so that only the sclerae are seen. There is often divergent squint. Papilledema is not often present because of the relief of pressure on the optic discs by the enlargement of the head, but optic atrophy may be noted. If there is complete atresia of the foramina of Luschka and Magendie there may be bulging of the posterior or occipital portion of the skull, which transilluminates light. There may be associated signs of cerebral palsy (spastic paraplegias, ataxias) and evidence of failure of psychomotor development. Signs of pressure such as vomiting and convulsions may also occur. The symptoms and signs vary depending on when the hydrocephalus began, pre- or postnatally, and the rapidity with which the enlargement of the head compensates for the increasing pressure. They will also depend on the etiological factor itself.

DIFFERENTIAL DIAGNOSIS: It is extremely important to make a diagnosis of hydrocephalus as early as possible, so that if surgery is to be done, relief may be obtained before too much damage to the brain has occurred. This will mean a consideration of those causes which may produce a large head in infancy, such as subdural hematoma, which is particularly amenable to surgery, the prognosis likewise depending on early recognition. Subdural punctures which are negative will rule out subdural hematoma. There may be anomalies of bone such as spina bifida or cranium bifidum, which should suggest accompanying hydrocephalus. Other conditions such as achondroplasia or platybasia may be associated with or should be differentiated from hydrocephalus. In addition, there are macrocephaly, rickets, gargoylism, hypertelorism, and hydranencephaly. Hydrocephalus may be a manifestation of a variety of conditions which have to be differentiated, such as bacterial meningitis, syphilis, toxoplasmosis, thrombosis of the dural sinuses, aneurysm of the vein of Galen, brain abscess, and brain tumor. All of these conditions and their relation to hydrocephalus are discussed in their respective sections of the book. In later childhood, brain tumor must be differentiated from the previously mentioned gliosis of the aqueduct or from gliosis of the subarachnoid space surrounding the medulla and cervical cord with secondary obstruction of the 4th ventricle.

MANAGEMENT: A complete history is taken. In this way an etiological factor may be obtained, e.g., toxoplasmosis, meningitis. Physical examination will reveal the presence of the enlarged head, distended scalp veins, widened fontanel, abnormal suture separation, and accompanying anomalies, e.g., spina bifida (myelomeningocele).

X-ray films will reveal signs of pressure, such as suture separation, thinning of the bones of the vault, and increased size of the skull. At the same time, calcification is noted in the case of toxoplasmosis, and other cranial defects previously mentioned will be seen.

The next procedure should be bilateral subdural punctures. If these are negative, a needle is inserted into the lateral ventricle and 1 cc. of neutral phenolsulfonephthalein is injected. This dye should normally be recovered through a lumbar puncture needle within ten to fifteen minutes. Allow the spinal fluid to drop into a tube containing several drops of N/10 NaOH or gauze containing ammonia. If at the end of a few hours the spinal fluid appears clear, showing no passage of dye, a non-communicating type of hydrocephalus should be suspected.

At the same time as the dye is injected into the lateral ventricle, all urine is collected by means of a permanent catheter. Fluid should be given by mouth and subcutaneously during the procedure to insure good urinary output. When no dye has appeared in the spinal needle, the output of dye in the urine will be extremely small, perhaps 5 per cent (normal 25-40 per cent in two hours; 50-70 per cent in 12 hours). If the dye, after some delay, appears in the lumbar puncture needle and is accompanied by a reduced percentage of dye in the urine, it suggests that there is communicating hydrocephalus. It has also been pointed out that some obstructive cystic lesions of the 4th ventricle allow dye but not cerebrospinal fluid to pass in sufficient amounts. There is some correlation between the extent of the pathology (ventricular dilatation) and the amount of dye output in the urine; the greater the degree of pathology, the less the output.

Ventriculography is then performed. This procedure will demonstrate enlargement of the ventricles, whether or not symmetrical, and any alteration in the cisterns. If the lateral and 3rd ventricles are dilated, the aqueduct may be obstructed. If only both lateral ventricles are dilated and not the 3rd, the latter may be obstructed. If one lateral ventricle is dilated, the foramen of Monro on that side is blocked. A large collection of air in the 4th ventricle suggests atresia of the Foramina of Luschka and Magendie. These findings are correlated with the dye studies.

In communicating hydrocephalus the entire ventricular system may be dilated. Interpretation will require the services of a roentgenologist and neurosurgeon. The fluids collected by ventricular and lumbar puncture are analyzed for appearance, pressure, cell count, bacterial culture, chemistry, and Wassermann.

TREATMENT: There are occasional instances in congenital hydrocephalus when successive measurements of the circumference of the skull indicate no undue increase in size. Along with this observation, it is noted that the infant has had no clinical evidence of any further increase in intracranial pressure. In other words, for reasons unknown, equilibrium between production and absorption has been reached. For the vast majority of cases, however, surgery is required. When there is obstruction within the 3rd ventricle or aqueduct of Sylvius, ventriculo-cisternostomy (Torkildsen procedure) is preferred. This form of non-communicating hydrocephalus is usually caused in children by stenosis of the aqueduct and tumors involving the aqueduct and 3rd ventricle, such as craniopharyngioma, dermoid, and gliomas of the brain stem. When there is obliteration of the Foramina of Luschka and Magendie, the cyst membrane enclosing the fluid in the dilated 4th ventricle is removed allowing for egress of the spinal fluid to the subarachnoid pathways. In these pathways, however, there are usually associated abnormalities, such as failure of development, so that an additional lumbar subarachnoid-peritoneal or ureteral shunt will be needed to relieve increased intracranial pressure. If there is patency of the ventricular system, but obstruction exists in the basilar cisternae or surface pathways, then arachnoid-ureterostomy is done. This means sacrificing one kidney, making sure first that both are normal, and connecting the polyethylene tube from the lumbar subarachnoid space to the ureter. If in addition to the above, there is obstruction of the posterior fossa and spinal subarachnoid space, as is the case in meningitis, then ventriculo-ureterostomy is performed. Other surgeons have utilized the peritoneal cavity instead of the ureter for these shunts. Recently a new technique of ventriculo-auriculostomy has been utilized. In this procedure the cerebrospinal fluid is shunted from the lateral ventricle into the right auricle. The tube enters the right auricle by way of the common facial and right internal jugular veins. This tube has a silicone rubber valve which allows cerebrospinal fluid to enter the auricle when the pressure in the tube is over 3 cm. of water. Thus far the results appear favorable, but the postoperative length of time is too short to draw any final conclusions.

Another recent report refers to the use of ventriculo-subdural drainage from the lateral ventricle to the overlying subdural space. One must be sure there is no subdural block due to adhesions.

PROGNOSIS: The outlook has been poor in the past. This is due to the presence of associated anomalies in many cases and to the fact that mental impairment has already occurred in most instances. It is to be hoped that with early recognition and newer surgical techniques the prospects will be improved.

Adams, R. D., Schatzki, R. and Scoville, W. R.: Arnold-Chiari Malformation; Diagnosis, Demonstration by Intraspinal Lipiodol and Successful Surgical Treatment, New England J. Med. 225:125, 1941.

Bering, Jr., E. A.: The use of Phenolsulphonphthalein in the Clinical Evaluation of Hydrocephalus. J. Neurol. 13:587, 1956.

Bickers, D. S. and Adams, R. D.: Hereditary Stenosis of the Aqueduct of Sylvius as a Cause of Congenital Hydrocephalus. Brain 72:246, 1949.

Chambers, W. R.: Hydrocephalus Consequent to Cranium Bifidum. A.M.A. J. Dis. Child. 88:466, 1954.

Dandy, W. E.: Experimental Hydrocephalus, Ann. Surg. 70:129, 1919.

————, W. E. and Blackfan, K. D.: An Experimental and Clinical Study of Internal Hydrocephalus. J.A.M.A. 61:2216, 1913.

Flexner, L. B.: Some Problems of Origin, Circulation and Absorption of Cerebrospinal Fluid. Quart. Rev. Biol. 8:397, 1933.

Forrest, D. M., Laurence, K. M. and Macnab, G. H.: Ventriculo-subdural Drainage in Infantile Hydrocephalus. Analysis of Early Results. Lancet 272:1274, 1957. 273:827, 1957.

Fowler, F. D. and Alexander, J. E.: Atresia of the Foramina of Luschka and Magendie. A.M.A. J. Dis. Child. 92:131, 1956.

Hirano, A. and Terry, R. D.: Aneurysm of the Vein of Galen. J. Neuropath. and Exper. Neurol. 17:424, 1958.

Ingraham, F. D. and Matson, D. D.: Neurosurgery of Infancy and Childhood. Hydrocephalus, p. 117. Springfield, Ill., C. C. Thomas, 1954.

Kahn, E. A. and Luros, J. T.: Hydrocephalus from Overproduction of Cerebrospinal Fluid. J. Neurosurg. 9:59, 1952.

Matson, D. D.: Hydrocephalus in a Premature Infant Caused by Papilloma of the Choroid Plexus. J. Neurosurg. 10:416, 1953.

———, D. D.: Prenatal Obstruction of the Fourth Ventricle. Am. J. Roentgenol. 76:499, 1956.

Presentation of Case: New England J. Med. 256:417, 1957.

Pudenz, R. H., Russel, F. E., Hurd, A. H. and Sheldon, C. H.: Ventriculo-auriculostomy. A Technique for Shunting Cerebrospinal Fluid into the Right Auricle. J. Neurosurg. 14:171, 1957.

Russel, D. S.: Observation on the Pathology of Hydrocephalus. Special Report Series Medical Research Council. London No. 265, 1949.

———, D. S.: Hydrocephalus. A. Res. Publ. Ass. Nerv. Ment. Dis. Proc. 34:160, 1954.

Sweet, W. H., Brownell, G. L., Scholl, J. A., Bowsher, D. R., Benda, P. and Stickley, E. E.: The Formation, Flow and Absorption of Cerebrospinal Fluid. Newer Concepts Based on Studies with Isotopes. A. Res. Publ. Ass. Nerv. Ment. Dis. Proc. 34:101, 1954.

Weed, L. H.: Meninges and Cerebrospinal Fluid. J. Anat. 72:181, 1938.

HYDRANENCEPHALY

In hydranencephaly the cerebral hemispheres are destroyed and converted into thin-walled, translucent, sac-like chambers filled with cerebrospinal fluid. The skull and meninges are intact. Before the dura is opened, the outline of the brain is normal and fills the cranial cavity. When the membrane (leptomeninges) is punctured, allowing the cerebrospinal fluid to escape, it is observed that there are no cortical hemispheres.

There are two forms described by Lange-Cossack. In the larger group there is destruction of the cerebral cortex, white matter, basal ganglia, thalamus, hypothalamus, and occasionally parts of the upper midbrain. The lower brain stem, cerebellum, and spinal cord are grossly intact. In a smaller group, the thalamus, hypothalamus, corpus striatum, midbrain, and some of the gyri at the base of the brain are intact. In some instances the aqueduct or ventricular foramina are closed suggesting a preceding hydro-cephalus with resultant cortical atrophy.

CLINICAL PICTURE: In the severe cases following birth there may be difficulty in sucking or swallowing, poor temperature regulation, episodes of asphyxia, and abnormalities of movement, posture, and muscle tone. The head may appear normal. These infants die within a month. They represent the group with major brain pathology. In others, there may be little symptomatology early. However, within a few weeks the head begins to increase rapidly in size and there are failure of psychomotor development, paralysis, and seizures.

DIAGNOSIS: The diagnosis is made clinically by transilluminating the head in a dark room. The light should be directed through a cone embracing the occiput. There will appear a reddish glow over the head, and if the pupils have previously been dilated, the beam of light will shine through them. The electroencephalogram shows a flat tracing with absence of electrical activity. Ventriculog-raphy shows no contour to the ventricles. In extreme hydrocephalus, transillumination of the skull may present a similar picture.

In all instances of retarded development, whether or not the head is enlarged, the transillumination procedure should be performed.

ETIOLOGY: Since the brain has been fully formed, it is felt that the agent producing hydranencephaly acts during the middle or latter part of pregnancy. Wolf feels that hydranencephaly is a pathological process, similar in kind, but of a more severe degree than multiple cystic encephalomalacia. The latter he relates to anoxia. Most authors feel that hydranencephaly is not due to hydro-cephalus.

PROGNOSIS: The outcome is fatal. A case of Hamby's lived 26 months.

TREATMENT: There is no therapy.

Hamby, W. B., Krauss, R. F. and Beswick, W. F.: Hydranencephaly, Clinical Diagnosis. Pediat. 6:371, 1950.
Lange-Cosack, H.: Die Hydranencephalie (Blasenhirn) als Sonderform der Grosshirnlosigkeit. Arch. für Psychiat. und Nervenkrankeiten. Anatomical Section 117:1-51, 1944. Clinical Section 117:595-640, 1944.
Levin, J. C.: Value of Transillumination in Diagnosis of Hydranencephaly. J. Pediat. 50:55, 1957.

Olive, J. T. and DuShane, J. W.: Hydranencephaly, Am. J. Dis. Child. 85:43, 1953.

Wolf, A. and Cowen, D.: The Cerebral Atrophies and Encephalomalacies of Infancy and Childhood. A. Res. Publ. Ass. Nerv. Ment. Dis. Proc. 34:199, 1954.

MONGOLISM

Mongolism, which derives its name from the peculiar appearance of the facies, is a prenatal developmental disorder associated with mental deficiency. It occurs at the rate of one in every 500 births. In institutions for the mentally defective it comprises ten per cent of the population.

CLINICAL PICTURE: The condition can usually be recognized at birth. The most apparent feature is the mongoloid appearance of the face due to the maldevelopment of the basilar bones of the skull, which gives the typical facies and orbital slant. The head is smaller than average, the skull brachycephalic in type and the hair coarse and scanty. The eyes appear to slant upwards and have narrow palpebral fissures; epicanthus is prominent; conjunctivitis and cataracts may occur. The ears may be malformed, the nose short and flat. The tongue is protruded and in time shows fissuring. There is a narrow posterior pharynx which, together with the presence of adenoid tissue, leads to mouth breathing and frequent respiratory infections. The teeth usually have poor alignment and appear small. The neck is characteristically bulging and short, with extra skin folds in the postero-lateral regions. Due to the marked general muscular hypotonia, the abdomen is protuberant, and umbilical hernia is often present. The mongoloid children are short in stature. The hands and feet are short and stubby, with widely spaced first and second digits, and there are abnormal creases in the palmar and plantar surfaces with only one transverse straight line across the palm and sole instead of two. The fifth or little finger curves inward and is very small. There may be maldevelopment of the middle phalanx. There is marked hypermobility of the joints with relaxation of the ligaments, so that the arms and legs may be placed in many abnormal positions. The genitalia are undeveloped. The heart may show congenital septal defects.

LABORATORY: There are a variety of skeletal deformities which may be seen by the X-ray, such as hypoplasia of the base of the skull and of the nasal bones (acromicria), decrease in the size of the osseous orbits, and dysplasia and hypoplasia of the phalanges.

There is undergrowth of the tubular bones in the extremities and of the vertebral bodies which accounts for the shortness of stature.

In the pelvis small acetabular angles, large ilia, and elongated tapering ischia are seen.

There is an increase in serum lipoproteins and urinary beta-aminoisobutyric acid.

PATHOLOGY: The brain weight is lower than average. A small frontal lobe, cerebellum, and brain stem may be seen. There are poverty of cells and failure of gyral development. The remaining pathological features are concerned with the developmental defects in the skeletal system and the associated anomalies previously mentioned.

ETIOLOGY: The cause of mongolism is as yet unknown. There are two conflicting theories and each has supporters with evidence to substantiate its claims. Certain facts are definite. It is agreed that mongolism occurs more often in women who give birth to a baby at an advanced maternal age. The risk of having a mongol baby increases in any woman over forty, perhaps six per cent. Therefore, those who believe that the cause of mongolism is environmental maintain that the older women have more chances for intrauterine abnormality, e.g., retroverted uterus, which could influence pre-natal development of the fetus. The occurrence of the bony deformities of the skull, cardiac defects, and cataracts would point to a noxious agent acting on the fetus at about the 8th week of gestation (Ingalls). Recently there have been reports of a much higher incidence of congenital leukemia with mongolism as compared to the general population, with the implication that the same stress effects on the fetus at the sixth to ninth week of gestation that produce mongolism also affect the hemopoietic system and bone marrow to produce leukemia later. Benda maintains that development in mongolism begins normally but fails to be completed perfectly. He feels that there is a deceleration of fetal growth with a disturbance of central growth regulation due to adverse factors in the neofetal and fetal period (congenital acromicria). On the other hand, Penrose feels mongolism is due to a single recessive gene. The condition occurs twenty-five times as often in families where mongolism has previously occurred as compared to the general population. Jervis has reported that in the case of twins, one or both with mongolism, twenty concordant pairs were monozygotic, whereas sixty-two of sixty-six discordant pairs were dizygotic.

Wright includes mongolism under disorders of possible metabolic origin because of the presence of metabolic (enzymatic) abnormalities.

Mental Development. The mongolian infants are always retarded mentally. The majority are in the middle or imbecile level. Some reach higher (moron) and others lower (idiocy) levels. They usually are able to walk, although the onset is delayed to about three years. Similarly, there is retardation in the onset of speech though eventually they do learn to converse to some extent. The children are usually pleasant, like music, and are easy to get along with. They will always require supervision and special types of education.

DIFFERENTIAL DIAGNOSIS: The major differential is from cretinism. Mongolism can usually be recognized at birth. Cretinism generally becomes apparent at about one to two months. The mongol has the brachycephalic skull with slanted eyes and epicanthic folds. The cretin has a dry, pale, cool, mottled skin, and the X-ray shows evidence of delay in ossification and epiphyseal dysgenesis. In the mongol, the X-ray shows evidence of hypoplasia of the basilar and nasal bones. In the cretin, I^{131} uptake, PBI and BEI are all diminished. Finally, if in doubt, thyroid may be given and the effects noted after a few weeks. There will be none in mongolism.

TREATMENT: There is no therapy which has proved to be of value. Benda has recommended calf pituitary substance plus thyroid and B_{12}. Glutamic acid has also been tried. The life expectancy for these children has increased with the advent of the antibiotic drugs. They should be cared for at home during infancy. Later in childhood the question of placement may be settled. The question of other children usually does not occur when the mother is elderly at the time of birth of the mongol baby. However, mongolism may occur in a young mother also. In this instance the risk of a repetition should be discussed with the parents, who can then decide their course.

Benda, C. E.: Research in Congenital Acromicria (Mongolism). Quart. Rev. Pediat. 8:79, 1953.
Böök, J. A. and Reed, S. C.: Empiric Risk Figures in Mongolism. J.A.M.A. 143:730, 1950.

Caffey, J. and Ross, S.: Mongolism (Mongoloid Deficiency) During Early Infancy. Some Newly Recognized Diagnostic Changes in the Pelvic Bones. Pediat. 17:642, 1956.

Ingalls, T. H.: Pathogenesis of Mongolism. Am. J. Dis. Child. 73:279, 1947.

Jervis, G. A.: A Note on the Etiology of Mongolism. Quart. Rev. Pediat. 8:126, 1953.

Krivit, W. and Good, R. A.: Simultaneous Occurrence of Mongolism and Leukemia. Report of a Nationwide Survey. A.M.A. J. Dis. Child. 94:289, 1957.

Merrit, D. H. and Harris, J. S.: Mongolism and Acute Leukemia. A.M.A. J. Dis. Child. 92:41, 1956.

Penrose, L. S.: Maternal Age in Familial Mongolism. J. Ment. Sc. 97:738, 1951.

Sobel, A. E., Strazzulla, M., Sherman, B. S., Elkan, B., Morgenstern, S. W., Marius N. and Meisel, A.: Vitamin A Absorption and Other Blood Composition Studies in Mongolism. Am. J. Ment. Def. 62:642, 1958.

Stern, J. and Lewis, W. H. D.: Serum Proteins in Mongolism. J. Ment. Sc. 103:222, 1957.

Walker, N. F.: The Use of Dermal Configurations in the Diagnosis of Mongolism. J. Pediat. 50:19, 1957.

Wright, S. W. and Fink, K.: Excretion of Beta-Aminoisobutyric Acid in Normal, Mongoloid and Non-Mongoloid Mentally Defective Children. Am. J. Ment. Deficiency 61:530, 1957.

———, S. W., Tarjan, G., Lippman, R. W. and Perry, T. L.: Etiologic Factors in Mental Deficiency. A.M.A. J. Dis. Child. 95:541, 1958.

MICROCEPHALY

(True, Primary, Genetic Micrencephaly)

These terms are used to express the type of microcephaly which is of genetic origin. The skull is smaller than the average and is of a peculiar configuration, with a receding forehead and a flat occiput. There is associated mental deficiency.

Clinical Picture: There are variations in the size of the head. At birth, a circumference below 33 cm. is considered suspect. The normal measurement is 33.5 to 37 cm. Most microcephalics do not reach beyond 43 cm. as adults, but Tredgold has reported some of 48 cm. and has stressed that it is the shape of the head which is significant rather than size. In the vast majority, however, the head is smaller than the average for the general population, and at a year is only 35 cm. (average 45 cm.). The head is cone-like or bird-like in appearance because of the flat occipital region and recessive frontal. There are reduced volume and deficient development of the skull, all secondary to the retarded growth of the brain. The second feature is the underdevelopment of the body. These children are of small stature and underweight. As adults they rarely reach five feet in height. The face, however, appears full compared to the head. All of the physical activities, such as walking and speech, are delayed. Seizures are present in about fifteen per cent of the cases. Occasionally there is spasticity with hyperactive tendon reflexes, presumably due to impaired development of the pyramidal pathways. The electroencephalogram shows some abnormalities, especially reduction in voltage, but there is nothing diagnostic. Most microcephalics are imbeciles, some idiots. They are generally restless, have a poor span of attention, and are usually affable.

PATHOLOGY: There are general hypoplasia of the cerebral hemispheres and a paucity of cells. The weight of the brain is only a few hundred grams (normal weight is 300 grams at birth and 1,000 grams at three years). The occipital and frontal lobes are shrunken. There is marked undifferentiation of the gyri; in some cases there is microgyria. False porencephaly and dilatation of the ventricles may be present due to cerebral atrophy. The pyramidal tracts and most of the spinal cord are poorly developed.

DIAGNOSIS: The diagnosis is based on the characteristic appearance of the skull, mental deficiency, nanosomia, associated at times with convulsions, and a hypofunction of the pyramidal system. Böök, Schut, and Reed have used the term "genetic micrencephaly" and have indicated that this term be applied where there are frequent occurrences of similar cases in the same sibship and an absence of exogenous etiology. The differential diagnosis must be made from several other conditions in which a small head may be present, especially craniosynostosis. In this condition the sutures close prematurely, preventing the brain from growing. There may be a history of failing vision and examination of the optic discs may reveal papilledema. X-ray makes the diagnosis, since it reveals premature closure of the sutures and density at the suture lines. In mongolism there is a decrease in the size of the head, but the differential is obvious by the visual mongoloid features.

In exogenous or secondary microcephaly the etiology is prenatal or natal, but non-genetic. Evidence has been presented in the discussion of mental deficiency to show that pelvic irradiation of the pregnant mother by X-ray or radium, prenatal viral infections, toxoplasmosis, or anoxia in the first trimester of pregnancy may produce microcephaly.

In these cases there are usually associated neurological lesions and anomalies of other organs.

ETIOLOGY: Microcephaly occurs in 1 to 25,000-50,000 of the general population, and is transmitted as a simple recessive. There is a heterozygous expression of the gene for this syndrome, manifesting itself by intellectual impairment.

PROGNOSIS: Most of the patients have poor resistance to infection and in the past died in childhood. With the advent of antibiotics, life is prolonged.

TREATMENT: There is no specific treatment. These children should be institutionalized.

Böök, J. A., Schut, J. W. and Reed, S. C.: A Clinical and Genetical Study of Microcephaly. Am. J. Ment. Def. 57:637, 1953.
Fois, A. and Rosenberg, C. M.: The Electroencephalogram in Microcephaly. Neurology 7:703, 1957.
Murphy, D. P., Shirlock, M. E. and Doll, E. A.: Microcephaly Following Maternal Irradiation for the Interruption of Pregnancy. Am. J. Roentgenol. 48:356, 1942.
Tredgold, A. F.: Mental Deficiency, ed. 8. Bailliere, Tindall and Cox, 1952.

CRANIOSTENOSIS

Craniostenosis refers to the premature closure of one or more cranial sutures. In contradistinction to microcephaly, where the skull bones unite to form a small head following the failure of normal brain development, there is primary union of the bones which prevents the growing brain from expanding. In addition to the peculiar appearance of the skull, there are accompanying signs of increased intracranial pressure. The differential is of practical importance, since relief of pressure and the probability of improvement may be offered in craniostenosis, provided the condition is recognized early in infancy and surgical relief is obtained.

ETIOLOGY: The condition may be genetically transmitted, probably as a recessive condition. The presence of the condition in other members of the family, and its association with anomalies of other organs, especially syndactylism, offers support for this point of view. On the other hand, sporadic cases do occur. Craniofacial dysostosis (Crouzon's Disease), a coronal synostosis plus deformity of the facial bones, is transmitted as an irregular dominant in which one-half the cases are sporadic.

Cranial Types (*Pathology*). Normally the cranial bones are separated from each other at birth. Both the anterior and posterior fontanels are open. The latter is usually no longer felt after six weeks; the anterior does not close until during the second year. In utero there is a fibrous union between the membranous bones at their borders that begins at about the sixth month. After birth, the borders between the bones (sutures) become dentated and fusion gradually begins. This is a slow process because allowance must be made for the growth of the brain, which during the first year more than doubles in volume. Furthermore, within the first two years the major increase in the circumference of the skull occurs.

The only suture to close shortly after birth is the metopic, uniting the frontal bones. The others do not close completely until later in life. When, therefore, the sutures are united in fetal life or shortly after birth, we have the condition of synostosis or premature fusion to an extreme degree. Associated anomalies are often present, especially syndactylism associated with acrocephaly, spina bifida, and cleft palate.

CLINICAL PICTURE: The various cranial deformities depend on the sutures involved. The expansion and shape of the skull is axial to the closed sutures (Virchow). When the sagittal suture closes prematurely, there is greater expansion antero-posteriorly because the coronal and lambdoidal sutures allow it; thus there is an elongated and narrow skull (scaphocephaly). With premature closure of the coronal suture, the sagittal and squamosal sutures allow for expansion laterally, and the forehead is flat and wide (acrocephaly). Premature fusion of the coronal, plus possibly squamosal on one side causes flattening of that side of the forehead (plagiocephaly), producing an asymmetrical skull. Finally, with premature fusion of all the cranial sutures, the head expands upward toward the anterior fontanel forming a tower skull; the base of the skull becomes deeper, the sinuses undeveloped or obliterated, and the orbits shallow (oxycephaly). The facial bones may also become fused, and when associated with acrocephaly the condition is referred to as Crouzon's syndrome. Protrusion of the lower lip, exophthalmos, hypertelorism, and divergent strabismus may also be present in Crouzon's syndrome.

As we have previously indicated, it is the effects of the premature synostosis of the cranial bones, resulting in increased intracranial pressure, which are of greatest importance. Therefore, craniostenosis requires early recognition in order to avoid irrevocable changes. Increased intracranial pressure results in papilledema and optic atrophy, usually secondary. In some instances exophthalmos is present. There may be extraocular disturbances such as nystagmus or divergent strabismus. These effects are due to downward pressure on the bony plates of the orbits. In untreated cases blindness may result. With involvement of the coronal suture particularly, and especially in the oxycephalic type where the other sutures are also synostosed, there are associated anomalies of the extremities, such as symmetrical syndactylism of the hands and feet.

LABORATORY: X-ray is extremely helpful in showing which sutures are prematurely closed and in revealing evidence of increased intracranial pressure. Abnormalities of the facial bones and other anomalies of the extremities can be seen. The vault shows convolutional markings which have a wavy appearance.

DIAGNOSIS: The most important consideration is early recognition, preferably within the first six months. When there appears to be any peculiarity in the shape of the head, a palpable ridge over the closed sutures, failure of the baby to see well, or exophthalmos, an X-ray should be obtained.

In microcephaly there are no papilledema or exophthalmos. Mental development is obviously retarded. There may be spasticity with seizures. Skull X-ray is negative for stenosis. The pressure on the orbits and the brachycephalic type of skull may produce confusion with hydrocephalus; however, in the latter, the suture lines are separated, fontanels widely open, and air injection in the ventricles plus dye studies will confirm the presence of hydrocephalus. Occasionally, early brain tumor must be considered because of papilledema, but here the signs of craniostenosis will reveal the diagnosis.

TREATMENT: Therapy is surgical. Several methods have been developed through the years. These are reviewed by Ingraham and Matson. They point out that because new bone grows rapidly from the outer layers of the dura as well as from the periosteum, artificial defects which have been created to keep the bones apart are quickly obliterated by new bony unions. They therefore use polyethylene film. This is divided into strips, 2½ cm. wide and 15-25 cm. in length, which are placed over the inner and outer bone surfaces following craniectomy. A modification of this technique is the use of Zenker's solution which is painted on the exposed dura.

PROGNOSIS: If the surgical procedure is done in the first few months, the cosmetic effects are good, mentality is preserved, and the prognosis is excellent. If done later, there are still some good effects, but the chances for changing the skull contour after two years are poor and there may be mental retardation.

Anderson, F. M. and Johnson, F. L.: Craniosynostosis: Modification in Surgical Treatment. Surgery 40:961, 1956.

Faber, H. K. and Towne, E. B.: Early Operation in Premature Cranial Synostosis for the Prevention of Blindness and other Sequelae. J. Pediat. 22:286, 1943.

Grieg, D.: Oxycephaly. Edinburgh M. J. 33:189, 1926.

Hope, J. W., Spitz, E. B. and Slade, H. W.: The Early Recognition of Premature Cranial Synostosis. Radiology 65:183, 1955.

Ingraham, F. D., Alexander, E. and Matson, D. D.: Clinical Studies in Craniosynostosis. Surgery 24:518, 1948.

————, F. D. and Matson, D. D.: Neurosurgery of Infancy and Childhood. Springfield, Ill., C. C. Thomas, 1954.

King, J. E. J.: Oxycephaly. Ann. Surg. 115:488, 1942.

Park, E. A. and Powers, G. F.: Acrocephaly and Scaphocephaly with Symmetrically Distributed Malformations of the Extremities. A Study of So-called "Acrocephalo-syndactylism." Am. J. Dis. Child. 20:234, 1920.

MACROCEPHALY

In this condition there is an enlarged brain associated with mental deficiency. Macrocephaly occurs more often in males. There appears to be some familial inheritance, possibly recessive, since more than one case may occur in some families, or there may be a history of mental disease or epilepsy.

CLINICAL PICTURE: The head appears large at birth. As the months go by, it is observed that the size of the head appears to be increasing excessively. The fontanels remain open. The rest of the body develops poorly. There are weakness of the musculature, mental impairment, visual disturbances, and seizures, more noticeable with the passage of time. The spinal fluid is normal.

PATHOLOGY: The brain is large and weighs far in excess of the normal at birth. The gross appearance is relatively normal except for the size. The cortex is thick. There are a paucity of nerve cells and a proliferation of glial tissue in the subcortical white matter.

ETIOLOGY: The cause of this condition is unknown.

DIAGNOSIS: The combination of enlarged head, mental deficiency, lack of normal physical development, and convulsions must be differentiated from the more common entities such as hydrocephalus and subdural hematoma. This can be done by bilateral aspiration for subdural hematoma. If this test is negative, then ventriculography should be performed to rule out hydrocephalus. The latter will show distended ventricles, whereas they are normal in macrocephaly.

PROGNOSIS: This is poor. Death occurs from intercurrent infection.

TREATMENT: There is no specific therapy. The general principles of management as discussed under mental deficiency should be applied. These children should be institutionalized.

Korbin, M. A.: Macrocephaly: Report of a Case Verified by Ventriculography and Autopsy. Bull. Los Angeles Neurol. Soc. 19:178, 1954.

HYPERTELORISM

This condition, described by Grieg, is characterized by the great distance between the eyes caused by a congenital craniofacial abnormality which involves the sphenoid bone, particularly that part which originates from cartilage. The lesser wings of the sphenoid bone are overly large whereas the greater wings are underdeveloped and small.

The appearance is characteristic. The skull is of a brachycephalic type, with a flattened occipital region and pronounced bulging of the frontal eminences. The nose is relatively small, but has a broad, depressed bridge and a median groove leading up the frontal bone from its root. The orbits are widely separated. Mental retardation is usually present.

ETIOLOGY: The disease may be transmitted genetically either as a single dominant gene or as a recessive; the exact nature is not clearly defined. In some families there is a dominant strain, but milder cases occur sporadically with less pronounced mental involvement. Hypertelorism is often associated with other congenital defects, such as cleft palate. Yannet has noted malformation of the heart in a number of cases.

DIAGNOSIS: The diagnosis is usually made from the characteristic appearance of the patient and the use of X-ray to bring out the abnormality of the sphenoid bones.

TREATMENT: There is no specific therapy, since there is an absence of increased intracranial pressure.

Curtin, J. M.: Hypertelorism. Irish. J. Med. Sci. 6. S. :121, 1953.
Grieg, D. M.: Hypertelorism: Edinburgh M. J. 31:560, 1924.

CONGENITAL FACIAL DIPLEGIA

Paralysis of the facial nerve, when it is congenital, is usually bilateral. In a few instances it occurs alone, but in the majority of cases there are associated anomalies which involve the other cranial nerves, especially the sixth (Möbius Syndrome).

CLINICAL PICTURE: In the newborn period it is noted that the baby does not suck well. The face has a masklike expression which is noticeable when the baby attempts to cry because there is no movement of the facial muscles. There are no wrinkles. There may be incomplete closure of the eyelids during sleep. The vast majority of these children have a combination of other cranial nerve involvement and other associated defects. Hence, there may be inability to adduct the eyes or ptosis of the lids due to involvement of the third nerve. With sixth nerve paralysis there is complete loss of abduction in both eyes. The Möbius syndrome consists of sixth and seventh nerve involvement, with associated congenital anomalies of the extremities, possibly of the brachial musculature, and other cranial nerve palsies. Three cases of Möbius syndrome were reported by Nisenson and his associates. One infant, at one week of age showed bilateral club feet, webbing of the toes, masklike facies, and tongue atrophy on the right side. There was also inability to adduct or abduct the eyes, indicating involvement of the third, sixth, seventh, and twelfth nerves. In two other children, of three and six years, there were deformities of the extremities, bilateral coxa valga, and equinus. In both these children there was inability to close the eyelids completely, and the eyes rolled upward (Bell's phenomenon) when the attempt was made. In older children, in addition to the masklike facies, speech is poor due to inability to use the lips properly. Intellectual level in these children is normal. There may be unilateral facial paralysis of the lower part of the face, but this is rare.

PATHOLOGY: There is absence or hypoplasia of the cranial nerve nuclei, especially the sixth and seventh. The nerves are small or absent, and the muscles fail to develop.

ETIOLOGY: There is no evidence of a familial or hereditary background. However, in four cases reported by Henderson of facial diplegia with no associated defects, two or more members of the family were affected. There are two theories as to the origin of the condition. According to one, the primary disturbance is an agenesis of the cranial nerve nucleus and its nerve (ectoderm). The other holds that there are primary aplasia of the muscles with secondary failure of the nerves to develop, and degeneration of the cranial nuclei through disuse (mesodermal).

DIAGNOSIS: The differential diagnosis must be made from acquired facial paralysis. The latter is unilateral, due usually to obstetrical trauma. There is injury to the nerve, either from forceps used on the face, or compression in utero of the shoulder against the head, or the face against the bony pelvis, especially the sacral prominence. There are no associated paralyses of other nerves. Pseudobulbar palsy, due to birth injury involves not only the facial nerve, but also the other nuclei of the bulb, so that there are palatal, pharyngeal, and tongue palsies. It is not accompanied by anomalies of the extremities. Facial paralysis may occur with congenital malformations of the external ears, mastoid, and temporal bone, accompanied by loss of hearing. This is a peripheral type of facial paralysis.

PROGNOSIS: The paralysis usually remains unchanged.

TREATMENT: There is no specific therapy.

Henderson, J. L.: The Congenital Facial Diplegia Syndrome: Clinical Features, Pathology, and Etiology. Brain 62:381, 1939.
Murphy, J. P. and German, W. J.: Congenital Facial Paralysis. Arch. Neurol. and Psychiat. 57:358, 1947.

Nisenson, A., Isaacson, A. and Grant, S.: Masklike Facies with Associated Congenital Anomalies. (Möbius Syndrome.) Report of Three Cases. J. Pediat. 46:255, 1955.

Paine, R. S.: Facial Paralysis in Children. Review of the Differential Diagnosis and Report of Ten Cases Treated with Cortisone. Pediat. 19:303, 1957.

CONGENITAL PTOSIS

Congenital ptosis is not infrequently seen in children. It is due to oculomotor paralysis, resulting in an inability of the levator palpebrae superioris to raise the upper eyelid. It is generally unilateral.

While the oculomotor nerve also supplies the superior, medial, and inferior recti muscles as well as the inferior oblique, these muscles are usually not affected. There may be dilatation of the pupil.

The ptosis is corrected surgically.

Rodin, F. H. and Barkan, H.: Hereditary Congenital Ptosis. Am. J. Ophth. 18:213, 1935.

MARCUS GUNN PHENOMENON

(JAW WINKING)

This condition consists of congenital partial ptosis of one eyelid when at rest. However, when the jaw is opened, the apparently paralyzed lid is *reflexly* elevated, usually above the level of the other normal eye. This phenomenon, described by Marcus Gunn, occurs in two per cent of congenital ptosis, affects males more often, and usually involves the left upper eyelid. It is considered an inherited blight and is noted in infancy.

TREATMENT: Surgical correction is usually not necessary unless the phenomenon is very unsightly. Smith and Gans suggest that the cause lies in the fact that the levator palpebrae muscle is connected not only with the third nucleus, but also with the external pterygoid portion of the fifth nucleus. Therefore, if surgical therapy is needed, section of the levator and utilization of the superior rectus to raise and control the upper lid may be performed or the motor root of the trigeminal nerve may be cut.

Smith, E. E. and Gans, M. E.: Jaw Winking (Marcus Gunn Phenomenon). J. Pediat. 50:52, 1957.

Congenital Hereditary Nystagmus

Congenital idiopathic nystagmus is observed from birth in those families where it has previously appeared. In others, it is usually recognized within a few months.

CLINICAL PICTURE: The nystagmus is usually bilateral. The movements are synchronous, mainly horizontal or rotary in direction, and pendular in type. When the infant looks to one side, there may be a more rapid component in the direction of the gaze. There are oscillatory head movements, such as head nodding, which keep pace with the nystagmus.

Some defective vision is present in these infants, but otherwise the eyes are normal. There are no neurological disturbances or defects of other systems.

With the passage of time the head movements become less noticeable or disappear, but nystagmus persists, though less marked, and vision remains defective.

ETIOLOGY: Congenital nystagmus is inherited as an irregular dominant condition. Both sexes are affected, males somewhat more frequently than females, and either sex may transmit the disease. Movements of the head are frequent, but pigmentary defects are rare (Nettleship).

Another form shows recessive sex-linked inheritance in which nystagmus occurs in males only, but is transmitted by females. In this type, head nodding is not as frequent, but there are pigmentary defects such as a red-green color blindness in some families.

Very rarely, a simple recessive form may be present which may be associated with parental consanguinity.

Congenital nystagmus is thought by some to be due to a disease of the central nervous system. An anomaly of the vestibulo-oculomotor apparatus is suggested. Others have considered it as a heredodegenerative familial disease. In two families with sex-linked hereditary nystagmus, reported by Lein, Stewart, and Moll, no evidence could be found of a generalized neurological disorder.

DIAGNOSIS: Nystagmus may appear in a number of diseases of the eye. These must be differentiated and include albinism, opacities of the media, macular changes, and defects of the optic nerve. Congenital nystagmus differs from these in being hereditary, appearing shortly after birth, and being free of associated neurological or ocular disease.

Congenital nystagmus must also be separated from spasmus nutans. The latter is characterized by involuntary head nodding and nystagmus. The onset is later than in congenital nystagmus, between four and twelve months, rarely eighteen months. Head nodding may proceed in an anterior-posterior or up and down direction, or laterally from side to side. It may be intermittent or constant. Duke-Elder refers to these movements as affirmation or negation, respectively. The movements are observed only when the child is sitting up and disappear with the eyes closed or in sleep. The nystagmus may be vertical, horizontal, or rotary, and is often more marked in one eye. The optic discs are normal. The cause is unknown. Some have suspected poor illumination and poor nutrition. The condition disappears by the end of the second year. Congenital nystagmus differs from spasmus nutans in its earlier onset, hereditary history, and persistence throughout life.

TREATMENT: There is no treatment for congenital nystagmus. Together with the defective vision it persists throughout life. The head nodding disappears.

Duke-Elder, W. S.: Congenital Idiopathic Nystagmus. Textbook of Ophthalmology, vol. IV. St. Louis, C. V. Mosby Co., 1949.

Lein, J. N., Stewart, C. T., Moll, F. C.: Sex-Linked Hereditary Nystagmus. Pediat. 18:214, 1956.

Nettleship, E.: On Some Cases of Hereditary Nystagmus. Tr. Ophth. Soc. United Kingdom 31:159, 1911.

CONGENITAL HYPERTROPHY OF THE MUSCLES WITH MENTAL DEFICIENCY

(WRESTLER'S SYNDROME)

The syndrome of congenital hypertrophy of the skeletal musculature with rigidity and mental deficiency was described by DeLange. The peculiar appearance is noted at birth. The infant has a short thick neck, broad shoulders, and symmetrical hypertrophy of the muscles including biceps, triceps, and quadriceps. The muscles feel as hard as stone and are markedly rigid. The infant looks like a wrestler. The back may be arched and opisthotonic. There are no cranial or peripheral nerve paralyses. An additional important feature is an enlarged, thickened tongue. Buchanan has reviewed the literature in his article.

PATHOLOGY: In DeLange's case the brain showed microgyria, porencephaly, large numbers of cavities in the central white matter, and ganglion cell defect in the corpus striatum. Marshall's case showed somewhat similar findings.

ETIOLOGY: According to DeLange, this disease is due to a disturbance of the basal ganglia. Others have viewed the condition as related to hypothyroidism, pointing to the improvement which followed therapy in their cases, both with respect to intellect and lessening of rigidity. In Marshall and Hodes' case, there was no evidence of adrenal or thyroid pathology.

DIAGNOSIS: The major diagnostic points are the wrestler's appearance, thick tongue, hypertrophy of the muscles, rigidity, and mental deficiency.

Cretinism should be eliminated through metabolic studies, including radioactive iodine (I^{131}) uptake, blood cholesterol, and bone age X-rays. Thomsen's disease and myotonic dystrophy should be differentiated.

PROGNOSIS: The outlook is poor, unless there is a basis for therapy due to diminished thyroid activity.

TREATMENT: There is no specific therapy, unless hypothyroidism is present.

Buchanan, D.: Clinical Conference. A Case for Diagnosis. Pediat. 18:1013, 1956.

DeLange, C.: Congenital Hypertrophy of the Muscles, Extrapyramidal Motor Disturbances, and Mental Deficiency. A Clinical Entity. Am. J. Dis. Child. 48:243, 1934.

———, C.: Two Cases of Congenital Anomalies of the Brain. Am. J. Dis. Child. 53:429, 1937.

Marshall, R. and Hodes, H. L.: Congenital Muscular Hypertrophy with Mental Deficiency (DeLange's Disease). J. Mt. Sinai Hosp. 22:119, 1955.

CHAPTER 4

INBORN ERRORS OF METABOLISM

PHENYLPYRUVIC OLIGOPHRENIA

Phenylketonuria is the result of an inborn error in the metabolism of phenylalanine and consists of a severe mental deficiency associated with the excretion of phenylpyruvic acid in the urine.

ETIOLOGY: The abnormality is inherited as a recessive condition, being transmitted by a single autosomal gene. The parents of these children are apparently normal in most instances, but parental consanguinity occurs in fifteen per cent. The condition is present in 0.5 to 1 per cent of institutional defectives, and at the rate of about 4 per 100,000 in the general population.

CLINICAL PICTURE: The children are usually blond and fair skinned. They may show an eczematoid dermatitis. Both sexes are equally affected. There are no distinct racial characteristics, though the disease is most frequent in the "Nordic" type. Otherwise the general physical examination is not distinctive. The neurological examination reveals in some cases a poor short-stepped gait, active tendon knee reflexes, spasticity, and tremors. In others, there are ataxia, rigidity, or poor posture so that the patient is stooped over appearing to have a pithecoid stance. Seizures are frequent in infancy. Speech is absent in many cases. The optic discs are normal. Some develop psychotic manifestations including untidiness, lack of awareness of their surroundings, marked hyperirritability, restlessness, and temper tantrums. Various hand postures and aimless movements of the fingers such as pill-rolling are described. The electroencephalogram is often abnormal. The IQ, in most, is of the idiot and imbecile level. However, several cases of near-normal intelligence have been reported.

PATHOLOGY: There is no distinctive pathology, but some demyelinization has been noted.

71

BIOCHEMISTRY: The chemical nature of the problem is the accumulation of phenylalanine in the blood because its normal transformation into tyrosine is blocked; as a result it is deaminated by the kidney. There is an enzymatic deficiency for this conversion, the specific enzyme being found normally in the liver. Phenylalanine appears in the urine in abnormal amounts. Phenylpyruvic acid, phenylactic acid, and phenylacetylglutamine, derivatives of phenylalanine, also appear in excess in the urine. It is felt that the excess phenylalanine in the plasma may prevent normal cerebral development because of its toxicity to cortical tissue. The normal blood level of phenylalanine is 1-2 mg. per 100 ml. In phenylketonuria levels of 20-60 mg. per 100 ml. occur. Phenylalanine also appears in excess in the spinal fluid.

DIAGNOSIS: Phenylketonuria should be suspected in the presence of mental deficiency, behavior retardation, and convulsions, or where there is an aromatic odor to the urine; the clinical impression is confirmed by laboratory tests. The diagnosis is made by testing for phenylpyruvic acid in the urine. The unknown urine (5cc) is acidified by adding 0.1N HCL. Then add a few drops of 5% ferric chloride solution, and the color turns deep bluish-green. This reaction is not present in normal urine. In the newborn, 5% ferric chloride may be added to the acidified diaper, and the bluish-green color should appear. The test may, however, be negative, for it often takes several months for the abnormal metabolites to be present. Hence, it should be repeated at three months of age.

TREATMENT: The treatment is to provide a diet low in phenylalanine. A protein hydrolysate free of phenylalanine is used. Proprietaries for this purpose with instructions for supplementing the diet are available. With this procedure the urine becomes free of phenylpyruvic acid in two to three weeks. The plasma phenylalanine level drops to normal later, usually after several months. Since phenylalanine is an essential amino acid required for growth, it cannot be omitted completely. According to Paine and Hsia the optimal dietary phenylalanine level for an infant of six months is approximately 25 mg./kg./day or 500 mg. per square meter per day. This will maintain a normal plasma phenylalanine level of about 1.5 mg. per 100 cc. The diet should be maintained for several years, perhaps until myelinization of the central nervous system is completed. Fruits, vegetables, and milk may be added in small amounts as indicated.

PROPHYLAXIS: In any baby who appears not to be developing satisfactorily, the diaper or fresh urine should be tested with a few drops of ferric chloride. As we have previously emphasized, when there is suspicion, repeat the test at intervals and check with a serum phenylalanine.

The parents of a child with phenylketonuria should be informed of the possibilities of recurrence in future offspring since there is genetic transmission. With each pregnancy the risk is twenty-five per cent. Members of such a family should be warned against consanguinous marriages.

PROGNOSIS: The outlook is good, especially when the diagnosis is made in infancy or early childhood. In the newborn the mental changes may be entirely prevented. Treatment in young children causes them to become brighter, the IQ may reach normal levels, behavior improves, seizures disappear, and the electroencephalogram returns to normal. Treatment begun in later childhood improves the child's behavior so that he reacts better to the family situation. However, there may not be so decided an effect on intellectual improvement.

Recent reports of several untreated patients with near normal or normal intelligence make it necessary to exercise caution in determining whether improvement is entirely due to therapy. Further observation with controlled studies will be needed.

Bickel, H.: The Effects of a Phenylalanine-free and Phenylalanine-poor Diet in Phenylpyruvic Oligophrenia. Exp. Med. Surg. 12:114, 1954.

Horner, F. A., Streamer, C. W., Clader, D. E., Hassel, L. L., Binkley, Jr., E. L. and Dumars, Jr., K. W.: Effect of Phenylalanine-Restricted Diet in Phenylketonuria II A.M.A. J. Dis. Child. 93:615, 1957.

Hsia, D. Y. Y. and Driscoll, K. W.: Detection by Phenylalanine Tolerance Tests of Heterozygous Carriers of Phenylketonuria. Nature 178:1239, 1956.

————, D. Y. Y., Knox, W. E. and Paine, R. S.: A Case of Phenylketonuria with Borderline Intelligence. A.M.A. J. Dis. Child. 94:33, 1957.

————, D. Y. Y., Knox, W. E., Quinn, K. V. and Paine, R. S.: A One Year Controlled Study of the Effect of Low-Phenylalanine Diet on Phenylketonuria. Pediat. 21:178, 1958.

Jervis, G. A.: Phenylpyruvic Oligophrenia (Phenylketonuria). A. Res. Publ. Ass. Nerv. Ment. Dis. Proc. 33:259, 1954.

Knox, W. E. and Hsia, D. Y. Y.: Pathogenetic Problems in Phenylketonuria. Am. J. Med. 22:687, 1957.

Kretchmer, N. and Etzwiler, D. D.: Disorders Associated with the Metabolism of Phenylalanine and Tyrosine. Pediat. 21:445, 1958. (Review Article.)

McLester, J. S. and Darby, W. J.: Nutrition and Diet in Health and Disease, ed. 6. Philadelphia, W. B. Saunders Company, 1952.
Meister, A.: Phenylpyruvic Oligophrenia. Pediat. 21:1021, 1958.
Paine, R. S.: The Variability in Manifestations of Untreated Patients with Phenylketonuria (Phenylpyruvic Aciduria). Pediat. 20:290, 1957.
———, R. S. and Hsia, D. Y. Y.: The Dietary Phenylalanine Requirements and Tolerances of Phenylketonuric Patients. A.M.A. J. Dis. Child. 94:224, 1957.
Rose, W. C.: Amino Acid Requirements of Man. Federation Proc. 8:546, 1949.
Wright, S. W. and Tarjan, G.: Phenylketonuria. A.M.A. J. Dis. Child. 93:405, 1957. (Complete Review of Literature.)

GALACTOSEMIA

Galactosemia is due to an inborn error of metabolism of galactose, perhaps inherited as a recessive condition. The accumulation of galactose is toxic to the tissues resulting in a clinical picture of retarded growth and mental development.

Galactose and glucose result from the hydrolysis of lactose in the intestine. In normal metabolism galactose is phosphorylated to galactose -1- phosphate (Gal-1-P) by the enzyme galactokinase and ATP (adenosine triphosphate). Gal-1-P is subsequently converted to glucose-1-phosphate (Gl-1-P).

1. Gal-1-P + UDPGl (uridine diphosphate glucose) $\rightleftharpoons$ Gl-1-P + UDPGal

2. UDPGal $\rightleftharpoons$ UDPGl

According to evidence presented by Isselbacher, Kalckar, and their associates, galactosemia represents the congenital absence of a specific enzyme, P-Gal transferase. The lack of this enzyme causes failure of conversion of the Gal-1-P to Gl-1-P in equation I. Isselbacher further feels that the toxic effect on the nervous system and other tissues may be due to the accumulation of Gal-1-P, either directly or indirectly. Others have suggested that the hypoglycemia which occurs with the administration of galactose and limitation of glucose may be the cause. The enzymatic defect is probably not complete as children appear to develop tolerance to galactose as they get older, or they may develop an alternate pathway for the utilization of galactose.

CLINICAL PICTURE: The infant appears normal at birth. After a period of several days feeding with milk, the baby develops vomiting, diarrhea, loss of weight, and lethargy. Soon there are jaundice, and an enlarged liver and spleen. Ascites and edema may be present. Cataracts are also seen at this time in over half the cases. If unrecognized and galactose intake continues, convulsions and mental retardation may occur. In another group of cases, the development of symptoms may be slower. There is a period of months during which vomiting, retarded mental development, and hepatomegaly occur.

LABORATORY: The blood glucose level is diminished and galactose increased. Total fasting blood sugar is normal. Mellituria is present. Paper chromatography demonstrates galactose in the urine.

When a reducing substance is present in the urine (Benedict's Test), test for glucose (Tes-tape ®). If negative, carry out the above tests for galactose.

DIAGNOSIS: The failure of a newborn baby to do well nutritionally, or the presence of jaundice or mellituria should suggest galactosemia. Consideration of erythroblastosis fetalis, sepsis, or birth injury because of jaundice or seizures would also require elimination of galactosemia. The diagnosis is confirmed by an elevated galactose level in the blood and an abnormal galactose tolerance test.

PROGNOSIS: If the condition is recognized early, the outlook is good for a return to normal. If unrecognized, the infants either die or remain physically and mentally retarded.

TREATMENT: Milk and milk products should be eliminated immediately. Lactose-free milk or special food mixtures should be substituted. The diet should be restricted as to lactose for several years; milk may then be added slowly.

Hartmann, A. F., Grunwaldt, E. and James Jr., D. H.: Blood Galactose in Infants and Children. J. Pediat. 43:1, 1953.
Holzel, A., Komrower, G. M. and Schwarz, V.: Galactosemia. Am. J. Med. 22:703, 1957.
Isselbacher, K. J., Anderson, E. A., Kalckar, H. M.: The Specific Enzymatic Defect in Galactosemia. A.M.A. J. Dis. Child. 92:458, 1956.
———, K. J., Anderson, E. P., Kurahashi, K. and Kalckar, H. M.: Congenital Galactosemia, a Single Enzymatic Block in Galactose Metabolism. Science 123:635, 1956.

Kalckar, H. M., Anderson, E. P. and Isselbacher, K. J.: Galactosemia, a Congenital Defect in a Nucleotide Transferase. Biochim. Biophys. Acta, 20:262, 1956.

Ritter, J. A. and Cannon, E. J.: Galactosemia with Cataracts. New England J. Med. 252:747, 1955.

Sidbury, Jr., J. B.: The Biochemical Pathogenesis of Galactosemia. A.M.A. J. Dis. Child. 94:524, 1957.

HEPATO-LENTICULAR DEGENERATION

(WILSON'S DISEASE)

This condition, originally described by Wilson in 1912, consists of degenerative changes in the basal ganglia and cirrhosis of the liver. It is a progressive disease, familial in character. In many cases there is a greenish-yellow or brown pigmentation of the cornea (Kayser-Fleischer ring). Included as a subentity of this disease is the pseudosclerosis of Westphal and Strümpell.

CLINICAL PICTURE: The onset is usually in late childhood and early adult life. There are a variety of motor phenomena. Tremor develops early. It may be present at rest, but is intensified by activity. At times a peculiar tremor of the upper extremities is noted in the form of an up and down movement of the arms, best brought out by having the arms extended. This tremor is similar to the flapping of a bird's wings, referred to as "wing beating." Rigidity of the muscles is a feature. There is marked hypertonicity with lack of relaxation, resulting in a fixed smile, wide open mouth, and dribbling of saliva (Parkinsonian rigidity). There is difficulty with speech, chewing, and swallowing due to muscle spasm. Involuntary movements including the dystonic type may occur, and there are emotional changes with sudden fits of laughter. Seizures may develop. There are no sensory changes. The reflexes are usually normal. There are usually no clinical symptoms of liver damage (cirrhosis). Occasionally, however, there have been reports including fever, jaundice, ascites, and liver atrophy, in some instances preceding the onset of nervous disease symptoms. Bone lesions including degenerative changes, fragmentation, and fracture may occur.

The greenish-yellow or brown pigmentation on the posterior surface of the cornea near the scleral junction may be seen by the naked eye, but is best brought out with the slit lamp (Kayser-Fleischer ring). This is present in about ninety per cent of patients, and is highly diagnostic.

LABORATORY: The spinal fluid is normal. Serum copper is usually decreased (N 90-125 mcg./100 ml.), but urinary copper excretion is markedly increased (N-25 mcg./24 hrs.). A combination of low serum copper plus high urinary excretion is very diagnostic. Serum ceruloplasmin is decreased (N-30 mcg./100 ml.). There is a marked increase in excretion of amino acids in the urine.

PATHOLOGY: The major changes occur in the basal ganglia, particularly the putamen, which may show cavitation. The caudate nucleus, globus pallidus, and ansa lenticularis may show moderate changes, such as a shrinkage or degeneration of neurons and cells. There is marked glial proliferation. The liver shows nodular cirrhosis. The spleen is enlarged. There are excessive amounts of copper in the liver, basal ganglia, and cerebral cortex, as well as in other tissues.

ETIOLOGY AND PATHOGENESIS: Hepato-lenticular degeneration is a familial disease with a high consanguinity rate, which appears to be inherited as a recessive condition.

The following data have been accumulated in Wilson's disease. There is usually a deficiency in ceruloplasmin, a copper-binding globulin. More than 90% of copper in plasma is normally present in ceruloplasmin. In Wilson's disease the non-ceruloplasmin plasma copper is excessively increased. There is an abnormality in copper metabolism, evidenced by its increased absorption through the gut, high urinary excretion, the marked increase and retention of copper in the brain and liver, and a low serum copper. Finally, there is marked aminoaciduria considered to be secondary to a disturbance in kidney function, brought about by the copper metabolic derangement. There is no elevation of plasma amino acids.

It is suggested that there is a genetic disturbance causing diminished synthesis of ceruloplasmin. There is also an increased absorption of copper from the gut which is either excreted in the urine or enters other tissues such as the brain and liver. This explains the excess unbound copper in the tissues, the kidney damage, and the excessive urinary copper excretion. The excess copper diminishes the brain oxygen uptake by interfering with the oxidative enzymes. The explanation is not complete in that it does not clarify the increased absorption of copper from the gut and the lack of improvement after giving ceruloplasmin. Furthermore, in some instances the ceruloplasmin level in the serum has been normal. Others postulate a fundamental genetic defect in protein metabolism. These proteins have a high affinity for copper, resulting in excess tissue deposits.

DIAGNOSIS: The diagnosis is based on the familial incidence and evidence of basal ganglia pathology (tremors, rigidity, dystonia) and corneal pigmentation (Kayser-Fleischer ring). At times there may be clinical symptoms of cirrhosis of the liver.

The differential must be made from postencephalitic Parkinson's and the dystonic syndromes, such as musculorum deformans.

The laboratory data with respect to copper and ceruloplasmin may be of help. The differential may be extremely difficult unless the liver pathology or corneal ring is obvious.

PROGNOSIS: The disease is slowly progressive. There may be remissions, but all cases are fatal. Death usually occurs within five years of the onset. Time will decide whether therapy with penicillamine, BAL, or versene has affected the outlook.

TREATMENT: Various forms of therapy have been tried to remove the excess copper from the tissues including BAL, versene (method described in the chapter on lead), and a high protein diet. Recently penicillamine has been utilized and appears to be the best agent thus far. It produces a rapid and marked excretion of copper in the urine. It is given orally in gelatin capsules, before meals, about 300 mg. three times a day.

In addition to the penicillamine, oral potassium sulphide may be used to decrease the absorption of copper from the intestine. The diet should be low in copper. To counteract possible mineral depletion, these should be added to the diet, including calcium, iron, magnesium, cobalt, and zinc. Vitamins should also be supplied.

Complications may occasionally occur with penicillamine. Prothrombin time should be checked. Hepatic necrosis and alopecia have been reported.

Therapy is given continuously in order to maintain a constant excretion of the excess copper. It is suggested that one begin with penicillamine. If unsuccessful, turn to BAL or versene. In using BAL one should be careful of toxic reactions, such as skin rashes, increased neurologic signs, or coma.

Bearn, A. G. and Kunkel, H. G.: Abnormalities of Copper Metabolism in Wilson's Disease and their Relationship to the Aminoaciduria. J. Clin. Invest. 33:400, 1954.

Fister, W. P., Boulding, J. E. and Baker, R. A.: The Treatment of Hepatolenticular Degeneration with Penicillamine, with Report of Two Cases. Canad. M.A.J. 78:99, 1958.

Scharenberg, K. and Drew, Jr., A. L.: The Histopathology of Wilson's Disease. J. Neuropath. and Exper. Neurol. 13:181, 1954.

Scheinberg, I. H. and Gitlin, D.: Deficiency of Ceruloplasmin in Patient with Hepatolenticular Degeneration (Wilson's Disease). Science 116:484, 1952.

————, Harris, R. S., Morell, A. G. and Dubin, D.: Some Aspects of the Relation of Ceruloplasmin to Wilson's Disease. Neurology, Supplement No. 1 8:44, 1958.

Uzman, L. L. and Hood, B.: The Familial Nature of the Amino-Aciduria of Wilson's Disease. (Hepatolenticular Degeneration). Am. J. Med. Sc. 223:392, 1952.

————, L. L.: Studies on the Mechanism of Copper Deposition in Wilson's Disease. A.M.A. Arch. Neurol. & Psychiat. 77:164, 1957.

————, L. L. and Jakus, M. A.: The Kayser-Fleischer Ring. A Histochemical and Electron Microscope Study. Neurology 7:341, 1957.

Walshe, J. M.: Penicillamine, a New Oral Therapy for Wilson's Disease. Am. J. Med. 21:487, 1956.

Wilson, S. A. K.: Progressive Lenticular Degeneration; a Familial Nervous Disease Associated with Cirrhosis of the Liver. Brain 34:295, 1912.

Zimdahl, W. T., Hyman, I., Stafford, Jr., W. F.: The Effect of Drugs upon the Copper Metabolism in Hepatolenticular Degeneration and in Normal Subjects. J. Lab. and Clin. Med. 43:774, 1954.

HARTNUP DISEASE

This condition, named after the family in which it was first described, is a hereditary disorder consisting of a pellagra-like skin rash, temporary cerebellar ataxia, constant renal aminoaciduria, and other bizarre biochemical features.

In the study of the family it was noted that there were eight siblings of a first-cousin marriage. Of these eight, four showed abnormal chemical findings, particularly the excretion of large amounts of amino acids and indole compounds. The parents were normal. The birth histories were also uneventful.

CLINICAL PICTURE: There is the tendency to develop a rough, reddened skin from exposure to moderate sunlight. The exposed parts, the face, neck, hands, and legs, are especially affected, more so in summer. The rash in two of the siblings appeared to be similar to pellagra. Ataxia of the cerebellar type and a coarse nystagmus appear with the rash. The ataxia is temporary and intermittent in contradistinction to the insidious onset and progressive nature of the hereditary cerebellar ataxias. Mental retardation was noted in some of the older siblings. There are a high-stepping gait, increased muscle tone, and hyperactive reflexes. The optic discs are normal. There are no sensory changes.

LABORATORY: There is a gross renal aminoaciduria. In addition to the amino acids there is also increased urinary excretion of indole-3-acetic acid, indican, and indole-3-acetylglutamine. The feces contain excess amounts of protoporphyrin.

Blood chemistry is normal.

DIAGNOSIS: This is made on the basis of a photosensitive, pellagra-like skin rash together with cerebellar signs. Analysis of the urine confirms the diagnosis through the presence of excessive amounts of amino acid and indole compounds.

ETIOLOGY: The authors have considered that this disease may be a biochemical disorder of a genetic nature due to abnormality of nicotinic acid utilization (deficiency of nicotinamide). There is a block in the conversion of tryptophan to nicotinic acid. It is suggested that under abnormal conditions such as excessive sunlight exposure, dietary deficiencies, or infection, extra demands for nicotinic acid are not met. The clinical features are secondary to the metabolic disorder and are not as constant or diagnostic. Other conditions similar to pellagra and corrected by nicotinic acid therapy have shown on paper chromatography similar patterns and indole metabolites.

PROGNOSIS: The clinical symptoms are apt to disappear except for the mental retardation.

TREATMENT: Nicotinamide should be tried in the early phases of the disease.

Baron, D. N., Dent, C. E., Harris, H., Hart, E. W. and Jepson, J. B.: Hereditary Pellagra-like Skin Rash with Temporary Cerebellar Ataxia, Constant Renal Amino-Aciduria and Other Bizarre Biochemical Features. Lancet 2:421, 1956.

AMINOACIDURIA

In this chapter on "Inborn Errors of Metabolism," we have had occasion to discuss several conditions in which aminoaciduria occurs. These include phenylketonuria, Wilson's disease, Hartnup disease, and galactosemia. We shall mention several other diseases of the central nervous system which are associated with aminoaciduria.

Menkes and his associates described four siblings who showed cerebral symptoms within the first week of life, after a normal birth. Westall reported a similar case. These babies refused to feed, there was an absent Moro, and then spasticity, coma, and death, which occurred within three months in Menkes' cases, and in twenty months in the one of Westall. The outstanding finding was an odor to the urine similar to maple syrup. Westall found an increase of valine, leucine, and isoleucine in the blood and urine and felt that the condition was due to an enzymatic defect involving these branched-chain amino acids.

Thelander and Imagawa reported a group of children with aminoaciduria and congenital defects including hypertelorism, stunted growth, and mental retardation.

Aminoaciduria also occurs in lead intoxication.

For a general discussion of aminoaciduria refer to the articles of the Harrisons, Lowe, and Snyderman.

Harrison, H. E. and Harrison, H. C.: Aminoaciduria in Relation to Deficiency Diseases and Kidney Function. J.A.M.A. 164:1571, 1957.

Lowe, C. U., Terrey, M. and MacLachlan, E. A.: Organic-Aciduria, Decreased Renal Ammonia Production, Hydrophthalmos, and Mental Retardation: A Clinical Entity. A.M.A. Am. J. Dis. Child. 83:164, 1952.

Menkes, J. H., Hurst, P. L. and Craig, J. M.: A New Syndrome: Progressive Infantile Cerebral Dysfunction Associated with an Unusual Urinary Substance. Pediat. 14:462, 1954.

Snyderman, S. E.: Metabolism of Amino Acids—A Review. Pediat. 21:117, 1958.

Thelander, H. E. and Imagawa, R.: Amino Aciduria, Congenital Defects, and Mental Retardation. A Preliminary Report. J. Pediat. 49:123, 1956.

Westall, R. G.: Maple Sugar Urine Disease. A.M.A. J. Dis. Child. 94:571, 1957.

CHAPTER 5

PRENATAL INFECTIONS

MATERNAL RUBELLA

The relationship of maternal rubella to congenital defects in the offspring was suggested by Gregg in a report of seventy-eight cases. Since that time a number of papers have been published on the subject. They confirm the fact that there is a definite causal relationship between maternal rubella and the development of congenital defects in the embryo, when the maternal disease is contracted in the first trimester of pregnancy. The major anomalies appear to be congenital cataract, heart disease, mental deficiency, and deafness. In addition, spastic diplegia, athetosis, epilepsy, and microcephaly may be noted. Spontaneous abortions and stillbirths also occur.

The reports on the percentage of babies who were injured because of the mother's having been infected with rubella vary considerably. In the early papers, Swan noted a very high correlation and in other papers which followed, figures anywhere from fifty per cent to one hundred per cent were given. On the other hand, Lundstrom studied 1067 cases of rubella selected from an epidemic in Sweden in 1951 in which there were 19,000 cases. This study had the advantage of observation during the actual occurrence of the German measles, whereas many of the previous studies had used a retrospective approach. He found that seventeen per cent of the babies of mothers who had rubella during the first four months of pregnancy developed congenital anomalies as compared to six per cent of the controls, or a ratio of about 3:1. There was also a greater incidence of stillbirths, neonatal mortality, and immaturity as compared to the controls. After the fifth month, rubella in the pregnant mother was harmless to the baby. Recently Greenberg and his associates reported that the incidence of congenital deformities among the live-born babies of women with rubella during the first trimester of pregnancy was 9.7 per cent.

If the pregnant mother is exposed to rubella in her first trimester and is relatively old, with little or no expectation of further pregnancies, she should get gamma globulin, and take the risk. If the pregnant woman is young, with possibilities for future pregnancies, she should be advised of the risk to the baby, and she and her husband should be given all the data. If they have decided to go through with the pregnancy in any event, the mother should be given gamma globulin. Certainly where there is doubt of exposure, or if the diagnosis is questionable, gamma globulin should be given to the mother and continuation of the pregnancy advised. Finally, the best procedure for the future is to allow exposure to German measles for all susceptible girls in their childhood.

Beswick, R. C., Warner, R. and Warkany, J.: Congenital Anomalies Following Maternal Rubella. Am. J. Dis. Child. 78:334, 1949.

Greenberg, M., Pellitteri, O. and Barton, J.: Frequency of Defects in Infants Whose Mothers Had Rubella During Pregnancy. J.A.M.A. 165:675, 1957.

Gregg, N. M.: Congenital Cataract Following German Measles in Mother. Tr. Ophth. Soc., Australia 3:35, 1942.

Ingalls, T. H. and Purshottam, N.: Fetal Risks from Rubella During Pregnancy. New England J. Med. 249:454, 1953.

Krugman, S. and Ward, R.: The Rubella Problem. J. Pediat. 44:489, 1954.

Lundström, R.: Rubella During Pregnancy: Its Effect Upon Perinatal Mortality, Incidence of Congenital Abnormalities and Immaturity. Acta. Pediat. 41:583, 1952.

Swan, C., Tostevin, A. L., Moore, B., Mayo, H. and Black, G. H. B.: Congenital Defects in Infants Following Infectious Diseases During Pregnancy, with Special Reference to Relationship Between German Measles and Cataract, Deaf-mutism, Heart Disease, and Microcephaly; and to Period of Pregnancy in which Occurrence of Rubella Is Followed by Congenital Abnormalities. M. J. Australia 2:201, 1943.

Wesselhoeft, C.: Rubella (German Measles) and Congenital Deformities. New England J. Med. 240:258, 1949.

TOXOPLASMOSIS

Toxoplasmosis is a generalized infectious disease, which in infants and children is congenital. It is produced by the protozoan Toxoplasma gondii, and manifests itself essentially through involvement of the central nervous system. In a series of papers, Wolf, Cowen, and Paige established the disease in man as a fetal encephalomyelitis with a prenatal inception and showed its etiological agent to be the protozoan toxoplasma. Since that time several hundred cases have been reported and the disease is not considered rare.

CLINICAL MANIFESTATIONS: Clinical signs of the disease may develop in the neonatal period or in later infancy or childhood. Both of these types are congenital. Since infection occurs in utero, there may be occasional cases of stillbirth, or instances in which the newborn baby is obviously ill when born. If neither of these conditions pertains the clinical picture will usually unfold within the next few days or weeks. The head may appear enlarged, suggesting hydrocephalus, or the reverse, microcephaly may occur. There may be convulsions, spasticity, petechial and purpuric rash, jaundice, fever, hepatosplenomegaly, microphthalmia, and chorioretinitis. X-ray of the skull will invariably show cerebral calcification diffusely scattered through the cortical areas and often abnormalities in the shape of the skull. The most significant features are the chorioretinitis, which is most often bilateral and is often accompanied by optic atrophy and microphthalmia, and the central nervous system manifestations. In the latter may be grouped cerebral calcification, hydrocephalus or microcephalus, and encephalitic signs such as seizures, spasticity and psychomotor retardation. The spinal fluid may be xanthochromic with marked elevation of protein and cellular increase, mostly lymphocytes. Blood eosinophilia may be present. During later infancy or childhood a similar picture may be seen. The disease may also take the form of an acute encephalomyelitis. On the other hand there are occasional cases of mild neonatal toxoplasmosis.

There is another type which occurs in older children and adults. This is probably acquired, but the mode of infection is as yet unknown. Primarily the clinical picture includes a maculopapular eruption and fever which together may simulate "spotted fever," pneumonia, splenomegaly, and occasionally signs of encephalitis. Chorioretinitis is absent. The outlook for recovery is generally good.

PATHOLOGY: In the brain are granulomas containing toxoplasma, which become calcified or necrotic. Toxoplasma may also invade the walls of blood vessels. The ventricles may be distended with hydrocephalus occurring secondary to occlusion of the aqueduct of Sylvius. There is evidence of encephalomyelitis. The eyes may show lesions in the retina, consisting of chorioretinal degeneration, which is focal and bilateral. The macula and peripheral parts of the retina are involved. Optic atrophy may be present.

DIAGNOSIS: The diagnosis of toxoplasma infection must always be considered in any infant who has evidence of hydrocephalus or microcephalus, seizures, or evidence of psychomotor retardation. In all these instances an X-ray of the skull should be requested for evidence of cerebral calcification. Furthermore, the fundi should be examined since chorioretinitis is invariably present. At times, the first presenting complaint may be failure of vision and the baby is brought to the ophthalmologist. The presence of chorioretinitis and optic atrophy will suggest the diagnosis. It should be emphasized that the presence of any single clinical feature requires confirmation with serologic tests or demonstration of the parasite. Cytomegalic inclusion disease should be ruled out.

1. Dye Test or Cytoplasm Modifying Test. Various dilutions of the patient's serum are incubated with mouse peritoneal exudate (containing live toxoplasma) which has been suspended in fresh negative human serum. Methylene blue is added. The test depends on the fact that if antibody is present, the cytoplasm of the toxoplasma will NOT stain; only the nuclear endosome takes the dye. With this test, antibodies in the patient's serum can be detected two weeks after infection with toxoplasma. The antibody titer lasts through most of the normal life span, remaining high the first two years of the infection and declining gradually. Diagnostic dilutions for active infections range between 1:256 to 1:16,000.

2. Complement Fixation. This test is also useful. However, it develops a positive more slowly than the dye test (one month after infection) and tends to disappear sooner, after two to four years. Therefore, this test cannot be used alone for diagnostic purposes.

There is a toxoplasmic skin test, but this is not of diagnostic value. The demonstration of parasites by examining slides of cerebrospinal fluid sediment should be attempted. The best technique for laboratory diagnosis is combined dye and complement fixation. A positive dye test plus negative complement fixation early in the disease of an infant means active toxoplasmosis. In infants over four months, a positive dye test in the mother and child is also diagnostic of active infection.

TREATMENT: Therapy consists of the use of sulfadiazine and pyrimethamine.

PROGNOSIS: The outlook is poor. Death occurs in some within a period of but a few weeks. The vast majority of survivors exhibit evidence of mental retardation, hydrocephalus or microcephaly, convulsions, chorioretinitis, and psychomotor disturbances, which persist in a chronic form.

PROPHYLAXIS: A mother may be advised to have another baby immediately irrespective of whether she has previously born a child with toxoplasmosis or has a high titer. No therapy is needed for the mother.

Eichenwald, F. F.: The Laboratory Diagnosis of Toxoplasmosis: Annals of the New York Acad. Sci. 64:207, 1956.

Eyles, D. E.: Newer Knowledge of the Chemotherapy of Toxoplasmosis. Annals of the New York Acad. Sci. 64:252, 1956.

Feldman, H. A.: The Clinical Manifestations and Laboratory Diagnosis of Toxoplasmosis. Am. J. Trop. Med. 2:420, 1953.

Kayhoe, D. E., Jacobs, L., Beye, H. K. and McCullough, N. B.: Acquired Toxoplasmosis; Observations on Two Parasitologically Proved Cases Treated with Pyrimethamine and Triple Sulfonamides. New England J. Med. 257:1247, 1957.

Koch, F. L. P., Wolf, A., Cowen, D., Paige, B. H.: Toxoplasmic Encephalomyelitis: Significance of Ocular Lesions in the Diagnosis of Infantile or Congenital Toxoplasmosis. Arch. Ophth. 29:1, 1943.

Sabin, A. B., Eichenwald, H., Feldman, H. A. and Jacobs, L.: Present Status of Clinical Manifestations of Toxoplasmosis in Man: Indications and Provisions for Routine Serologic Diagnosis J.A.M.A. 150:1063, 1952.

Stillerman, M.: Mild Neonatal Toxoplasmosis. A.M.A. J. Dis. Child. 93:563, 1957.

Wolf, A., Cowen, D., Paige, B. H.: Fetal Encephalomyelitis: Prenatal Inception of Infantile Toxoplasmosis. Science 93:548, 1941.

CYTOMEGALIC INCLUSION DISEASE

Generalized cytomegalic inclusion disease is a viral infection, occurring especially in infancy. Viruses are isolated from human tissue culture including the submaxillary gland and kidney of infected infants and from the adenoid tissue of older children. Transmission occurs prenatally and postnatally.

PATHOLOGY: Intranuclear and cytoplasmic inclusions are seen in all the organs of the body, producing in the brain a meningoencephalitis. Rarely, hemorrhages in the brain may also occur.

CLINICAL PICTURE: The nervous system manifestations do not occur as a primary disease, but rather in association with the general picture of cytomegalic inclusion disease. The newborn infant, usually under 2500 grams, exhibits jaundice, hepatosplenomegaly, and petechiae within the first twenty-four hours after

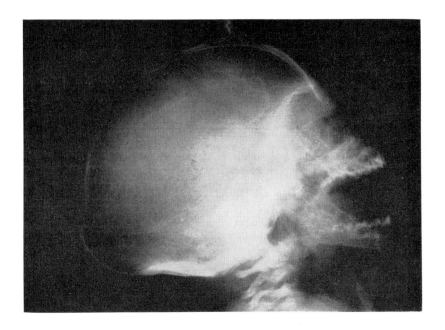

7. Cytomegalic inclusion disease. Roentgenogram shows calcification in periventricular tissue about the lateral ventricles. The latter are markedly dilated.

birth. The picture is similar to erythroblastosis. There may then follow lethargy, twitching, or convulsion. Microcephaly or hydrocephaly may be noted. In a recent case the onset of symptoms first occurred at six weeks. Both chorioretinitis and cerebral calcification were present.

LABORATORY: The spinal fluid is normal. The blood may show hemolytic anemia or thrombocytopenia. X-ray of the skull may show cerebral calcification. In a number of cases a line of calcification outlines the lateral ventricles. In the urine are inclusion bodies in the tubular epithelial cells.

DIAGNOSIS: Cytomegalic inclusion disease must be differentiated from hemolytic disease of the newborn, other viral diseases e.g. herpes simplex, sepsis in the newborn due to E. coli or staphylococcus, toxoplasmosis, neonatal hepatitis, congenital syphilis, and galactosemia. It should be strongly suspected in the presence of microcephaly and X-ray evidence of calcification lining the lateral ventricle. However, toxoplasmosis may present similar findings. The diagnosis is made by careful examination of fresh urinary sediment. Tubular epithelial cells with characteristic inclusions are seen. (Papanicolaou stain). This is specific. Inclusion bodies may also be observed in the gastric washings. The virus may be grown in tissue culture from the patient's urine.

PROGNOSIS: The disease is mostly fatal. Some children have survived with mild motor and mental retardation.

TREATMENT: Cortisone may be used. The rationale is that steroids have been successful in other hemolytic anemias and in thrombocytopenia. Both are present in this disease.

Birdsong, McL., Smith, D. E., Mitchell, F. N. and Corey, Jr., J. H.: Generalized Cytomegalic Inclusion Disease in Newborn Infants. J.A.M.A. 162:1305, 1956.
Blanc, W. A.: Cytologic Diagnosis of Cytomegalic Inclusion Disease in Gastric Washings. Am. J. Clin. Path. 28:46, 1957.
Guyton, T. B., Ehrlich, F., Blanc, W. A. and Becker, M. H.: New Observations in Generalized Cytomegalic-Inclusion Disease of the Newborn. Report of a Case with Chorioretinitis. New England J. Med. 257:803, 1957.
McElfresh, A. E. and Arey, J. B.: Generalized Cytomegalic Inclusion Disease. J. Pediat. 51:146, 1957.
Medearis, Jr., D. N.: Cytomegalic Inclusion Disease. Pediat. 19:467, 1957.

Sackett, Jr., G. L. and Ford, M. M.: Cytomegalic Inclusion Disease with Calcification outlining the Cerebral Ventricles. Am. J. Roentgenol., Radium Therapy and Nuclear Medicine. 76:512, 1956.

Weller, T. H., Macauley, J. C., Craig, J. M. and Wirth, P.: Isolation of intranuclear inclusion producing agents from infants with illness resembling cytomegalic inclusion disease. Proc. Soc. Exper. Biol. and Med. 94:4, 1957.

Congenital Neurosyphilis

Congenital syphilis, caused by the Treponema pallidum, occurs in infancy by passage of the spirochete through the placenta to the fetus, usually during the latter months of pregnancy.

General Features of Congenital Syphilis. In early congenital syphilis the baby may be born prematurely. However, there is usually no evidence of abnormality until about two to ten weeks after birth. There are often signs of rhinitis or snuffles, which may be accompanied by bleeding from the nose. Skin eruptions are noted, usually maculopapular in appearance. There are scaling or desquamation of the feet and osseous lesions such as osteochondritis, epiphysitis, periostitis, and rarely dactylitis. Other signs which may be present include, condylomata, hepatosplenomegaly, jaundice, anemia, mucocutaneous fissures, malnutrition with edema, generalized glandular enlargement, and pseudoparalysis of the arms due to epiphysitis (Parrots). Along with these general features of early congenital syphilis there are often signs of involvement of the central nervous system. These include convulsions, signs of meningitis (neck stiffness, bulging fontanel), hydrocephalus, and paralyses.

In late congenital syphilis there may be clinical signs of meningovascular neurosyphilis (hyperactive reflexes, convulsions, paralysis, optic atrophy, mental deterioration) and an abnormal spinal fluid. Other signs include interstitial keratitis, Hutchinson's teeth, 8th nerve deafness (rare), bone changes, chorioretinitis, saber shin, subcutaneous gummata, and saddle nose.

PATHOLOGY: In early congenital syphilis the pathology in the central nervous system consists chiefly of meningitis. Secondary hydrocephalus may result. There is also evidence of involvement of the blood vessels with infiltration of the walls (endarteritis). Only occasionally are there lesions within the brain cortex. In late congenital syphilis there are more frequent lesions. There is evidence of meningitis. Encephalitic lesions are of a vascular type. There is blood vessel damage and also degeneration of nerve cells. Miliary gummata are present. There are parenchymatous changes with diffuse degeneration of the cortex and destruction of nerve cells (juvenile general paresis). The spread of the meningeal inflammation to the nerve sheaths accounts for the neuritis of the various nerves, especially the 2nd, 3rd, 4th, 6th, and 7th. The spinal cord is not so frequently involved as the brain. When this does occur there is degeneration of the posterior roots and posterior columns.

Clinical Features of Congenital Neurosyphilis. The central nervous system may be involved along with the general spirochetemia in congenital syphilis; therefore, it is involved early or it escapes entirely. If the spinal fluid Wassermann is negative during infancy, neurosyphilis will not develop (Jeans).

The clinical manifestations of neurosyphilis depend on the fact that the infection is first blood borne. The spirochetes get into the cerebrospinal fluid, invade the pia so that the meninges and their blood vessels are involved, and finally enter the parenchyma of the brain. There may be a few mild signs of meningeal involvement which then subside for a long interval before late features appear; the spinal fluid, however, may be positive. This is referred to as the asymptomatic stage (no symptoms but positive cerebrospinal fluid). Therefore, the spinal fluid should be checked in every case of congenital syphilis. On the other hand, instead of subsiding, the illness may advance during the acute stage to death (rare) or immediately develop meningovascular syphilis with late features.

SPECIAL FEATURES: Meningitis occurs in 40 per cent of infants under one year of age. Hydrocephalus is present in one-third of all cases. Cranial nerve involvement includes especially the 7th, with facial palsy. Argyll-Robertson pupil (complete loss of reaction to light and normal response to accommodation—convergence) when observed is usually bilateral. This sign is not exclusively diagnostic of neurosyphilis, but is highly suggestive. Deafness may be present, due either to 8th nerve involvement or to temporal bone syphilis. There may also be optic atrophy. Jeans found optic atrophy associated with chorioretinitis in ten of twenty-one cases.

Juvenile general paresis is rare. The onset occurs between ten and twenty years of age. There is progressive, rapid deterioration affecting behavior and mentality. Physically, there are disturbances of speech, tremors, memory defects, palsies with motor disability, and seizures. Psychologically there may be anxiety, delusions of grandeur or persecution, depression, anti-social behavior, and finally in about five years complete idiocy and death. It affects those previously normal or those with mental deficiency.

Juvenile tabes dorsalis is uncommon. The onset takes place in puberty with incontinence of urine, optic atrophy, and meningo-myelitis.

It should be stressed that while a series of individual clinical manifestations has been described, they are not clearly separable and many of them exist together. Furthermore, the picture in ac-quired neurosyphilis, which is extremely rare in children, is similar to the congenital, except for the signs of syphilis where the primary infection has occurred.

A comment is needed concerning the presence of mental de-ficiency in congenital syphilis. There may be associated micro-cephaly or idiocy. The question to decide, if possible, is whether syphilis produced the mental and physical deficiency or whether it was grafted on a congenitally maldeveloped infant. The incidence of mental deficiency due to congenital syphilis is about three per cent of all mental defectives with the probability that this will be lowered due to premarital tests and antibiotic therapy given before and during pregnancy.

LABORATORY DIAGNOSIS:

1. Routine prenatal serological tests on the mother (Hinton, Kolmer, Venereal Disease Research Laboratory Slide-flocculation).

2. Blood Wassermann test on baby (also check with Kahn, Mazzini, or any of the above).

If negative, repeat at four months, for the baby may not have developed antibodies.

3. Spinal fluid: The spinal fluid Wassermann is positive in con-genital neurosyphilis. This is the most important test. The cell count may be normal or there may be some increase (50-200), mostly lymphocytes. Occasionally the cell count is markedly increased in acute meningitis. The sugar is normal unless there is acute menin-gitis. Protein is increased.

As previously stated, the spinal fluid should be examined in every patient with congenital syphilis. This will detect the asymptom-atic types in infancy.

4. X-ray of the bones: There may be periostitis or epiphysitis which is very diagnostic.

PROGNOSIS: This depends on the promptness with which the diagnosis is made. The earlier treatment is begun, the better the outlook. However, one of the difficulties is that the nervous system may be involved by the time a diagnosis can be made and that the brain is being infected during its developmental period. At least, if treatment is begun during the meningeal vascular phase or asymptomatic period, there may be a good chance to prevent the paretic phase. Any of the residuals such as hydrocephalus or mental defect are liable to remain, irrespective of therapy.

TREATMENT: The best therapy is prevention. Detection of the pregnant syphilitic mother and therapy with penicillin will almost always prevent congenital syphilis. Nelson and Struve found in 1220 children of 423 mothers with a history of infection with syphilis that congenital infection occurred in 13.4 per cent in untreated mothers, in 5.8 per cent in inadequately treated mothers, and there was no congenital syphilis if there was even one course of therapy given to the mother.

Infants and children should receive a total dose of 100,000 units of penicillin per kg. of body weight. Procaine penicillin G in oil with 2% aluminum monostearate in doses of 150,000 to 300,000 units may be injected every two to four days until the total dosage is completed. The spinal fluid should be checked every six months. If therapy is efficacious, the white cell count will return to normal in three to six months, the total protein in one to one and one-half years, and the spinal fluid Wassermann in five to ten years. Therapy is continued until the cells and protein are normal. In older children, penicillin is given parenterally, a total of six to twelve million units in fourteen to twenty-one days.

Jeans, P. C. and Cooke, J. W.: Prepubescent Syphilis. Clin. Pediat. Vol. XVII, New York D. Appleton & Co. 1930.

Nelson, N. A. and Struve, U. R.: Prevention of Congenital Syphilis by Treatment of Syphilis in Pregnancy. J.A.M.A. 161:869, 1956.

Platou, R. V.: Treatment of Congenital Syphilis with Penicillin. Advances in Pediatrics, New York, Interscience Pub. 4:39, 1949.

Rose, A. S.: Neurosyphilis-Pathogenesis, Classification and Present Day Treatment. The Medical Clinics of North America. W. B. Saunders Co. 1141, 1952.

Thomas, E. W.: Current Status of Therapy in Syphilis. J.A.M.A. 162:1536, 1956.

Vandow, J. E. and Sobel, N.: The Present Status of the Diagnosis and Treatment of Syphilis. New York State J. Med. 56:2796, 1956.

CHAPTER 6

CEREBRAL PALSY

Cerebral palsy is a term applied to the disability of a child who is suffering from neuromuscular dysfunction due to brain impairment. While the motor disturbance is obvious, there are other evidences of brain damage which are also associated with the cerebral palsied child. These comprise sensory changes; speech, visual and auditory disturbances; impairment in growth, intellectual alterations, including a lowered mental level and perceptual difficulties; convulsions, emotional and behavioral changes. Any, or all of these, may be present along with the motor disability. In most instances the clinical condition is apparent by two years of age.

There are about 250,000 cases of cerebral palsy in the United States. The incidence has been estimated by Levin et al as 5.9 per 1,000 live births and the prevalence rate 152 per 100,000 population. The problem of the actual number of cases of cerebral palsy and its incidence is still being studied as there is lack of correlation between the various reports in the literature. (Refer to Kurland's article.)

The pathology which produces the brain damage originates primarily before birth (prenatal), or during labor (natal); occasionally after birth (postnatal). The etiological factors are varied and not, as yet, clearly defined.

The definition excludes progressive neurological diseases of the cortex. If the condition is progressive, search should be made for brain tumor, unrecognized subdural hematoma, hydrocephalus, or some degenerative disease as Schilders and treatment directed toward these conditions specifically. When the hydrocephalus, etc. has been controlled, then habilitation of the cerebral palsy condition can be instituted. Obviously a degenerative condition will progress, uninfluenced by any corrective measures of the type used in cerebral palsy therapy. Also excluded by common understanding are neuromuscular disturbances occurring in the adult, although

93

the latter may develop hemiplegia and other forms of palsy secondary to cerebrovascular accidents.

Cerebral palsy is a life time problem. Since it is usually neither fatal nor completely cured, plans must be made which envisage a complete therapeutic program of habilitation looking toward adult life. These problems will be discussed subsequently.

CLASSIFICATION OF CEREBRAL PALSY (MOTOR)

(As adopted by the American Academy for Cerebral Palsy—Nov. 1954)

(A) SPASTIC
(B) ATHETOTIC
    1. Tension
    2. Non-Tension
    3. Dystonic
    4. Tremor
(C) RIGIDITY
(D) ATAXIC
(E) TREMOR
(F) ATONIC
(G) MIXED

(A) SPASTIC (SPASTICS)

This type makes up about 50 to 60 per cent of all children with cerebral palsy. The muscle is hyperirritable to stimuli and there is hyperactivity of the stretch reflex or a lowering of the threshold needed to produce it. This means that when the muscle is passively flexed and extended, or suddenly elongated, there is increased resistance to this manipulation. The muscle contracts, becomes stiff and hypertonic and movement is slowed. There are associated hyperactive deep tendon reflexes, Babinski sign, and ankle clonus. In some instances, the effect of the hyperactive stretch is such that manipulation of one muscle causes not only spasticity of the muscle itself, but also overflow, thus producing spasticity of other muscles in addition. It is obvious that this will interfere with the ability of the child to carry out his daily living functions, such as walking, feeding, speech, etc.

Spasticity is due to an upper motor neuron lesion and has been considered to be an expression of the removal of inhibition on the lower spinal reflex area by virtue of damage to the cerebral cortex (Pre-Rolandic area) and basal ganglia. According to Magoun, however, spasticity does not depend on a release phenomenon in which the spinal reflex may become exaggerated. He feels rather that with the removal of the suppressor area, stimuli from the cortex may exert an augmented influence. The pathways for these cortical stimuli include extrapyramidal connections with the reticular formation of the brain stem and reticulospinal fibres to the cord. Electromyography may record an abnormal tracing with decreased action amplitudes.

(B) ATHETOTIC (ATHETOIDS)

These children make up the next largest group, 25 per cent, and with the spastics comprise most of the cerebral palsied population. Athetotic refers to involuntary, uncontrollable, bizarre movements involving particularly the extremities, as well as the facial and trunk muscles and those of speech. The reflexes are normal. The movements lack a fixed amplitude, rhythmicity or direction. The electromyographic tracing is usually normal, although voluntary relaxation cannot be obtained.

1) Tension—When this is present, there is tightness of the muscle but no active stretch reflex.

2) Non-Tension—The muscle has very little tone—almost flaccid. This is especially noted in infancy.

3) Dystonic—This refers to slow, turning movements, especially of the trunk muscles. Dystonia is usually associated with marked hypertonicity. The face and trunk may assume tonic postural positions, with rotation of the extremities producing distorted attitudes. The movements are not continuous, but postural changes and abnormal positions occur constantly throughout the day.

4) Tremor—In the tremor athetoid, there are abnormal, uncontrollable, involuntary movements, involving antagonistic groups of muscles of the extremities, for example the flexors and extensors. These movements are, however, irregular, uneven, and lack smoothness. Thus they are not truly tremors, but rather tremor-like movements.

While the sub-types of athetosis previously discussed have been accepted by the American Academy for Cerebral Palsy, Phelps has described other clinical varieties of athetosis. One of these involves slow rotary movements of the muscles of the hands and feet. The feet produce circular motions, while the hands pronate and supinate. Another is the neck and arm type which involves the muscles of the neck, arm, and shoulder girdle, but not the lower extremities. The movements are dystonic, or rotary or tremor-like. Emotional release may occur with any of the rotary or tremor-types depending on the amount of tension present. In the emotional release type, there may be laughing, crying or anger with minimal stimulation needed to provoke the reaction. In some instances the emotional reaction is unrelated to the circumstances of the moment.

It should be noted that athetosis is referred to as a tension type when this overshadows or masks the accompanying rotary, tremor-like, or dystonic movement. The tension state is only a temporary condition and as it is reduced with treatment the true type of athetoid movement is uncovered.

(C) RIGIDITY

In this type there is resistance of both the extensors and flexors to passive movement of the muscles, especially in slow motion. There is no active stretch reflex. The muscle is so hypertonic that there is a loss of contractility or movement. The tightness of the muscle has been described as similar to the feeling attained in attempting to bend a lead-pipe. Reflexes are usually normal and there are no involuntary movements. Where there is periodic inter-ruption of rigidity, it is referred to as intermittent.

(D) ATAXIC

Lack of muscular coordination is present. There is disturbance of the sense of balance. Hypotonia is associated.

(E) TREMOR

There are involuntary movements involving antagonistic groups of muscles. They are apt to be rapid, rhythmical, of regular amplitude and frequency. They may be intentional, that is, present on voluntary effort (cerebellar) or appear when the extremity is at rest (extrapyramidal).

(F) ATONIC

This refers to a lack of muscle tone or marked hypotonia, but accompanied by active tendon reflexes and a hyperactive stretch reflex. There are no involuntary movements of the muscles.

(G) MIXED

These are types in which there may be spasticity and athetosis combined in the same child, or various forms of athetosis may occur in the same patient at different times.

In addition to the classification based on motor disturbances, cerebral palsy may also be described according to the parts of the body involved (topographical). In quadriplegia, all extremities are affected, the legs more so than the arms in the diplegic type. Hemiplegia refers to one side of the body, including an arm and leg; paraplegia includes only the lower extremities. Triplegia, usually involves both legs and an arm, and monoplegia refers to a paralysis of one limb. In double hemiplegia, one side is affected more than the other and the arms more so than the legs.

CLINICAL SYNDROMES

(A) Spastic Group

This group, as we have previously stated, comprises the majority of patients in the cerebral palsy population, perhaps 50 to 60 per cent. Pathology is present in the cerebral cortex, involving the pyramidal tract and extrapyramidal system. The areas in the cortex which are especially damaged include area 4, the motor area, which contains the large cells of Betz, lies just anterior to the Rolandic fissure, and gives rise to the origin of the pyramidal tract. This is known as the precentral area. Recent experimental work in animals suggests that fibres to the pyramidal tract also come from the parietal, temporal and occipital lobes. Just anterior to area 4 are, in order, areas 4S and 6. These have extrapyramidal associations with the basal ganglia and lower centers. Area 4S is known as a suppressor area. When damage occurs in the motor area or pyramidal tract alone, flaccidity results with mild spasticity. However, the adjacent areas are almost always involved in cerebral palsy since most cases belong to the spastic group. Neural mechanisms for the development of spasticity have been previously discussed. The various types of spasticity include quadriplegia, hemiplegia, paraplegia, monoplegia, triplegia.

Spastic Quadriplegia. In this form there is most often marked spastic paralysis of the lower extremities. The upper limbs are also involved but to a lesser extent. In the older literature, this is called spastic diplegia and presents a picture similar to the original type of cerebral palsy known as Little's Disease. When the child is held up by the examiner, the typical "scissor gait" is noted. This consists of the child standing on his toes with ankle equinus, the limbs markedly spastic in extension, with adduction of the thighs and internal rotation of hips. The tendon reflexes are increased, Babinski sign is present, and there is a hyperactive stretch reflex. There may be varying degrees of severity. In the more marked there is also mental deficit and seizures. The combination of mental retardation, spasticity, and seizures is associated with an abnormal electroencephalogram in a high percentage of such children, especially if the recording is made during sleep. The pattern of the EEG is usually of the major type of seizure; the 3 per second spike and wave (petit mal) type is absent or rare. In the mild types, the arms may hardly be affected and the child begins to walk at about the age of four years; however, all movements are awkward. Speech is delayed and also imperfect. Prematurity is present in a good number of these children.

Some of the very severe cases are seen immediately following birth; there are difficulty with feeding, poor sucking and swallowing, and attacks of cyanosis. Convulsive twitching and lethargy may be noted. As the weeks go by delayed development is observed. The head is not held up and is "floppy." The baby may be hypotonic at this time and show a lack of movements. Later, at about six months, the hypotonia is replaced by spasticity of the back and extremities and the head is retracted, a picture of decerebrate rigidity. Convulsions may be present. The severely damaged infants exhibit a disturbance of their regulatory mechanisms and as a result may run high fevers. They take little nourishment and usually die in infancy. The majority, however, continue to develop spasticity, with some muscle groups showing contraction resulting in shoulder adduction, flexion of the elbows, pronation of the forearms, and flexion of the wrists and fingers. The lower limbs are stiff and rotated inward with hips flexed, knees adducted, heels off the floor. The Moro and tonic neck reflexes persist beyond the period when they should have disappeared, which is about three to four months. In the severe spastics, their persistence together with other data such as pneumoencephalographic evidence of cortical atrophy and a lowered I.Q. is an indication that the brain is so badly damaged that the infant will not walk. In addition to diplegia, there are other cases of spastic quadriplegia in which the arms are more involved. There may be mixed types in which athetosis is also present. In these, also, the arms show a more marked involvement.

"High Spinal Spastic"—while the spastic group has been described as being due to cortical brain damage, Fay has called attention to a group of spastics, whose pathology is located in the cervical cord at the level of the junction between the skull and atlas. They are due to birth injury of the cervical spine, producing displaced fractures and dislocation with resulting pressure on the pyramidal tract. The diagnosis is based on the presence of spastic quadriplegia in a child who has normal mentality and no seizures or athetosis. It is confirmed by X-ray evidence of anterior displacement of the atlas, axis, or 3rd cervical vertebra. Fay feels that decompression helps these patients.

INFANTILE SPASTIC HEMIPLEGIA

This subgroup comprises the most frequent type of cerebral palsy. It forms about one-half of the total spastic population, or about one-third of the total number of cerebral palsy cases.

CLINICAL PICTURE: Since in the majority of these infants, sixty-five per cent, the cortical pathology occurs at birth, there is noted early in infancy a lack of use of the arm and leg on one side. The clinical picture is most frequently due to birth trauma associated with a vascular lesion such as the occlusion of the middle cerebral artery. Cyst formation occurs in the cerebral hemisphere, often communicating with the ventricle. The symptoms and signs following delivery include lethargy, inability to suck, seizures, cyanosis, weak cry, or comatose state. The management of the acute stage is described in the chapter on birth trauma. A similar type of hemiplegia is observed in those children whose onset is postnatal. In the latter there may be a preliminary period of flaccidity, immediately following the cortical insult, e.g., trauma or convulsion, but this subsequently changes to spasticity. In the postnatal group there is often a sudden onset with high fever, convulsion, and coma. After the return of consciousness, the hemiplegia is observed. Improvement may occur, occasionally with complete recovery. If not, the picture of hemiplegia remains, with the initial flaccid muscles becoming spastic. Most of the children are in the two to six year age group. In the literature they are referred to as cases of "acute infantile hemiplegia."

In the fully developed picture of infantile spastic hemiplegia, including both those of natal and postnatal origin, there is slight flexion of the arm, marked flexion deformity of the hand, and extension with equinus of the foot. Spasticity is marked, especially in the affected arm. The limbs are underdeveloped and there is shortening. The pelvis may be tilted as a result. Atrophy and growth disturbance of the muscles may be due to involvement of the post-central gyrus as well as the precentral areas. The facial muscles on the same side are but slightly affected. Function on the affected side is poor. In addition to the motor effects, there are sensory changes, including loss of proprioception and discrimination of form (astereognosis). The tendon reflexes are hyperactive, the Babinski sign present. The EEG shows abnormal patterns, but usually diffuse and general in children, rather than focal. Convulsions and mental defect may occur. In one study the average range of mental level was twenty points below normal. In older children with a right hemiplegia, there may be an associated aphasia. In addition to the lack of intellectual development, there are behavior and emotional disturbances, which may become marked.

ETIOLOGY AND PATHOLOGY: The brain shows marked cortical atrophy on the side opposite the hemiplegia. Abnormalities associated with prenatal pathology such as a true aplasia or porencephaly rarely occur. In the majority the damage occurs at birth due to trauma associated with intracranial vascular occlusion of an artery. Prematures and infants of excessive birth weight are especially vulnerable. Postnatal factors are next in frequency. In the latter, the pathology is most often of a vascular nature. The hemiplegia may occur in a variety of infectious diseases. There may be acute encephalitis, meningitis, or acute hemorrhagic encephalitis of the Marie-Strümpell type. In pertussis, intracerebral hemorrhage may occur. There may be hemorrhage from trauma to the head or vascular thrombosis associated with blood diseases such as sickle cell anemia. The outcome depends upon the extent of damage and the underlying cause. Infantile hemiplegia is also associated with the Sturge-Weber syndrome (vascular abnormality with cerebral calcification and skin nevus).

Double Hemiplegia. In this type, while all the extremities are affected, one side has a greater degree of hemiplegia than the other and the arms are more involved then the legs. It is usually associated with mental deficiency and pseudobulbar palsy. Pseudobulbar palsy consists of disturbances in speech, chewing and swallowing and facial expression. Jaw reflexes are increased. There may be emotional outbursts of laughing and crying. The pathology involves cortical or subcortical areas, or the internal capsule. As a result, both corticobulbar pathways which serve the medullary nuclei are affected.

Monoplegia. This is rarely seen in a pure form. There are usually other parts of the body that are very slightly involved as well as the one outstanding paralyzed limb. Where the upper limb is palsied (usually spastic) there is also associated weakness of the lower side of the face on the same side (monoplegia faciobrachialis).

Triplegia. This usually involves both legs and one arm. If there is a hemiplegia, the affected arm will show the characteristics previously described.

B. ATHETOTIC GROUP

The clinical picture is referable to involvement of the basal ganglia and extrapyramidal system. The motor cortex and its relay system (pyramidal) are intact. A variety of syndromes has been included in this group, such as congenital double athetosis, congenital double chorea, choreoathetosis, torsion spasm, hemiballismus (sudden, violent, spasmodic movements of wide amplitude, involving one side of the body). The baby may be brought to the physician between five to six months because the parents note something is wrong with its progress. The major initial complaints are concerned with a delay in motor development, e.g., failure to hold the head up at the normal age, defective grasp, or inability of the baby to sit up unsupported at the expected age. To a lesser degree there is noted inability to respond to normal stimuli, difficulty in sucking and swallowing, and inability to follow objects. On examination there is noted a decrease in muscle tone (hypotonia). The athetoid movements are seen replacing hypotonia at about one to two years. They are accompanied by speech difficulties (dysarthria), and in the Rh type of athetosis associated with kernicterus, partial deafness with loss of hearing in high range frequencies may be an added feature. There is persistence of tonic neck and Moro reflexes in about 25 per cent of the patients. These interfere with feeding or dressing and create anxieties, especially fear of falling due to loss of balance. These children may also exhibit an extensor thrust reflex. They will assume various postural attitudes. There is delay in onset of walking. Deformity occurs in a number of these children, in some due to their involuntary movements, in others because of joint fixation; for example, "wheelchair" flexion contractures of the hip and knee. Other deformities include torticollis, scoliosis, dislocation of the hip, and subluxation of the temporo-mandibular joint. As in the spastics, various parts of the body may be involved. In the athetoid with quadriplegia the arms especially show the abnormal movements. Convulsions are much less frequent in this group than in the spastics; the I.Q. is somewhat higher. Consistent with these findings, the EEG is less likely to be abnormal than in the spastic group. Associated with the dysarthria there are grimacing, drooling, and difficulty in chewing and swallowing due to the ceaseless involuntary movements. Hand function is interfered with because of overextension of the fingers and their abnormal activity. All these involuntary movements disappear during sleep. Clonus and the Babinski sign are usually absent. There are neither active stretch reflex nor hyperactive tendon reflexes. These children show marked lack of weight gain and poor nutrition in early infancy and childhood. In the cerebral palsy clinics one often sees combinations of spastic quadriplegia with athetosis. These are mixed types and have the characteristics of both.

The etiology is believed to be birth injury, with asphyxia and resultant anoxia. Kernicterus due primarily to Rh incompatibility, has been a factor in about three per cent.

C. RIGIDITY

This type is usually due to severe brain damage, which is likely to be widespread, involving the cerebral cortex and basal ganglia. The muscles are extremely tight and hypertonic, cannot be flexed, and are in a state of contraction. The feel of the muscles has been compared to that of a lead-pipe. The child lies in an opisthotonic position in the very severe cases. There is no active stretch reflex or hyperactive tendon reflexes. The outlook is poor, except in the intermittent type, where the brain is not so badly damaged and the mental level is higher.

D. ATAXIC

As in the other forms, the signs of trouble are first noted in the developmental areas. There is failure to hold the head up, sit up, stand, or walk without swaying. Later it is observed that the child walks on a broad base, with the feet spread apart, because of a lack of equilibrium. There is evident muscular incoordination when the child attempts to write, or to feed himself, or throw a ball. All these motor faculties are delayed. When the baby holds out his hand, a tremor may be noted. This becomes more marked with time and increases with excitement. Nystagmus may be seen. Reflexes are physiological and mentality is usually normal, although Yannet found 10 cases of ataxia amongst 31 cases of hypotonic cerebral palsy in mental defectives. There may be combinations of ataxia and diplegia, either spastic or atonic. The pathology is in the cerebellum or its pathways. Generally defective development is at fault. However, in this group especially if the condition is progressive, one must keep in mind the possibility of tumor or a heredodegenerative disease.

Occasionally cases of acute cerebellar ataxia are reported. These occur suddenly without apparent cause, in children usually under five years of age who have previously been well, or in the course of an acute infectious disease. There are staggering, uncertain gait, intention tremor, nystagmus and muscular incoordination. Fever is absent. The spinal fluid is normal, but late in the disease there may be a rise in the protein. Most cases recover, but occasionally one remains chronic. These cases must be differentiated from posterior fossa tumor, labyrinthine ataxia, and acute demyelinating diseases.

E. TREMOR

Tremor is present in lesions of the basal ganglia or cerebellum. It is rhythmical, with regular amplitude and frequency. It is seen both at rest (basal ganglia) or with activity (cerebellar), especially in the latter, as in using the hands for writing or dressing. A familial tremor has been described, its appearance originating in childhood and dominantly transmitted. There are usually no other neurological findings and the condition remains static.

F. ATONIC DIPLEGIA

This is a rare form. There is extreme hypotonicity or loss of muscle tone (atonia). Although there is marked weakness, the deep tendon reflexes are active and there is also a good stretch reflex. Mental deficiency is marked in most of the reported cases. When the child is suspended by the axilla, the lower extremities may become rigid. Although there is no loss of power to perform movements, these children usually do not stand or walk. Electrical reactions are normal. Ultimately the hypotonia may change to spasticity during the second year, with the arms more markedly involved (double hemiplegia). The etiology is thought to be either neonatal asphyxia with cerebral anoxia or prenatal in origin. Differential diagnosis must be made from amyotonia congenita, where the tendon reflexes are usually absent or markedly diminished and mentality is normal. Muscular dystrophy usually sets in at a later age, and creatine-creatinine determinations indicate a creatinuria and diminished output of creatinine. A muscle biopsy may also help diagnose dystrophy. Weakness due to rickets may be differentiated by X-rays of the bones and serum calcium and phosphorus determinations. Cretinism is recognized by the clinical appearance of the infant including the dry mottled skin and thick tongue and a low I ^{131} uptake. Mongolism is differentiated by the appearance, X-ray showing hypoplasia of the skull bones (basilar), and general acromicria. Atonic diplegia will be recognized and differentiated from the above groups if the examiner keeps it in mind. The demonstration of hyperactive stretch and tendon reflexes indicating cortical involvement, usually serves to distinguish this from the other conditions mentioned.

ETIOLOGY: Since cerebral palsy embraces a varied number of clinical conditions, there is no clearly accepted etiology for the disease. At the same time, it appears to be quite clear that most cases are not genetically produced. The etiology may be divided into those factors operating prenatally, paranatally and postnatally. Obviously, this is only a working classification, for often the etiology cannot be definitely determined. In other instances more than one condition is at fault; there may be prematurity with toxemia in the mother and a difficult labor. Yet, listing the factors which may produce cerebral palsy and the time when they operate does have a practical advantage: it aids the physician in estimating prognosis and in the advice he may offer the parents concerning future pregnancies. It also stresses the significance of obstetrical etiology.

I. *Prenatal Factors.*

1. Hereditary (Genetic)—The clinical conditions include congenital cerebellar ataxia and familial tremor. These are nonprogressive.
2. Environmental or Acquired:
    a. Infection, e.g., neurotropic virus infecting embryo: toxoplasmosis, or rubella
    b. Maternal toxemia of pregnancy or maternal trauma (fetal cerebral hemorrhage)
    c. Nutritional and vitamin deficiency of the mother
    d. Rh, ABO incompatibility (Kernicterus after birth)
    e. Radiation of maternal pelvis, especially in early months of pregnancy (gonadal irradiation)
    f. Syphilis
    g. Metabolic (maternal diabetes)

h. Improper fetal implanation, placental infarct, premature separation of placenta, maternal anemia or carditis, maternal hypotension, all leading to fetal anoxia.

II. *Natal and Paranatal.*

Birth Injury	Anoxia—Excessive anesthesia during labor, oversedation (barbiturates),
	Cord abnormalities (twisted around neck of baby or prolapsed)
	Obstruction of fetal airway and atelectasis
	Placenta previa

Trauma and Hemorrhage—Malposition
Disproportion between head and pelvis
High forceps
Breech presentation

Anoxia and traumatic hemorrhage may be combined.

Prematures are especially vulnerable

III. *Postnatal.*
a. Meningitis and encephalitis
b. Skull fracture with hemorrhage
c. Lead encephalopathy
d. Residual effects following tumor of brain, hydrocephalus
e. Vascular (embolism or thrombosis)

In the above list, the most frequent etiological factors fall into the antenatal and birth period. It has previously been indicated that about eighty-five per cent of cerebral palsy occurs from damage produced at these times. Prematurity is a tremendous hazard, as it means the infant is much more vulnerable to the effects of anoxia and hemorrhage. Over a third of all cerebral palsied children are born prematurely. The natal factors are essentially obstetrical. Eastman has indicated that the obstetrical factors of significance in the etiology of cerebral palsy include primarily premature births and also trauma, uterine bleeding after the twentieth week, intrauterine infection, and anesthesia accidents. To reduce the factor of prematurity he stresses the importance of rest for the expectant mother in the last trimester of pregnancy and long-acting progesterone for uterine bleeding. Other obstetrical aids include the desirability of spontaneous delivery and the routine use of oxygen for the mother during at least the latter portion of the second stage of labor.

PATHOLOGY AND PATHOGENESIS: As indicated in the discussion of etiology, there is similarly no common pathology in cerebral palsy. The present feeling is that the damage to the brain is the result primarily of anoxia and also hemorrhage, irrespective of the etiological mechanism involved.

Some of the pathological lesions resulting from anoxia are diffuse atrophy of the cerebral cortex with loss of nerve cells, scars, focal cortical necrosis, and gliosis. Stagnant anoxia consequent upon venous engorgement, according to Schwartz, explains bilateral lesions of the cerebral cortex or basal ganglia. These areas are drained by the sagittal sinus or great vein of Galen. Atrophic lobar sclerosis (ulegyria) in which there is focal cerebral cortical atrophy and scarring, and mantle sclerosis consisting of focal cyst formation in the cortex and superficial white matter are attributed to anoxia. Wolf and Cowen feel that vascular abnormalities such as occlusion of the venous sinuses or leptomeningeal vessels or emboli may be at fault. They also include infection and birth trauma. In another group in which there are multiple cysts and cavities in the central and subcortical white matter of the cerebral hemispheres (porencephaly of the white matter) they feel that birth trauma leading to circulation abnormalities causing asphyxia and anoxia have produced the pathological changes. Status marmoratus (hypertrophied myelinated nerve fibres) and status dysmyelinisatus (demyelination of nerve fibres) have been noted in anoxia associated with severe jaundice. This pathology has been seen in the basal ganglia, corpus striatum and globus pallidus especially and attempts have been made to correlate this with the athetoid syndrome. In other instances, there may be evidence in the reaction of the brain tissue that inflammation has been present or that hemorrhage has occurred either in the vein of Galen or its tributaries or in the subdural space. The effects of intracranial hemorrhage as a result of birth trauma are also significant in the production of cerebral palsy especially in the spastic group. These mechanisms have been fully discussed under birth injury. Postnatal pathology revolves essentially about the effects of meningitis and encephalitis and trauma to the head.

In summarizing the discussion of etiology and pathology, we

repeat that these are varied. Stress has been laid on prenatal and natal factors resulting in anoxia and hemorrhage. Attempts have been made to associate spasticity with hemorrhage, athetosis with anoxia, cerebellar defects with congenital lesions due both to genetic factors and secondary to anoxia, but the demarcation is certainly not so clear. At the present time it does not seem that the clinical types of cerebral palsy can be accurately correlated either with specific etiological factors, definite areas of anatomical involvement, or a single type of pathology. What is becoming increasingly evident is that research into the factors producing cerebral palsy, epilepsy, congenital anomalies, and mental deficiency is shedding light on agents common to all these conditions.

DIAGNOSIS: The printed forms which are used in our Cerebral Palsy clinic at the Long Island College Hospital are referred to as a systematic method of obtaining data on which a diagnosis may be made. This plan can be followed by the doctor in his office or by the student or interne in the hospital clinic. The purpose of the questions is twofold: first to aid in making a diagnosis and second, if the diagnosis is cerebral palsy, to use the data for information as to etiology and management. Parenthetically, the type of approach and data which is obtained through the use of this form should be applied to the work-up of any neurological complaint for which a child is presented for diagnosis and management.

Family History. Page 1 of the chart stresses the family history. Here information is obtained relative to the age of the parents (elderly mother in monogolism), race (Hebrew in amaurotic idiocy) or any consanguinity. Abortions or miscarriages, if frequent and spontaneous, raise the question of maternal diabetes, syphilis, or nephritis. A genetic or hereditary factor is looked for in the familial diseases.

Prenatal. Page 2—Pregnancy—Stress should be placed on the mothers condition. Any infections—e.g.: Rubella, toxoplasmosis, syphilis, diabetes, nephritis, toxemia, bleeding, X-ray therapy in the first trimester especially, hypertension.

Paranatal. Complete description of the labor. Isoimmunization; drugs used; type of delivery, breech? Instruments used—mid or high forceps; malposition, prolonged labor, cord around infant's neck or prolapsed; twins; premature rupture of membranes—Caesarian Section, Why? Was prematurity present? Was the baby born anoxic? Might there have been intracranial hemorrhage or asphyxia? Any jaundice and time of onset? Resuscitation—the time before the cry of the baby was heard; any special therapy for the baby after birth? Any congenital defects noted? Condition of mother during and after the labor?

Postnatal. Pages 2 and 3. Any injuries to the baby or diseases of the C.N.S.—e.g., meningitis, encephalitis, other severe illness, e.g., sepsis, pertussis, intoxications as lead encephalopathy. Disturbance of feeding—convulsions—operations. Immunizations—any severe reactions as post-vaccination encephalomyelitis, or encephalopathy following pertussis immunization. Laboratory—X-rays of skull for cerebral calcifications, increased pressure, fractures; long bones and wrists for lead, hypothyroidism. EEG—especially for cortical localization, if seizures are present. Pneumoencephalogram. Blood count, blood chemistry, lumbar puncture, subdural tap; fundoscopic for papilledema or optic atrophy. Psychometric evaluation and psychiatric study including an estimate of the child's personality, emotional reactions, concepts of his illness and also interviews with the parents.

History of Presenting Condition. Page 4. Maturation Status—including speech, sight and hearing.

Physical Examination. Page 5. The physical examination is especially useful in demonstrating the presence of cerebral palsy. The various types can usually begin to be recognized about the sixth month and thereafter: the spastics, with hypertonicity and stiffness especially of the lower extremities, hyperactive stretch reflex, the marked adductor spasm, hyperactive tendon reflexes; the hemiplegic with limited movement of one side and shortening of the arm. The athetoid movements especially in the hands and upper extremities are noted toward the latter part of the first and early second year. There are also poor sucking movements, drooling, dysarthria, and facial grimaces. It should be emphasized that while these motor patterns are useful in the early diagnosis of cerebral palsy, they may change later in childhood before becoming finally fixed. Thus atonia in infancy may become spastic or athetoid later on. Moro, tonic-neck, and rooting reflexes should disappear after three or four months. Their persistence beyond this period together with other indices of cerebral palsy would suggest severe brain damage.

The ocular movements should be observed for early evidence of strabismus, usually internal. Nystagmus may be present, especially in some forms of congenital ataxia. Disturbances in gaze, either lateral but especially supravergence, may be noted. These are detected by observing that the child utilizes his head and neck to look upward to a greater degree than usual to accommodate for the paralysis of upward gaze. The ocular defects are not related to any specific type of cerebral palsy. Each child should be given a complete ophthalmological study.

Hearing difficulties should be checked by the use of special tests by the otologist. Every child should be given a complete hearing evaluation. This is referred to more fully in the discussion of kernicterus and deafness.

DIFFERENTIAL DIAGNOSIS: With the preceding data, including family history, maternal condition during pregnancy, the labor and postnatal condition of the child, the developmental history of the infant, and the physical examination (including accessory examinations such as psychological, X-rays, blood studies, electroencephalography, pneumoencephalography when needed, speech, visual, and hearing tests), we are in a position to make a differential diagnosis of cerebral palsy and classify it as to motor type, topographic involvement, etiology, and the severity of the degree of involvement.

In the differential diagnosis, the presence of hyperactive stretch and deep tendon reflexes, Babinski sign, and clonus, cause little difficulty in recognizing the spastic type of cerebral palsy. The rare spinal types previously discussed should be eliminated by the presence of a normal X-ray of the cervical region of the spine. The athetoids are also readily recognizable. Ataxia must be separated from the progressive types like Friedreich's or tumor. The rare atonic diplegia must be differentiated from poliomyelitis, muscular dystrophy, amyotonia, or cretinism. All the latter are associated with diminished or absent deep tendon reflexes and absence of stretch reflexes. In atonic diplegia there are active deep tendon reflexes and positive stretch. The greatest difficulty, in my experience, has been for students and physicians to differentiate in infancy developmental retardation due to mental deficiency from cerebral palsy. In both mental retardation and cerebral palsy there is delay in holding up the head, sitting up, speech, grasp, and reaching for objects. Therefore, if development in infancy is retarded, look for evidences of cerebral palsy, namely, atonia or spasticity, increased stretch reflexes, tremors, persistence of T.N.R. or Moro, abnormal movements, hyperactive deep tendon reflexes, or clenched fists beyond the period of three months. Later, either spasticity, athetosis or ataxia develops. If none of these or other rarer types are present, there is no cerebral palsy. One then looks for evidence of mongolism, cretinism, congenital deafness, blindness, etc. If no specific entity is found, there is likely to be familial mental retardation, mild birth injury, or an unknown cause.

It is finally important to stress that in cerebral palsy developmental retardation does not mean a low I.Q. necessarily, for since the tests used for estimating mental development are often based on motor activity, one cannot use these same tests for studying mental progress in a child who has a neuromuscular disturbance with limited motor function. This difficulty in estimating the I.Q. is overcome by a variety of psychometric techniques which take into account the neuromotor and other handicaps.

MANAGEMENT

While the diagnosis of cerebral palsy depends on the individual doctor, therapy in this disease is best accomplished by a "group approach." Intelligent management includes:

1. Care of the general medical problems (pediatric).
2. Supervision by an orthopedist or physiatrist or both of the specific program of habilitation—this includes the services of physical, occupational and speech therapists.
3. Affiliated consulting services: Otolaryngologist, Ophthalmologist, Dentist (Each child is sent to the CP Dental Clinic), Neurologist, Psychiatrist, Neurosurgeon.
4. Social Worker (who acts as liaison for the group—she interprets the ideas of the Cerebral Palsy unit to the parents and vice versa).
5. Special management of seizures (drug therapy).
6. Surgery.

The medical management includes pediatric care throughout infancy and childhood. These babies are often hypertonic, cry a good deal, are restless and irritable. They require close supervision of nutrition, including vitamins, and medication for sleep or relaxation. In the normal process of child development the fully dependent baby begins to assert its independence in the second and third

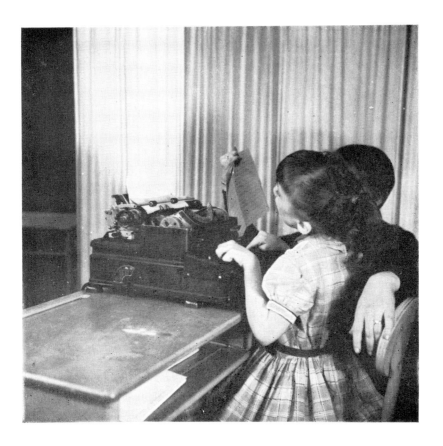

8. ADL (activities for daily living). Electric Typewriter.

years and gradually grows into a well organized adolescent, free, to a large extent, of excessive parental control. The cerebral palsied child, however, is dependent for many years on his parents, the mother particularly, for elemental tasks such as dressing, feeding, locomotion and toilet responsibilities. There are thus many emotional problems which arise due to this unnaturally prolonged close relationship, resentments on the part of the child and mother, guilt feelings on the part of the parents. The physician in charge of the medical program with the assistance of the social worker and psychologist will explain a good deal of this to the parents so that better understanding will bring with it better cooperation. In extreme situations the child and parents are referred to the psychiatrist. Muscular relaxation is gained through physical therapy; then by a means of functional and occupational therapy the aim is to secure voluntary muscle balance and control which will result in independent sitting, standing, walking, talking, dressing, self feeding, and care of bathroom duties. In other words, the objective in habilitation of the child with a neuromuscular disturbance, is to get him to perform the activities needed for daily living or ADL activities, as it is referred to. To do this, training must be directed towards speech, ambulation, maximum use of the hands, and correction of any deformities which are severely affecting the performance or appearance of the child.

The physical therapist functions in part through exercises and passive stretching. This is important in the spastic in order to avoid contractures and deformities of the joints. In the athetoid training is especially directed toward obtaining voluntary control of the muscles. Contractures are not so much of a factor. The ataxic child lacks balance and coordination and has lost kinesthetic sense. He must therefore be taught to use tactile and visual sensations in a functional position. Thus, instead of beginning treatment on a table as in the spastic or athetoid so as to obtain relaxation, the ataxic is taught balance and coordination exercises possibly given in front of large mirrors, and stress is laid on improvement of gait.

The occupational therapist lends her efforts particularly toward training the child in the daily living activities. This is carried out by repeated exercises. In this way the child develops voluntary muscular control and through repetition learns the developmental patterns needed for useful function. Rhymes and songs may occasionally accompany the exercises and are very useful in securing relaxation and rhythm.

In the hemiplegic attention is first directed toward establishing

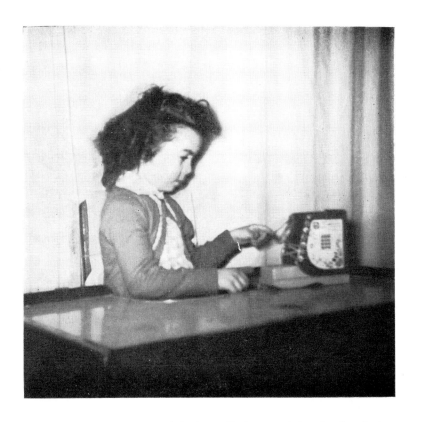

9. ADL (activities for daily living). Preliminary training for shoe lacing.

dominance of one side, before active therapy of the paralyzed arm is begun. In the presence of speech disorders and/or seizures it may be necessary to postpone occupational therapy and training of the handicapped arm. Otherwise these may be more aggravated. When the latter are under control, active therapy for the limb can be resumed.

Bracing is used in the spastic to avoid or correct deformity, of which the most common is pes equinus. In the athetoid bracing is used to control the overactive movements. Braces are also used for support as in teaching children to walk and to maintain posture, and they also prevent the deformity of flexion at the knee.

Crutches may be needed for ambulation. Wheelchairs are used for the child to get about until walking begins. He may not be able to get out of the chair; in that case it serves as his method of ambulation.

Seizures are treated by the use of anticonvulsants. (See Epilepsy.) Ataraxic drugs may be utilized when behavior as described in the chapter on "brain injured" children or the hyperkinetic type of reaction occurs. These drugs include Thorazine®, Serpasil ®, and the amphetamines. One should be careful if the child has seizures, since the phenothiazine derivatives such as chlorpromazine may enhance susceptibility to them.

Muscle relaxants such as Artane®, Tolserol ® or Prenderol ® are used in some spastics and athetoids. Artane® may also aid in reducing the amount of drooling. Zoxazolamine (Flexin®) may be tried in spasticity.

Toys are useful in both habilitation and education of the cerebral palsied child. He derives the same gratification as normal children. They help to develop motor skills, reaching for objects, manipulation, hand grasp, and hand-eye coordination. Blowing and sucking is useful in speech training. (For type of toys, see reference.)

Speech Therapy. Disturbance in speech is quite frequent in cerebral palsy. This is due in part to lack of synchronization between the movements of the thorax, diaphragm, and abdomen during inspiration and expiration. In addition, there is irregularity in breathing, with intrusion of inspiration, while exhaling for example. There are also lack of tongue control, expressed most commonly in an inability to elevate the tip of the tongue, and poorly coordinated jaw movements. Excessive stretch reflex of the muscles may cause them to tighten, e.g., masseter. Laryngeal spasm, interfering with speech, may also occur.

The objective in therapy is to develop intelligibility of speech for communication. It is therefore necessary to teach:

a. proper breathing and speech relationship.
b. correction of articulatory errors, omissions, substitutions.

It should be stated that prior to the onset of speech therapy, a complete hearing evaluation is made which includes audiometry. This is part of the general work-up of the patient.

Education. In the normal process of education the child is admitted to the school system at about five to six years of age. He has a reasonably average intellectual ability, sound body, and a wealth of experience gained through contact with his environment. To get this far he has been required to have a normally developing brain and neuromuscular apparatus and intact sensory-motor organs for vision, hearing, and speech. As a result he is able to develop abstract thinking, good concept formation, and proper speech. The cerebral palsied child, obviously, is totally different. Having a neuromuscular disturbance which limits his activity, he has not had the opportunity to develop the outside contacts, such as playing ball in the park or street, skating, going to the stores. He has specific sensory handicaps of vision and hearing. The ocular findings involve especially disturbances in muscle balance, with strabismus of frequent occurrence. Often, especially in the Rh group with kernicterus, there is nerve deafness, auditory aphasia, or both. Lack of control of the muscles (tongue, jaw, etc.) and poor breathing mechanisms produce difficulty with speech.

In addition, cerebral palsied children have the difficulties characteristic of the brain-injured child, namely disturbances of perception, visual, auditory, and tactile. They have a short attention span, are easily distractible, and perseverate. There may be sensory disturbances, often making it difficult to recognize the form and shape of objects as a book or pencil (astereognosis). The athetoids and ataxics also show marked incoordination.

Therefore, in teaching these children special techniques are used. Essentially this means using concrete materials which can be easily handled and visualized. Confusing backgrounds are eliminated and extraneous stimuli reduced.

SURGERY

In cerebral palsy surgery must be considered as an adjuvant in the total habilitation of the patient. Depending on the indications use is made both of orthopedic and neurosurgery.

Orthopedic Surgery. Orthopedic surgery may be employed to improve function by increasing the range or strength of motion, correct deformities, provide stability, or for cosmetic reasons.

The disabilities necessitating surgery arise basically from the dynamic imbalance about a joint due to the asymmetrical involvement of reciprocal motor units. The balance may be redressed by weakening or lengthening a spastic or hypertonic muscle as in the heel cord lengthening commonly employed for a persistent equinus limp. Another method of weakening the muscle is to reduce its motor power by a partial neurectomy as in the Stoffel procedure performed on the gastrocnemius.

On the other hand balance may be reestablished by selective tendon transplants which are particularly useful about the foot and ankle. In these procedures maximal use is made of the existing musculature but the line of pull is redirected into desirable channels of functional motion.

In flexion deformities of the wrist arthrodesis or fusion of the bones so as to place the wrist in extension provides more adequate function because the fingers may be used to better advantage. In addition the appearance is improved and the joint stabilized. A triple arthrodesis of the foot may be needed to produce stabilization when the lateral movements of the foot cannot be controlled.

Recently there has been a departure from the theory that very young children do not benefit from orthopedic surgery. Successful adductor tenotomies, obturator neurectomies and gastrocnemius resections have been performed on the nursery school-age child, thus ruling out the use of braces. All, or part, of these procedures may be done on any one child, according to the orthopedic decision.

Advocates of early surgery have found that with a good follow-up program there is lessened incidence of recurrence of the orthopedic problem, and six weeks after surgery is performed active gait training can be instituted. Good home programs and motivation on the part of the patient result in independent ambulation at an earlier date, completely eliminate the use of braces, and provide a more active existence for the child.

In any event, to obtain success following surgery prolonged physical and occupational therapy should be maintained, together with protective bracing when indicated.

Neurosurgery. Neurosurgery is used where the brain pathology can be removed or its effects overcome. This is obvious in subdural hematomas or hydrocephalus. The question of hemispherectomy is especially pertinent in the infantile hemiplegic group. The child, in addition to his paralysis, may have seizures and intellectual and behavioral disturbances. He is managed, as we have already outlined, in the manner of all cerebral palsied patients. However, in some cases, the seizures continue in spite of adequate drug therapy. If they become uncontrollable and result in marked interference with intellectual development and behavior, and pneumoencephalographic studies show cortical atrophy, hemispherectomy should be performed. In the birth injured group this should be done preferably during the first two years. Following surgery the seizures usually disappear. Function of the limb is not affected. It may be necessary to continue some drug therapy if the electroencephalogram is still abnormal. The reports thus far are encouraging: intellectual development improves, behavior is much more normal, and the children react better to their environment.

Recently attempts have been made to ameliorate the disabling effects noted in the extrapyramidal or basal ganglia group of cerebral palsy, namely in the child with involuntary movements or hyperkinetic disorders. These include choreoathetosis, rigidity, tremors, dystonia, and hemiballismus. Surgery has been used only in extremely severe cases with marked incapacities. Cooper has performed chemopallidectomy in the globus pallidus contralateral to the affected limb. Others like Wycis and Spiegel have used stereotaxic coagulation. Ultrasonic beams are also being directed towards the globus pallidus and thalamus. Myers has performed bilateral intermediate midbrain crusotomy.

It is too early to form a final judgment as to the efficacy of these procedures.

TEETH

As part of the management of every child with cerebral palsy, the teeth should be carefully examined and treated.

INTELLECTUAL LEVEL

The intellectual level of the patient with cerebal palsy is of extreme importance. Each child should be evaluated as part of the diagnostic study. It is realized that often the initial psychometric estimation must be interpreted in relation to the physical condition of the child at the time of examination and account taken of special disabilities, vision, hearing, speech. Some studies have shown that often the IQ is significantly higher on retest. This has been the experience in our own clinic in some cases.

In general, the data indicate that about 40 per cent of cerebral palsied children are in the normal group and 60 per cent in the subnormal range, with IQ's mostly between 55 and 70. It is therefore clear that a majority of the youngsters are educable to some degree.

PROGNOSIS: It has been our observation that where intellectual level is higher, there is a better outlook for improvement in cerebral palsy. The prognosis, however, is also affected by the severity of the motor involvement. Where there is mild to moderate disability and average or high IQ, there is the best chance for a good outcome. This includes about 40 per cent of cerebral palsied children. Where progress is not shown, even when these positive influences are present, social and emotional factors should be explored. If retrogression sets in, the possibility of some new factor such as brain tumor should be kept in mind.

In about 15 per cent physical disability is too severe to accomplish progress, even though the IQ is close to or normal. The remainder, 35 to 45 per cent, have a very low IQ and with their neuromuscular limitations have a poor prognosis.

To get better integration between the physical habilitation program and education of the cerebral palsied child, cerebral palsy school classes now function in New York City. These classes contain about twenty-five students each. Part of the day is spent on the physical therapeutic program and the other part on education. In this way there is a continuity of therapy established from the period of early diagnosis and care by the individual physician, to management by the cerebral palsy clinic, and then onto the school room. Thus the objective of trying to make each child as independent and useful as possible may be accomplished. Follow-up through a program of vocational training may be then carried out to help prepare the child for adult life.

The cerebral palsied child should be brought up at home where he will get the loving care of his family, and his program of therapy should be carried out as previously outlined. He can be transported to and from the clinic or school.

There are inpatient clinics, where the child with a satisfactory mental level, but who is severely handicapped, may receive more active treatment. He then may subsequently be sent home and attend the cerebral palsied classroom.

Where the child is severely handicapped and also markedly

mentally deficient, institutionalization should be carefully considered.

In the final analysis the problem of cerebral palsy is one of total habilitation of the child so as to make him useful to himself and to the community. If therapy is successful the child will not only improve physically, but his personality will also develop satisfactorily; this includes mental, emotional, and social maturity.

Batten, F. E. and Von Wyss, W. H.: The Atonic Form of Cerebral Diplegia. Brit. J. Child. Dis. 12:65, 1915.

Benda, C. E.: Developmental Disorders of Mentation and Cerebral Palsies, New York, Grune & Stratton, 1952.

Blumel, J., Evans, E. B. and Eggers, G. W. W.: Hereditary Cerebral Palsy— A Preliminary Report. J. Pediat. 50:454, 1957.

Bobath, K. and Bobath, B.: Diagnosis of Cerebral Palsy in Infancy. Arch. Dis. Child. 31:408, 1956.

Breakey, A. S.: Ocular Findings in Cerebral Palsy. A.M.A. Arch. Ophthal. 53:852, 1955.

Cooper, I. S.: Relief of Juvenile Involuntary Movement Disorders by Chemopallidectomy. J.A.M.A. 164:1297, 1957.

Cottom, D. C.: Acute Cerebellar Ataxia. Arch. Dis. Child. 32:181, 1957.

Courville, C. B.: Cerebral Palsy, Los Angeles, San Lucas Press, 1954.

Critchley, McD.: Observations on Essential (Heredofamilial) Tremor. Brain 72:113, 1957.

Deaver, G. G.: Rehabilitation of the Handicapped Child. Rehabilitation Monograph IX, Institute of Phys. Med. and Rehab., N. Y. Univ., Bellevue Med. Center, 1955.

Dekaban, A. S. and Norman, R. M.: Hemiplegia in Early Life Associated with Thrombosis of the Sagittal Sinus and Its Tributary Veins in One Hemisphere. J. Neuropath. and Exper. Neurol. 17:461, 1958.

Denhoff, E. and Jones, M. H.: Rehabilitation of Neuromuscular Disturbances, Summary of Round Table Discussion. Pediat. 20:165, 1957.

Eastman, N. J.: The Causes and Prevention of Cerebral Palsy. Pediat. Clin. N.A. Philadelphia, W. B. Saunders Co., Nov. 1957, P. 995.

Educational Advisory Board: Realistic Educational Planning for Children with Cerebral Palsy. Pamphlets 1 to 6, United Cerebral Palsy Assn., N. Y. C.

Fay, T.: Problems of Rehabilitation in Patients with Cerebral Palsy. Del. State Med. J. 18:57, 1946.

Fazekas, J. F., Shea, J. G., Ehrmantraut, W. R. and Alman, R. W.: Convulsant Action of Phenothiazine Derivatives. J.A.M.A. 165:1241, 1957.

Goldwyn, A. and Waldman, A. M.: Acute Cerebellar Ataxia in Children. J. Pediat. 42:75, 1953.

Ingram, T. T. S.: The Early Manifestations and Course of Diplegia in Childhood. Arch. Dis. Child. 30:244, 1955.

Klingman, W. O. and Hodges, R. G.: Acute Ataxia of Unknown Origin in Children J. Pediat. 24:536, 1944.

Koven, L. J. and Lamm, S. S.: The Athetoid Syndrome in Cerebral Palsy Part II, Pediat. 14:181, 1954.

Kurland, L. T.: Definitions of Cerebral Palsy and their Role in Epidemiologic Research, Neurology 7:641, 1957.

Lamm, S. S. and Koven, L. J.: The Athetoid Syndrome in Cerebral Palsy Part I, Etiology Pediat. 14:2, 1954.

————: The Intellectual Level in Cerebral Palsy. Cerebral Palsy Review 16:11, 1955.

————, and Fisch, M. L.: Intellectual Development of the Cerebral Palsied Child as a Factor in Therapeutic Progress. Amer. J. Ment. Def. 59:452, 1955.

Langdon, M., Ream, C. T. and Doebler, M. H.: Report of a Study on the Use of Toys in Work with Cerebral Palsied Children. Pub. by the National Society for Crippled Children, Chicago, Ill.

Lassek, A. M., Woolsey, C. N., Walker, A. E., Boshes, B. and Rose, A. S.: The Pyramidal Tract. Neurology 7:496, 1957.

Levin, M. L., Brightman, I. J. and Burtt, E. J.: The Problem of Cerebral Palsy. New York State J. Med. 49:2793, 1941.

Magoun, H. W.: Physiology of the Cerebral Cortex and Basal Ganglia in Relation to the Symptoms of Cerebral Palsy. Quart. Rev. of Pediat. 6:113, 1951.

Minear, W. L.: A Classification of Cerebral Palsy. Pediat. 18:841, 1956.

Myers, R.: Results of Bilateral Intermediate Midbrain Crusotomy in Seven Cases of Severe Athetotic and Dystonic Quadriparesis. Am. J. Phys. Med. 35:84, 1956.

Perlstein, M. A. and Hood, P. N.: Infantile Spastic Hemiplegia. Part I Incidence. Pediat. 14:436, 1954. III Intelligence Pediat. 15:676, 1955.

Phelps, W. M.: Description and Differentiation of Types of Cerebral Palsy. The Nervous Child 8:107, 1949.

————: Long Term Results of Orthopaedic Surgery in Cerebral Palsy. J. of Bone and Joint Surg. 39-A. No. 1:53, 1957.

Schachat, W. S., Wallace, H. M., Palmer, M. and Slater, B.: Ophthalmologic Findings in Children with Cerebral Palsy. Pediat. 19:623, 1957.

State Education Dept.: Teaching Aids for Children with Cerebral Palsy. Albany, The University of the State of New York, 1956.

Tizard, J. P. M., Paine, R. S. and Crothers, B.: Disturbances of Sensation in Children with Hemiplegia. J.A.M.A. 155:628, 1954.

Tobis, J. S.: Rehabilitation of the Handicapped Child. New York State J. Med., 56:2354, 1956.

Via, Jr., W. F. and Churchill, J. A.: Relationships of Cerebral Disorder to Faults in Dental Enamel. A.M.A. J. Dis. Child. 94: 137, 1957.

Winfield, D. L., Hughes, J. G. and Sayle, W. E.: Electroencephalography— Sleep Findings in Cerebral Palsy. Pediat. 15:88, 1955.

Wolf, A. and Cowen, D.: The Cerebral Atrophies and Encephalomalacias of Infancy and Childhood. A. Res. Publ. Ass. Nerv. Ment. Dis. Proc. 34:199, 1954.

Wycis, H. T. and Spiegel, E. A.: Treatment of Certain Types of Chorea, Athetosis and Tremor by Stereoencephalotomy. J. Internat. Coll. Surgeons 25:202, 1956.

Wyllie, W. G.: Acute Infantile Hemiplegia. Proceedings of the Royal Soc. of Med. (London) 41:459, 1948.

KERNICTERUS

The term kernicterus was introduced by Schmorl to describe the intense yellow discoloration which was observed with pathologic changes in the nuclear masses (Kern) of the basal ganglia in infants who had died with severe jaundice a few days after birth. With the development of knowledge concerning hemolytic disease of the newborn, it became apparent that kernicterus was most frequently associated with erythroblastosis fetalis, which is one of the major causes of jaundice in the neonatal period. There are other conditions which occasionally produce kernicterus including sepsis, congenital familial nonhemolytic jaundice, and physiologic jaundice of the newborn. These factors operate with greater effect in the presence of prematurity.

PATHOLOGY: In kernicterus there is a focal distribution of the yellow pigment due to localized changes in the various nuclear masses, especially in the basal ganglia including the globus pallidus, putamen, caudate, and thalamus. Other areas of nuclear staining are also noted, as in the Corpus Luysii, dentate and inferior olivary areas, medulla, and gray matter of the spinal cord. There is a diffuse involvement of the cerebral cortex with loss of nerve cells and fibrous gliosis. Crome has also shown a deficiency of myelin in the large radial bundles of the putamen and a mural fibrous gliosis of the entire ventricular system. In addition to the diminution of cells noted in the cerebral cortex, there is also a cell loss in the Purkinje group of the cerebellum, cranial nerve nuclei, and anterior horn cells of the spinal cord. The cells show evidence of degeneration with pyknotic and eccentric nuclei associated with glial proliferation.

The pigment which stains the nuclei is indirect bilirubin. Its source in erythroblastosis fetalis is the breakdown of the hemoglobin which follows hemolysis of the sensitized red blood cells. In the case of familial nonhemolytic jaundice, Najjar postulates that there is a deficiency of an enzyme which controls the conjugation of indirect reacting bilirubin. There is also a physiological disturbance of the liver which reduces its ability to excrete bilirubin, so that it accumulates to excess. Since recent evidence indicates that the excretion of direct bilirubin is the result of conjugation with glucuronic acid in the liver, the genetic deficiency in these children may lie in the impairment of their ability to make glucuronic acid conjugates. Bilirubin has been shown to be toxic to brain tissue.

There may be other factors which make these infants more suscept-ible, and anoxia may play a role. The problem remains as to whether the bilirubin is the primary cause of the brain damage or whether there is an underlying encephalopathy first with secondary stain-ing by bilirubin. Another possibility is that the functional maturity of the blood-brain barrier in preventing or allowing the excess bilirubin in the blood to pass to the cerebrospinal fluid and brain may be a factor in the development of kernicterus.

Finally, it is clear that kernicterus is a pathological diagnosis proven only at autopsy. In those who survive, the diagnosis is made on the basis of the clinical and laboratory picture.

ETIOLOGY: The major cause of kernicterus is erythroblastosis fetalis or hemolytic disease of the newborn. This disease includes in its mildest form congenital anemia, which does not produce kernicterus; hydrops fetalis, in which the fetus is born dead or so damaged that it dies before developing kernicterus; and the type with which kernicterus is especially associated, namely icterus gravis. In all these there is hemolysis of the red blood cells. This process is a consequence of immunization of the mother by in-herited factors in the fetal blood, the intrauterine passive transfer of the resulting maternal antibodies, and their specific reaction, both in utero and in the neonatal period. Rh incompatibility is the major factor and 90 per cent of mothers whose babies have erythro-blastosis are Rh negative. In a very small number of cases there may be other incompatibilities within the group comprising the Rh-Hr system. Finally there may be A-B hemolytic disease, in which there is incompatibility of the group A or B fetus with its mother.

Kernicterus also occurs with sepsis. Congenital familial non-hemolytic jaundice is another rare cause. Crigler and Najjar re-ported seven cases of genetic origin, all descended from the same forebears and occurring in three related family groups. In one of the marriages in the third generation there was consanguinity.

In some cases of physiological jaundice of the newborn the serum bilirubin level rises above 12 mg/100 ml in full term infants and 15 mg/100 ml in prematures. If the level is over 10 mg/100 ml on the first day, the question of exchange transfusion arises. In prematures under 2,000 grams the serum bilirubin continues to rise on the sixth day of birth instead of falling as in mature babies or those over this weight. It is thus obvious that the development of kernicterus, which in erythroblastosis fetalis occurs between the second to fifth day postpartem, may occur in the jaundice of prematures at a later period, up to about 10 days. Prematures are also susceptible to the development of kernicterus through the injection of excess Vitamin K intramuscularly following delivery and the use of Gantrisin® in the neonatal period.

CLINICAL PICTURE: In erythroblastosis fetalis, jaundice develops at or shortly after birth, usually within the first twelve to twenty-four hours. Associated with the jaundice there is hepatomegaly and splenomegaly, anemia, and finally the clinical picture of kernicterus. The latter appears between the second and fifth days. There are lethargy and restlessness, inability to suck well, high pitched cry, vomiting, absent or a poor Moro reflex, hypertonicity, opisthotonos, and convulsive twitchings. Many of these babies die; if they survive they may later show signs of cerebral palsy, which is the outstanding complication of kernicterus. The type of cerebral palsy which these children most frequently develop is athetosis. Occasionally they may develop spastic quadriplegia or rigidity, or a mixture of athetosis and spasticity. Some cases of atonic diplegia and hypotonia with ataxia have also been described. The complete discussion of the types is given in the chapter on cerebral palsy.

LABORATORY: Mother is Rh negative; Infant Rh positive.
Anti-Rh titre of mother is increased.
Coombs test on infant is positive.
There is anemia with lowered hemoglobin, increase in nucleated red blood cells, reticulocytes.
Rise in serum bilirubin.

If there is no Rh incompatibility, it may be an A or B type. In this case the mother is usual'y Rh positive and type O. Kernicterus is not common with ABO incompatibility since the hemolytic disease is usually milder than Rh disease.

DIAGNOSIS: If the picture of kernicterus develops, there must be a consideration of the possible causes. Of paramount importance is erythroblastosis fetalis. This is usually recognized during pregnancy by the presence of a rising anti Rh antibody titer in the blood of the Rh negative mother. After birth, the confirming tests reveal that the newborn baby is Rh positive and Coombs test positive. There are a low hemoglobin and elevated serum bilirubin. Clinically, the onset of jaundice within the first twenty-four hours is in keeping with the diagnosis and is an important diagnostic aid. If Rh disease is disproved, then ABO or intragroup incompatibility should be ruled out.

Jaundice due to sepsis may be proven by a positive blood culture. The congenital nonhemolytic jaundice with kernicterus is rare. There is a genetic background with a family constellation of cases. Prematures, if jaundiced, should be carefully followed by serum bilirubin determinations for excessive levels in the physiologic type. As previously emphasized, their onset of jaundice is later, from the fourth to tenth day. The amount of Vitamin K they have received should also be checked.

It is obvious that the cause of jaundice should be diagnosed, if possible, before the development of kernicterus. Other factors producing jaundice and requiring differentiation include cytomegalic inclusion disease, toxoplasmosis, congenital syphilis, congenital obliteration of the bile ducts, infants born of diabetic mothers, and infectious diarrhea with severe dehydration, especially in prematures.

TREATMENT: Replacement or exchange transfusion is the method of treatment since it will combat the development of kernicterus, which may have already begun during the first twenty-four hours following birth, by removing the sensitized red cells which are the source of bilirubin and also some of the excess bilirubin already present in the blood. It also regulates the infant's blood volume and increases the oxygen carrying capacity of the infant's blood. For details as to indications for exchange transfusion refer to the references.

PROGNOSIS: Death may occur at birth or shortly thereafter. In other instances complete recovery occurs. The prognosis may be based on the level of maternal antibody titer, cord-blood hemoglobin, and reticulocyte percentage. The important complication after the first days of survival is kernicterus. Allen and Diamond noted that before exchange, kernicterus occurred in 6 of 20 liveborns. In their last 125 cases there was no instance of kernicterus. Clinically, kernicterus accounts for about three per cent of the cerebral palsied population. Such children may develop motor retardation, extrapyramidal syndromes with athetosis, and a hearing loss. (See Cerebral Palsy.) The loss of hearing may be partial and the audiogram usually shows a high frequency type of nerve deafness. The deafness may be nuclear, involving the cochlear ganglion, or the auditory pathways to the subcortical areas may be affected. Since the Rh children with kernicterus behave as brain injured children, the question has been raised as to whether their lack of hearing may be due to aphasia or deafness or both. When there is doubt, use a hearing aid to see if improvement results. There is also interference with the development of speech. Byers states that 75 per cent of kernicterus survivors have an IQ of 70 or better and feels that the IQ may appear lower because of hearing loss and visual disturbances due to a dyskinesia of conjugate movements of the eyes. In this condition the head is moved upward to accomplish upward gaze (difficulty in supraversion) and may turn for lateral gaze, thus compensating for the incoordinated ocular movements. Since the latter can be moved at will or by labyrinthine stimulation (Byers), nuclear palsy is ruled out.

Kernicterus plays a very small role in mental deficiency. Yannet has reported cases of Rh isoimmunization leading to mental deficiency without evidence of kernicterus and cerebral palsy. On the other hand, Gerver and Day have reported only slight impairment of the intellectual level in children who have recovered from erythroblastosis without obvious motor damage and conclude that the prognosis in these children is good.

Allen, Jr., F. H. and Diamond, L. K.: Prevention of Kernicterus. J.A.M.A. 155:209, 1954.

Bound, J. P. and Telfer, T. B.: Effect of Vitamin K Dosage on Plasma-Bilirubin Levels in Premature Infants. Lancet 1:720, 1956.

Brown, A. K. and Zuelzer, W. W.: Studies in Hyperbilirubinemia. I Hyperbilirubinemia of the Newborn Unrelated to Immunization. A.M.A. J. Dis. Child. 93:263, 1957.

———— and Burnett, H.: Studies on the Neonatal Development of the Glucuronides Conjugating System. A.M.A. J. Dis. Child. 94:510, 1957.

Byers, R. K., Paine, R. S., Crothers, B.: Extrapyramidal Cerebral Palsy with Hearing Loss Following Erythroblastosis. Pediat. 15:248, 1955.

Childs, B. and Najjar, V. A.: Familial Nonhemolytic Jaundice with Kernicterus. A Report of Two Cases without Neurologic Damage. Pediat. 18:369, 1956.

Criger, Jr., J. F. and Najjar, V. A.: Congenital Familial Nonhemolytic Jaundice with Kernicterus. Pediat. 10:169, 1952.

Crome, L., Kirman, B. H. and Marrs, M.: Rhesus Incompatibility and Mental Deficiency. Brain 78:514, 1955.

Day, R.: Kernicterus Problem: Experimental in Vivo and in Vitro Staining of Brain Tissue with Bilirubin. Am. J. Dis. Child. 73:241, 1947.

————: Further Observations on the Toxity of Heme Pigments. Pediat. 17:925, 1956.

Ernster, L., Herlin, L. and Zetterström, R.: Experimental Studies on the Pathogenesis of Kernicterus. Pediat. 20:647, 1957.

Gerver, J. M. and Day, R.: The Intelligence Quotient of Children Who Have Recovered from Erythroblastosis Fetalis. J. Pediat. 36:342, 1950.

Gunson, N. J.: An Evaluation of the Immunohematological Tests Used in the Diagnosis of A B Hemolytic Disease. A.M.A. J. Dis. Child. 94:123, 1957.

Kelsall, G. A., Vos, G. H., Kirk, R. L. and Shield, J. W.: Prognosis of Hemolytic Diseases of the Newborn (Erythroblastosis Fetalis). Pediat. 20:221, 1957.

Meyer, T. C.: A Study of Serum Bilirubin Levels in Relation to Kernicterus and Prematurity. Arch. Dis. Child. 31:75, 1956.

Rosenthal, I. M., Zimmerman, H. J. and Hardy, N.: Congenital Nonhemolytic Jaundice with Disease of the Central Nervous System. Pediat. 18:378, 1956.

Silverman, W. A., Anderson, D., Blanc, W. A., Crozier, D. N.: A Difference in Mortality Rate and Incidence of Kernicterus among Premature Infants Allotted to Two Prophylactic Antibacterial Regimens. Pediat. 18:614, 1956.

Wheeler, W. E. and Ambuel, J. P.: The Efficient Use of Exchange Transfusions in the Treatment of Erythroblastosis. Pediat. Clin. N. A., Philadelphia, W. B. Saunders Co., 1957.

Yannet, H.: The Importance of the Rh Factor in Mental Deficiency. Bull. N. Y. Acad. Med. 20:512, 1944.

————, and Horton, F.: Hypotonic Cerebral Palsy in Mental Defectives. Pediat. 9:204, 1952.

CHAPTER 7

BIRTH INJURY

Potter has shown that the pathological processes which produce mortality in the intrauterine and birth period are anoxia, trauma, and prematurity. In the chapter on cerebral palsy the role of anoxia has been stressed; this may lead to focal or diffuse hemorrhages throughout the brain by increasing capillary permeability.

Here we shall emphasize the role of the trauma of labor as a cause of intracranial hemorrhage at birth, attempting a differentiation from prenatal anoxia, neonatal asphyxia, and hemorrhagic diseases of the newborn due to deficiency of Vitamin K, and possibly other factors. It should be emphasized, however, that intracranial hemorrhage and anoxia may be associated in the same infant. Furthermore, one may lead to the other and vice versa.

Cephalhematoma. This is a subperiosteal collection of extravasated blood overlying the bony skull due to the trauma of delivery. The blood never crosses a suture line since its accumulation is limited to the area enclosed by the periosteal attachment along the suture. The parietal area is most frequently involved, occasionally the occipital.

CLINICAL PICTURE: On palpation one feels a soft, fluctuating mass, which does not vary in size with crying. The mass cannot be reduced. There may be an accompanying caput succedaneum. If X-rays of the skull were taken in every instance, a certain number of cephalhematomas would be found to be associated with a fracture of the underlying bone. However, since there is usually no displacement of the bony fragments and because these infants do so well, an X-ray is usually not taken.

The swelling is noted shortly after birth. A few weeks later the edges of the cephalhematoma feel rigid and along with the soft

127

center give an impression of a depressed fracture. The blood within the mass then gradually disappears and a new line of bone forms over the subperiosteal mass, which eventually becomes the outer table of the calvarium. This process generally takes about four months.

The diagnosis is usually not difficult. The location, absence of symptomatology, and lack of pulsation or change in size on crying or pressure eliminate cervical meningocele, hydrencephalocele, or vascular tumor. Caput succedaneum is a diffuse edema not limited by suture lines to one bone; it subsides in a few days.

TREATMENT: The cephalhematoma should be allowed to disappear spontaneously. In some instances the large ones have been aspirated and antibiotics given to avoid infection, but this procedure is rarely necessary.

INTRACRANIAL HEMORRHAGE

The problem of cranial birth trauma due to mechanical injury with resultant intracranial hemorrhage is met in two forms. The first occurs immediately after delivery when it becomes apparent that the newborn baby is not doing well and the question of birth injury arises. The other situation in which the problem appears is when a child several years of age is brought to the physician because of failure of proper development. Among the causes to be considered in differential diagnosis is birth trauma associated with intracranial hemorrhage.

CLINICAL PICTURE: Immediately after birth the baby may present symptoms of delayed onset of respiration and crying. When these functions are established, they are likely to be irregular and weak; often the cry is of a shrill type and high pitched. There may be pallor, intermittent cyanosis, muscular twitching or convulsion, and inability to suck properly.

On examination there may be bulging of the anterior fontanel. The pupils may be irregular, often dilated. Ophthalmoscopic examination reveals retinal hemorrhages (15 per cent). In some babies one may note listlessness, apathy, inability to be aroused, and flaccidity of the musculature. Others are hyperirritable, exhibit increased muscular tonus, neck stiffness, and rigidity of the extremities. At this age it is difficult to make an anatomical diagnosis as to the location of the hemorrhage on the basis of symptomatology and physical signs.

The Moro reflex is sometimes absent immediately after birth if the hemorrhage is very extensive. However, even if present it usually disappears within the next few days.

PATHOLOGY: There are various forms of intracranial hemorrhage to account for the clinical picture.

(1) Subdural: This may be due to tears of cortical veins as they penetrate the meninges to enter the venous sinuses, especially the longitudinal.

(2) Tentorial tears with associated bleeding from small vessels within. If subtentorial, blood collects around the base (cerebellum) or if supratentorial, it traverses the occipital lobe.

(3) Rupture of the Vein of Galen with generalized bleeding subtentorially around the cerebellum, pons and medulla.

(4) Intraventricular, often associated with anoxia. This occurs especially in premature infants.

(5) Hemorrhages of the transverse, straight, or superior longitudinal sinuses.

(6) Intracerebral. These are small, punctate hemorrhages throughout the brain. There may be hemorrhage into the subarachnoid or subdural space, or intraventricular areas.

ETIOLOGY: A variety of factors associated with the labor have been advanced to explain birth injury associated with traumatic intracranial hemorrhage. These are related to the pressure on the infant's head as it passes through the maternal birth canal. They include such factors as contracted pelvis, enlargement of the fetal head, breech delivery, precipitate or prolonged labor, the use of high forceps, and prematurity. Intracranial hemorrhage also occurs in birth by Caesarian Section and in apparently normal deliveries.

There is a vast literature concerned with the relative importance of trauma (hemorrhage) versus anoxia as causes for brain damage. One may read the references following the chapter on cerebral palsy and those following this chapter for detailed discussion.

DIAGNOSIS: Having obtained a detailed history of the delivery, one should then perform a careful physical examination followed by lumbar puncture. An X-ray of the skull may aid in determining the site of hemorrhage and help to rule out fractures. The spinal fluid may be clear, xanthochromic, or bright red. If it is clear, there is no subarachnoid bleeding, but intracranial hemorrhage may still be present. There may be intracerebral or subdural hemorrhage, neither of which need be connected with the subarachnoid space. Very rarely an intraventricular hemorrhage which is blocked may also not communicate with the spinal subarachnoid space. If the fluid is xanthochromic it suggests that some old bleeding had occurred, with the color due to degraded red blood cells. There would be a positive benzidine test. Since it has been shown that following normal deliveries, with no signs of trouble in the infant, about seven per cent of newborn babies will have red blood cells or xanthochromia in the spinal fluid, this finding usually requires interpretation. If there is clinical evidence of a disturbed baby along with the presence of blood or xanthochromia in the spinal fluid, one may consider a diagnosis of subarachnoid hemorrhage. If xanthochromia is present after a week or so, it might also be due to a subdural hemorrhage. In this case, there may be increased spinal fluid pressure along with an excess of protein.

Frank blood obtained immediately after birth by lumbar puncture must first be differentiated from a traumatic puncture. If traumatic, the fluid collected in three separate tubes will show clearing with each successive tube due to greater dilution with spinal fluid. On standing, the supernatant fluid is clear. The first tube may even show clotting. In a nontraumatic puncture the spinal fluid appears the same in the succeeding tubes, the red blood cells are often crenated, the supernatant fluid gives a positive benzidine reaction, and the spinal fluid usually does not clot. Frank blood in the spinal fluid suggests subarachnoid hemorrhage. Particularly when prematurity is present, the possibility of intraventricular hemorrhage must be considered.

Types of Intracranial Hemorrhage

(1) *Subdural Hematoma.* This condition is rarely a factor in the neonatal period. It becomes a problem, however, in the subsequent months of infancy. In the occasional instance where it does produce the severe symptomatology previously described under intracranial hemorrhage immediately following delivery, the bleeding is usually bilateral, produces increased intracranial pressure with perhaps a bulging fontanel and loss of consciousness, and death usually results. We must consider subdural hematoma then under a variety of circumstances in which the baby following birth is not doing well. There is no sharply defined picture. The infant is likely to show a failure of weight gain, anemia, marked irritability, periods of vomiting, hemiplegia, convulsion, or fever. In two instances we have

seen babies with vomiting, fever, and diarrhea as the presenting complaint. In others there may be a large head. When this is present, one must consider a differential diagnosis from hydrocephalus. In both of these there may be cranial suture separation, bulging of the anterior fontanel, and dilatation of the scalp veins. Ophthalmoscopic examination usually does not reveal papilledema because the suture separation relieves pressure on the optic discs. However, retinal hemorrhages are often present in subdural hematoma. There are other causes for an enlarged head which should also be considered, such as toxoplasmosis, macrocephaly, achondroplasia, rickets, and finally congenital syphilis. Incidentally, a large head may also be a normal family characteristic.

LABORATORY: There may be some anemia, and tests for bleeding tendencies are usually negative. X-ray of the skull may sometimes show an old fracture or suture separation. The EEG may be abnormal. Transillumination of the skull is abnormal. (See section on Meningitis)

PATHOLOGY: The pathogenesis is concerned with the bleeding of cortical veins along the longitudinal sinus where they bridge the subdural space. Others have suggested that the origin of the hemorrhage may be from the deep capillaries of the dura matter. The bleeding is usually bilateral. The basic mechanism for the formation of subdural hematoma appears to be an effusion through damaged or irritated capillary walls. Gitlin feels that this explanation holds for all instances of subdural fluid whether due to traumatic hematoma, bacterial meningitis or the presence of subdural air. The hematoma becomes encapsulated by a membrane which grows from the inner area of the dura. Subdural hematoma experimentally may be associated with cerebral collapse. When it is remembered that the brain doubles its volume in about three to five months after birth and that the major portion of the expansion is completed in the first two years (80%) it is obvious that a space occupying lesion like a subdural hematoma must interfere with the normal growth of the brain. Therefore, if it is unrecognized and hence not removed, the result may be cortical atrophy with seizures, paralysis, and mental retardation.

DIAGNOSIS: The diagnosis is confirmed by doing subdural aspiration on both sides of the brain. Normally less than one cc. of clear fluid is obtained by inserting a needle at the extreme lateral angle of the anterior fontanel or in the coronal suture. In subdural hematoma the fluid will flow freely. About 10 cc. should be removed from one or both sides. The fluid is bright red or more frequently xanthochromic. It does not clot and is rich in protein. By taping the test tubes alongside the crib, one may compare the subsequent subdural fluids and note the diminution in intensity of color as improvement occurs. Spinal puncture should also be performed to observe whether there may be associated subarachnoid hemorrhage or a connection with the subdural space.

TREATMENT: There are two methods for the treatment of this condition. In one, subdural punctures are performed every other day and occasionally daily the first few days. The color of the fluid may clear and less may be obtained. The patient may show rapid improvement, eat well, start to gain weight, and seizures cease. After about ten days to two weeks if no more fluid is obtained, therapy is ended. The other method is based upon the theory that since there is an encapsulated membrane, burr holes should be made in the parietotemporal regions and exploration and removal of these membranes should be carried out. Otherwise, new pockets of subdural fluid will be formed. If there is bilateral subdural hematoma, the second side should be treated six to ten days after the first. Ingraham and Matson have operated on 350 cases with no mortality in the last 15 years. It would seem that both methods can be used with equally good results. In the first method, if improvement is not obtained within a few weeks, the burr hole technique may then be carried out with removal of the membrane. This is the procedure we have followed at the Kings County Hospital (State Univ. Div.). In the type of chronic subdural hematoma which is characterized by marked enlargement of the skull, drainage of the fluid and excision of the membrane may not be sufficient because the brain cannot expand enough to fill the entire cavity. In these cases Ransohoff uses a subdural-pleural shunt to completely evacuate the subdural fluid.

PROGNOSIS: This depends upon how much brain damage has occurred prior to therapy. Early recognition and treatment usually means a good prognosis. Favorable results leading to normal subsequent development have been reported in 70 to 80 per cent of the cases.

(2) *Tentorial tears involving small blood vessels* and

(3) *Torsion tears of the Vein of Galen* are associated with col-

lections of blood about the base of the brain, cerebellum, pons, and medulla. These are manifested by severe symptoms and signs of shock together with cardiac and respiratory disturbances. The lumbar puncture will show a bloody spinal fluid. These conditions are often fatal. If the bleeding is above the tentorium, the anterior fontanel may be tense or bulging with signs of increased intracranial pressure, including a slow cardiac or respiratory rate. There may be unequal pupils, retinal hemorrhages, and spastic or flaccid paralysis. The outlook here is also doubtful.

(4) *Intraventricular hemorrhage.* This occurs especially in prematures and should always be considered when the infant shows clinical evidence of cerebral pathology or respiratory disturbance. Serial determinations of the capillary hematocrit show a sharp decline. The diagnosis is confirmed by intraventricular puncture. We have had three cases in which results have been good following drainage of the blood.

(5) *Hemorrhages of the transverse, straight, or superior longitudinal sinuses.* These babies are usually stillborn.

(6) *The intracerebral hemorrhages* are considered to be due to anoxia rather than trauma. The history of the pregnancy and labor will aid in determining whether the bleeding is due to anoxia, trauma, or both. For detailed discussion refer to the chapter on cerebral palsy.

Hemorrhagic disease of the newborn and other blood dyscrasias can be diagnosed by signs of bleeding elsewhere, e.g., umbilicus, bowel, and skin, and by positive laboratory blood tests.

TREATMENT: The treatment of intracranial hemorrhage due to birth injury depends on general principles such as warmth to the baby and as little handling as possible. The head of the crib should be elevated slightly. Oxygen should be administered, first making sure of the patency of the airway. Two mg. of Vitamin K should be injected intramuscularly, and sedation such as phenobarbital (1 mg/kg. im.) should be given for seizures.

Lumbar puncture is performed for diagnosis, but thereafter it should be avoided except for special circumstances, such as the presence of a markedly bulging fontanel with obvious signs of increased intracranial pressure and increasing lethargy. The pressure is reduced by withdrawing the bloody spinal fluid slowly. Spinal puncture is then repeated as needed. When the lumbar puncture reveals normal spinal fluid, or when there is no clinical improvement following the withdrawal of bloody spinal fluid, or if the anterior fontanel remains bulging, subdural punctures bilaterally should be performed. If these are not revealing, then one may proceed with intraventricular punctures. Surgery is usually not indicated in the acute stage to stop bleeding. If there is a depressed fracture, the skull bone should be elevated to prevent compression of the brain and allow for expansion and growth.

PROGNOSIS: If death occurs it is usually in the first few days. Should the baby survive, the chances for a satisfactory recovery are good. Statistics may be found to show that the late results of recovered cases are poor in that sequelae such as lowered I.Q., paralysis, seizures, or behavior deviations may result. In other series the results are more favorable. Our own experience in recent years leads us to look upon the outcome of intracranial injury with hemorrhage with much more hope. Obviously each patient will have to be judged individually irrespective of statistics.

Bound, J. P. and Telfer, T. B.: Effect of Vitamin K Dosage on Plasma— Bilirubin Levels in Premature Infants. Lancet 1:720, 1956.

Caffey, J.: Some Radiological Features of Traumatic Lesions in the Growing Skull. A. Res. Publ. Ass. Nerv. Ment. Dis. Proc. 34:341, 1954.

Capon, N. B.: Intracranial Traumata in Newborn. J. Obstet. & Gynec. Brit. Empire, 29:572, 1922.

Girard, F.: Subdural Hematomas: Experimental Study. Acta. Pediat. 45:618, 1956.

Gitlin, D.: Pathogenesis of Subdural Collections of Fluid. Pediat. 16:345, 1955.

Haller, E. S., Nesbitt, R. E. L., Jr., and Anderson, G.: Clinical and Pathologic Concepts of Gross Intracranial Hemorrhage in Perinatal Mortality. Obst. Gynec. Surv. 11:179, 1956.

Matson, D. D.: Intracranial Hemorrhage in Infancy and Childhood. A. Res. Publ. Ass. Nerv. Ment. Dis. Proc. 34:59, 1954.

Meyer, T. C. and Angus, J.: The Effect of Large Doses of "Synkavit" in the Newborn. J. Arch. Dis. Child. 31:212, 1956.

Potter, E. L.: The Trend of Changes in Causes of Perinatal Mortality. J.A.M.A. 156:1471, 1954.

Ransohoff, J.: Chronic Subdural Hematoma Treated by Subdural-Pleural Shunt. J. Pediat. 20:561, 1957.

Silverman, W. A.: Care of the Premature. Report of a Round Table. Pediat. 21:857, 1958.

Streifler, M., Freundlich, E. and Beller, A. J.: Electroencephalography in Subdural Hematoma and Effusion in Infants. A.M.A. J. Dis. Child. 95:25, 1958.

SPINAL INJURY

ETIOLOGY: Crothers has pointed out that the spinal cord of infants at delivery is subjected to the unphysiological forces of traction. It is fragile and relatively inelastic. The cord is fixed by the brachial plexus above and by the roots of the cauda equina below. The spinal column on the other hand consists of a series of elastic rings, and the dura is strong and tough, so that any pull on the spinal column in the course of delivery, as in breech extraction, would produce damage primarily to the spinal cord. In this procedure the head is fixed in the pelvis and pull on the legs causes traction on the trunk, with the cord becoming hyperextended and receiving the brunt of the stretch. In head delivery, where the shoulder is fixed, lateral traction on the head to release the shoulder causes stretch or injury to the cords of the plexus or avulsion of the plexus from the cord and injury to the cord itself.

PATHOLOGY: As a result of the injury there are dural tears, hemorrhages into the cord, and extradural and subdural hemorrhages. There may be complete transection with subsequent degeneration of the cord. In very traumatic cases there are associated cervical fractures and dislocations.

CLINICAL PICTURE: This depends on the location of the lesion in terms of the delivery. Most of the cases of cord damage occur in breech extractions. If the lesion is high cervical, the baby dies quickly. If the injury to the cord is low cervical and/or high thoracic (majority) with involvement of the brachial plexus, the baby is at first quite unresponsive and in marked shock. There may be rapid, shallow respirations with paralysis of the intercostal muscles. The arms are flaccid, as well as the lower extremities. The abdomen bulges due to weakness of the musculature. There is bladder retention. Reaction to pain is absent and there is no sweating. Reflex action cannot be obtained. After the initial phase of spinal shock has subsided, reflex activity may begin to return. When cord damage involves the lumbar segment, there are wasting and paralysis of the lower extremities, loss of deep tendon reflexes, urinary and rectal retention, and trophic changes in the skin. In some cases with complete transection of the cord the muscles below the level may carry out reflex activity independently, but the infant will not survive.

In later childhood there are various deformities of posture and position, with atrophy or failure of development of those parts of the body previously involved by the damage to the cord. Spinal deformities result such as scoliosis or lordosis. Due to dural tears at birth, adhesions with a subsequent block of spinal fluid flow or changes within the cord, such as gliosis or syringomyelia may occur. When the brachial plexus or the cervical sympathetics have been involved, there will be evidence of an Erb's or Klumpke's paralysis or a Horner's syndrome.

LABORATORY: X-ray usually does not reveal a fracture of the spinal column. The spinal fluid may contain blood.

DIAGNOSIS: This depends on a history of a troublesome delivery, usually breech extraction or difficult head presentation. The paralysis is present from birth.

Differential from:

A. At birth:

1. Spina bifida occulta: In this condition there is likely to be dimpling of the skin with a hair tuft or mole over the lumbar spine. X-ray shows abnormality of the spine. There may also be other associated anomalies discovered by examination and X-ray.

2. Amyotonia: The weakness is more generalized. There is no disturbance of the sphincters. The labor is usually normal.

B. If the child is seen for the first time at a later age, one may need to differentiate:

1. Brain injury: There may be cranial nerve paralysis or spastic hemiplegia. The deep tendon reflexes are hyperactive and Babinski sign is present. If the mentality is lowered or there are seizures, the pathology is likely to be cortical.

2. Poliomyelitis: There is involvement of specific groups of muscles and a history of previous infection.

3. Spinal cord tumor—The spinal fluid shows the "block syndrome" of xanthochromia and high protein.

4. Infections about the cord are usually associated with fever and foci elsewhere. There may be a history of trauma. Lumbar puncture may reveal a "block syndrome" or pus.

PROGNOSIS: The outlook is poor. In most instances there are varying degrees of transection of the cord with paralysis of the limbs, inability to stand or walk, bladder disturbances, and death. If the patient survives, there are likely to be deformities in later childhood.

TREATMENT: Measures are taken for the special care of the infant, with particular attention to feeding, proper function of the bladder, and skin. The back is kept immobilized. The best treatment is prophylactic. The problems of abnormal presentation or labor should be anticipated, and measures such as Caesarian Section instituted.

PERIPHERAL NERVOUS SYSTEM

Birth injuries involve the peripheral nervous system producing:
  A. Brachial plexus pathology (Erb's, Klumpke's).
  B. Facial pathology.

A. *Brachial Plexus.* The cause of brachial plexus injury lies usually in the delivery of the after-coming head in breech extractions. The plexus is stretched by traction exerted on the shoulder or upper extremity. It may also occur in head presentations when the shoulder is being delivered because of the strenuous pulling away of the head and neck from the shoulder.

PATHOLOGY: The pathology consists of hemorrhage about the nerves of the plexus. When there is avulsion of the roots from the spinal cord, bleeding occurs in the subarachnoid space and the gray matter of the cord may be damaged. The nerve trunks may be torn.

CLINICAL PICTURE: The paralysis is noted immediately after birth. It is almost always unilateral. The picture presented depends upon the portion of the brachial plexus involved.
  Erb-Duchenne. This includes injury to the 5th and 6th cervical roots. As a result the infant lies with the arm and shoulder adducted and internally rotated, elbow extended, forearm pronated, and the wrist may be in flexion. There is mild weakness of the extensors of the wrists and fingers. There may be sensory loss over the outer arm and forearm, but in the newborn this is impractical to demonstrate.
  On examination there may be ecchymosis and swelling in the supraclavicular fossa. If the arm is lifted, then allowed to drop, it falls as though lifeless. The biceps reflex is absent. The Moro reflex on the affected side is also absent. If the phrenic nerve is involved (C4), there is paralysis of the diaphragm on the same side. By fluoroscopy there is a high diaphragm which rises on inspiration (reverse of the normal side) "see-saw." Hand grasp is retained.

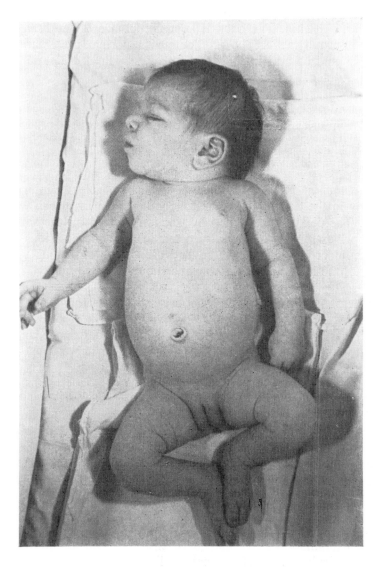

10. Erb's Palsy—left arm.

Klumpke: This type of paralysis is less common. It involves the lower nerve roots of the plexus, namely 7th and 8th cervical and 1st thoracic. The hand is edematous and paralyzed because of involvement of the intrinsic muscles and the flexors of the wrists and fingers. There is loss of the grasp reflex. There is also some sensory loss. With involvement of the 1st thoracic root we may have a homolateral Horner's syndrome consisting of miosis, enophthalmus, and ptosis of eyelid, due to injury to the sympathetic pathway. Occasionally the upper and lower roots of the plexus are all involved, producing complete paralysis of the entire arm, loss of all reflexes, and sensory loss almost to the shoulder. There may be associated fractures of the clavicle or shaft of the humerus.

DIAGNOSIS: This is usually obvious in the Erb-Duchenne type, which is the most frequent. The position of the arm and shoulder in adduction and internally rotated, the forearm extended and pronated, all are characteristic. X-ray of the shoulder should be taken. Fracture may accompany the paralysis or more often may cause the appearance of pseudoparalysis due to immobilization of the limb. The X-ray will rule out fractures of the clavicle or humerus, dislocation or epiphyseal separation of the humerus, and epiphysitis (traumatic or syphilitic).

Birth trauma (intracranial) will usually cause a hemiplegia rather than monoplegia. Spastic paralysis with hyperactive tendon reflexes and other evidence of brain damage are present.

PROGNOSIS: In the Erb type the chances for recovery are good. In the Klumpke type and in cases where all the roots are involved, the outlook is poor, for this usually means avulsion of the nerve roots from the cord.

TREATMENT: As soon as recognized a splint should be applied intermittently to keep the arm abducted and externally rotated. The elbow should be flexed 90 degrees, wrists extended upward (aeroplane splint). This is done to prevent deformity until recovery takes place. The paralyzed muscles are relaxed and the antagonists are stretched and not allowed to pull against the weaker muscles or plexus, thus avoiding deformity. This should be followed after a few weeks by physical therapy. Active surgery is rarely recommended. If there is no improvement in three to six months, however, neurolysis may be done to free the nerves from their scars. The outcome is problematical.

Phrenic nerve:
Injury may be associated with brachial plexus palsy, as the nerve is derived from the upper cervical roots. Cyanosis and difficult respiration are present. Examination also shows lack of abdominal bulging with inspiration and diminution of breath sounds on the affected side.

DIAGNOSIS: Fluoroscopy reveals elevation of the diphragm on the affected side and a normal diaphragm on the opposite side ("see-saw").

TREATMENT: Oxygen and antibiotics should be used.

PROGNOSIS: This is poor, as there is likely to be extensive cord and plexus damage along with the phrenic nerve paralysis. If there is no associated extensive damage, the outlook for slow recovery of the phrenic nerve paralysis alone is good.

B. *Facial Nerve.* Paralysis is usually due to birth injury resulting from forceps compressing the nerve or intrauterine pressure. It is a peripheral type of palsy and usually unilateral.

CLINICAL FEATURES: The paralysis is noted especially when the infant cries. Then the eye fails to close on the affected side and there is no movement of the facial muscles on that side. There is an absence of the nasolabial fold. The mouth is drawn to the normal side, whereas the paralyzed side droops.

DIAGNOSIS: Aplasia of the facial nerve is usually bilateral. The marks of the forceps blade should aid in distinguishing peripheral (facial) paralysis from intracranial birth injury with facial involvement. The latter would have other signs as well, such as spastic hemiplegia and seizures.

PROGNOSIS: The outcome is good and recovery usually occurs within several months. In rare instances, however, there is no recovery and a reaction of degeneration is present. In these, the nerve has probably been torn rather than compressed.

TREATMENT: The open eye should be washed daily and covered with an eye ointment. When there is an open laceration of the cheek and the nerve is divided, suture of the facial nerve should be done (Matson).

Byers, R. K.: Transection of the Spinal Cord in the Newborn. Arch. Neurol. and Psychiat. 27:585, 1932.

Crothers, B. and Putnam, M. C.: Obstetrical Injuries of the Spinal Cord. Medicine 6:41, 1927.

———— B.: Injuries of the Brain and Spinal Cord and Their Coverings; Edited by Samuel Brock, Baltimore. William & Wilkins, 1949, p. 503.

Feldman, G. V.: Radial Nerve Palsies in the Newborn. Arch. Dis. Child. 32:469, 1957.

Ford, F. R.: Breech Delivery in Its Possible Relations to Injury of the Spinal Cord. Arch. Neurol. and Psychiat. 14:742, 1925.

Ingraham, F. D. and Matson, D. D.: Neurosurgery of Infancy and Childhood. Springfield, Ill. Chas. C. Thomas, 1954, p. 201.

Smith, C. A.: Effects of Birth Processes and Obstetric Procedures upon the Newborn Infant. Advances in Pediatrics, Chicago, Year Book Pub. 3:1, 1948.

CHAPTER 8

INFECTIONS OF THE CENTRAL NERVOUS SYSTEM

MENINGITIS

Children who are ill with an acute bacterial infection of the central nervous system, such as meningitis, are apt to vary in the clinical picture they present.

The newborn, for example, may show signs of sepsis, including cyanosis, jaundice, and periods of irregular breathing. Elevation of fever may not be present, but this can be misleading unless one remembers that not infrequently infection may be present without accompanying rise of fever at this age. Obstetrical difficulties, an inflamed navel, or diaper area may be the source of infection. In the full term newborn and premature, E. coli is most often found.

During infancy the symptoms may be rather vague and difficult to group together. There can be marked irritability, convulsion, fever, vomiting, drowsiness, a vacant stare. A high pitched, weak cry may be noted. On examination, a bulging fontanel, if present, is helpful in diagnosis. Neck stiffness is also noted, and Kernig's sign is present. Occasionally, on percussion of the skull, a "cracked pot" tone may be observed suggesting increased pressure with ventricular distention. Not all of these symptoms and signs may be present at the same time in any one patient; hence, the physician must be on the alert for atypical and varied manifestations and keep meningitis as a factor in his mind at all times. It should be stressed that in studying an infant in whom fever is continuous and unaccounted for, a diagnostic lumbar puncture should be performed, even though there appear to be no signs of central nervous system infection.

In childhood the symptoms and signs suggesting meningitis are usually characteristic; hence the need for diagnostic lumbar puncture is recognized early.

The history of the illness, up to the time the doctor is first called to see the patient, should be carefully noted. If the onset of fever, drowsiness, headache, vomiting, and hyperaesthesia came on suddenly and is accompanied by a bulging fontanel or stiff neck, an acute meningitis or encephalitis should be considered. A more protracted onset, with loss of spirit, some drowsiness, perhaps change in disposition, then deepening stupor, is suggestive of tuberculous meningitis. A dimple or sinus tract along the midline of the back or the occipital region, which may be accompanied by a port wine stain, should be considered a potential portal of entry for the development of meningitis. The presence of a dermal sinus is especially significant and should be searched for where there is recurring meningitis. It must be eliminated surgically.

Where a petechial eruption or ecchymotic rash is present in conjunction with the symptoms and signs of meningitis, meningococcus bacteremia should be the working or initial diagnosis. The presence of a draining ear or the history of recent ear infection in conjunction with meningeal signs should make one suspicious of pneumococcus, streptococcus, or influenzal meningitis. Under these circumstances brain abscess must also be considered. If the child has recently had an infectious disease, or been exposed to one, or is in the early stages of the illness, the onset of symptoms such as headache, convulsion, and paralysis should suggest encephalitis associated with the primary illness, e.g., measles encephalitis.

The possibility of lead ingestion should always be ruled out when tuberculous meningitis and especially encephalitis is suspected. The season of the year is significant, since poliomyelitis is to be strongly considered during the summer. The parents should be asked whether the child was bitten (rabies), or had any injury (tetanus) recently, or been injected or vaccinated within a short period prior to the onset of symptoms (post-vaccination encephalitis).

In the preceding discussion some suggestions have been made which might aid in the early clinical differential diagnosis when infection of the nervous system is suspected. However, irrespective of the presumptive diagnosis based on the clinical picture, the major point is that these considerations lead to *prompt* lumbar puncture.

Lumbar puncture should always be preceded by examination of the fundi. In most instances these will appear normal and the spinal puncture may thus be safely performed. If, however, papilledema is present, and the clinical picture suggests generalized infection, lumbar puncture should still be done, allowing the cerebrospinal fluid to escape slowly. This will avoid the danger of sudden shock or even death, which may occur if there is a subtentorial (cerebellar) brain abscess or tumor and the cushion of cerebrospinal fluid beneath the tentorium is suddenly removed by rapid withdrawal of large amounts of spinal fluid. Should the symptoms and signs, such as headache, vomiting, and ataxia, suggest brain tumor, methods other than initial lumbar puncture may be used for diagnosis. These will be referred to later in the discussion of tumors.

The appearance of the spinal fluid should be noted as to clarity and the pressure measured. The fluid should be collected in three sterile test tubes containing 3 cc. to 4cc. in each.

Some of the spinal fluid (0.3 cc. to 0.4 cc.) from the first tube should be added to a blood agar plate and blood broth tube and incubated anaerobically in a jar with an atmosphere of approximately 10% CO_2. A similar amount of spinal fluid should be added to a Levinthal agar plate, a tube of Levinthal broth, and a Mac-Conkey plate (enteric group) and incubated aerobically.

If tuberculosis is in question, additional spinal fluid should be removed for special tests, as discussed under tuberculous meningitis.

SIX TUBE TEST FOR ESTIMATING SUGAR CONTENT OF SPINAL FLUID IN MILLIGRAMS PER 100 CU. CC.

Tube No.	Cerebrospinal Fluid cc.	Milligrams Sugar per 100 cc.					
		$>$50	40-50	30-40	20-30	10-20	$<$10
		Reduction of 1 cc. of Benedict's Solution					
1	0.05	+	0	0	0	0	0
2	0.1	+	+	0	0	0	0
3	0.15	+	+	+	0	0	0
4	0.2	+	+	+	+	0	0
5	0.25	+	+	+	+	+	0
6	0.0	0	0	0	0	0	0

Pipet 1 cc. of Benedict's qualitative solution into each of six test tubes. Into the first five introduce the amounts of spinal fluid indicated in the table with tube six as a control. Shake well. Immerse all tubes in boiling water and allow to boil actively for 10 minutes. Let cool before reading. Interpret reduction by means of the table. This test should be confirmed by quantitative analysis.

Some of the fluid in the second tube should be used for a total cell count and differential. Examine a wet mount of spinal fluid with low and high power for organisms. Centrifuge the remainder and make a slide of the sediment (Gram stain). Where organisms are seen suggesting meningococcus, pneumococcus, or influenza bacilli, the "Quellung" reaction may be carried out. A small loopful of spinal fluid sediment containing organisms is mixed with a large loopful of typing serum, to which mixture a small loopful of methylene blue is carefully added in order to stain the organisms in the preparation. Examine under oil immersion for capsular swelling.

The fluid from the third tube should be used for chemistry, including Pandy, protein, chloride, and sugar.

Acute Bacterial Meningitis. The spinal fluid will appear turbid and flow under increased pressure (.N 100-200 mm. water); the cell count usually will be in the thousands per cu. mm. with a high percentage of polymorphonucleated cells (85%); the direct smear and culture may reveal the organism. The protein will be slightly elevated, about 45-60 mg. per 100 ml., and the spinal fluid sugar is usually below 30 mg. per 100 ml.

In every case a blood culture should be taken, and also cultures of the nose, throat, and ears if the latter are draining pus.

If a petechial rash is present, the eruption may be aspirated and a direct smear (Gram stain) made. This may reveal a meningococcus.

When the anterior fontanel is patent, subdural aspirations may be done as any recovered fluid can be used for early diagnosis of the type of meningitis. This is particularly important today, when almost every type of infection in childhood is treated in the home with some antibiotic. As a result, if meningitis was not recognized, the treatment may not have been adequate, but is often sufficient to prevent a growth of any organisms from the spinal fluid or blood, whereas a positive result may at times be obtained from subdural fluid. Routine subdural puncture as an admission procedure has an even more important aspect than its use as an additional diagnostic method for the type of meningitis. Early recognition of subdural effusion means immediate aspiration with good prospects of eliminating this complication. Thus far in the pediatric service of the Kings County Hospital (State University Division), where we are doing subdural punctures routinely on admission of all meningitides with open fontanels, we have diagnosed six subdural effusions from a total of twelve cases. These effusions were xanthochromic in appearance, contained elevated protein, and treatment successfully eliminated the subdural complication. Our studies indicate that the procedure itself does not produce subdural effusion. Recently a technique using transillumination has been described for the diagnosis of collections of subdural fluid in infants under one year of age. A narrow cuff of opaque sponge rubber is placed about the illuminating surface of a standard two cell flashlight. This cuff is pressed against the cranial vault of the infant in a darkened room. Normally a rim of faint light about the rubber cone is seen, not exceeding 1.5 cm. When a subdural collection of fluid is present, the area of light about the rubber cone is brighter and extends for a distance of 2 to 12 cms. The only exception is a fresh subdural hemorrhage which requires about three days to show abnormal transillumination. This occurs when the fluid becomes xanthochromic.

This test may be used as a routine procedure in infants under a year for the detection of subdural fluid. Under these circumstances subdural punctures would then be done only in those cases which showed abnormal transillumination.

Incidentally the procedure may also be used to follow puncture and drainage of the subdural effusion, as the transillumination of the head returns to normal with successful therapy.

The principles involved in therapy are based on early clinical and bacteriological diagnosis and prompt and effective treatment so as to eliminate the organism as rapidly as possible.

I should like to stress that it is important for the physician who first sees the patient in the home to have a high degree of suspicion concerning meningitis and to keep in mind the lack of typical histories in infancy.

In the hospital, the interne who first sees the patient and performs a lumbar puncture should study the spinal fluid carefully and do the Gram stain of the sediment. This is extremely important today, for some of the spinal fluids, modified by therapy at home, may not show the classical innumerable white blood cells, but only a few hundred or so, thus simulating encephalitic or aseptic meningitis fluid. In some prematures and newborns there is no cellular increase with meningitis. Hence, because the spinal fluid may not be typical, smear and bacterial culture of the fluid should be carried out in every instance; the cell count and staining of the smear should be done immediately by the interne, who should not depend upon the laboratory, where many hours may elapse before the slide is examined, as in an admission at night. In H. influenzae type B and pneumococcus there may be direct typing of the organism through use of the "Quellung" reaction with type specific serum. This aids in early diagnosis. Initial therapy should be based on the identification of an organism in the slide. It is modified by the report of the culture which is obtained later. Here also specific typing of the organism may be performed.

Since many children admitted to the hospital have already had some drug or antibiotic therapy at home, no organism may be seen on smear or subsequently grow out on culture. For this patient, a combination of penicillin, chloramphenicol and sulfadiazine, according to the dosages listed in the treatment of the individual types of meningitis, is recommended.

Except for meningococcus meningitis, drugs in combination of at least two should always be used. In meningococcus, sulfadiazine alone is sufficient, though penicillin may be added if desired, especially in infants and severe cases in older children. The exception to using sulfadiazine alone is the child admitted with the Waterhouse-Friderichsen syndrome. In this instance there is shock with circulatory collapse and marked fall in blood pressure. Both sulfadiazine and penicillin should be given, and additional support in the form of intravenous fluids, blood, and drugs such as cortisone and norepinephrine should be offered. The last should be given intravenously, 5 mg/liter by drip. The eosinophil count may be of some value as a guide. In the normal child the eosinophil count is 100 to 200 per c/mm. When the adrenals are effective in acute meningitis counts of 0 to 25 per c/mm. are present (eosinopenia). If the adrenal gland is not functioning, as in the Waterhouse-Friderichsen syndrome, eosinophil counts nearer to 100 per c/mm. are found. The eosinophil count is, however, not completely reliable and other techniques such as the level of plasma corticoids may also be used. The normal blood plasma level is 12 micrograms per 100 ml. In ordinary meningitis or acute infection where the adrenal and pituitary are functioning, the level rises in response to stress. In the Waterhouse-Friderichsen syndrome there may be a low level, indicating the need for hydrocortisone. Hydrocortisone should be given immediately, 50 mg. intravenously by drip in 5% dextrose in saline and 100 mg. intramuscularly. Continue steroids daily, reducing the amounts, utilizing eospinophil counts and the return of blood pressure as a guide. When the organism is identified, sensitization tests should be carried out and the results checked with the drugs and antibiotics being used.

Except for the possible use of polymyxin in Ps. aeruginosa

(pyocyaneous) infection there appears to be no need for intrathecal therapy, and the potential dangers involved should cause this route to be by-passed.

If the patient is responding to treatment, a lumbar puncture done forty-eight hours after the initial spinal tap should reveal a clear fluid with few cells. The smear should show no organisms, and culture should be sterile. The spinal fluid sugar (quantitative) should rise to normal.

Should the fever persist, intense vomiting occur, focal neurological signs remain, or convulsion take place during convalesence, or if the spinal fluid examination does not indicate a return to normal, complications should be looked for. If the anterior fontanel is open, subdural puncture, bilateral, should be performed. If excess fluid is found, over 1-2 cc., this is pathological. The subdural fluid may be clear to xanthochromic, occasionally turbid with a high protein content of 0.5 to 3.5 gm. per 100 cc. and about 200 cells. At times culture of the fluid is positive, mainly influenza or pneumococcus. Treatment consists of puncture of the subdural space daily for about seven days with drainage of fluid up to 10 cc.; this is followed by removal of subdural fluid every other day. This technique usually is successful, but if the fluid continues to persist after about four weeks, then craniotomy with burr holes, as in the case of subdural hematoma, should be done.

GENERAL OUTLOOK: The immediate prognosis in meningitis is good. In general the mortality is highest in the newborn period and infancy. The outlook is poorer in those who already have evidence of cerebral damage when admitted to the hospital, usually due to a delay in diagnosis.

In those children who have had their onset of acute meningitis prior to two years of age, poorer progress, both mentally and physically, is noted much more frequently. Brain damage which results in motor impairment, mental retardation, and behavior disturbances, is more marked in the younger age group. This may be linked with undiagnosed subdural infection, the type of causative organisms, and failure of early diagnosis which results in hydrocephalus.

Meningococcus Meningitis. This is caused by the meningococcus (Neisseria intracellularis meningitidis), which is a gram-negative coccus, inhabiting the nasopharynx. It produces meningitis by way of the blood stream. Type I meningococcus is the most common one producing meningitis; it exhibits capsular swelling with type specific antiserum. Occasionally types II and IIA are cultured from the spinal fluid. Meningococcus menigitis may occur at any age, but is especially prevalent in the first and early years of infancy.

PATHOLOGY: Early in the disease there is a transient bacteremia which traverses the choroidal barrier and produces infection within the ventricles as well as in the meninges. When the organisms persist more actively in the blood stream (septicemic form), producing petechiae in the skin due to invasion of the blood capillaries, there may also be involvement of the joints, pericardium, eyes, and adrenals. In the last there may be necrosis of the adrenal cortex or severe hemorrhage in the gland (Waterhouse-Friderichsen syndrome).

The arachnoid and pia show inflammatory reaction with the presence of white blood cells and organisms. The blood vessels are engorged. There is exudate over the base of the brain especially, which may lead to a block of the flow of cerebrospinal fluid with resultant hydrocephalus. The convexity of the brain may also be involved. The brain tissue itself may show inflammatory areas with petechial hemorrhages or thrombosis of the arteries or veins. Exudate along the nerve sheaths causes cranial nerve palsies.

CLINICAL PICTURE: The onset of meningitis develops acutely with severe headache, vomiting, chills, high fever, hyperaesthesia and occasionally convulsions, especially in infancy. Examination reveals neck stiffness and Kernig's sign. In infants the anterior fontanel is tense and bulging. The spine may be rigid and together with a stiff neck may produce an opisthotonic position. In the septicemic form there is a petechial eruption on the skin and in some areas large pupuric spots. When the disease is ushered in overwhelmingly, the Waterhouse-Friderichsen syndrome may supervene with a picture of shock, including weak pulse and marked lowering of the blood pressure.

We have already commented on the difficulties of diagnosis in infancy where a picture of sepsis may be present without evident neurological signs. Marked irritability, evidence of hyperaesthesia, signs of sepsis with jaundice, or severe diarrhea, should create suspicion of meningitis.

The diagnosis may be confirmed by spinal puncture and examination of the fluid.

LABORATORY: The spinal fluid is turbid, under increased pressure, and with thousands of cells per cu. mm., polymorphonuclears predominating. The smear reveals gram-negative diplococci, both intra- and extracellular, suggestive of meningococcus. Final confirmation is based on a positive culture. The protein is increased, sugar and chloride diminished.

TREATMENT: Immediate treatment consists of the slow injection intravenously of sodium sulfadiazine, 50 mg./kg. as a 5% solution. This should be done after the lumbar puncture has been performed and spinal fluid has been withdrawn for the various tests. If the smear suggests meningococcus, a total daily dose of 200 mg./kg. of the drug (sodium sulfadiazine) should be calculated for infants and small children, and for older children about 100 mg./kg. per day. This should be administered subcutaneously as a 20% solution with saline or intravenously in 5% solution either every twelve hours or by constant drip. If there is no history of vomiting, the drug may subsequently be given orally q. 6 h. This should give a blood level of the drug of at least 10 mg./100 ml., which is satisfactory. If penicillin is desired, procaine penicillin 1,000,000 units, twice daily, intramuscularly, should be given for older children; for infants half the amount, for two successive days. A lumbar puncture performed forty-eight hours after the initial one should show a spinal fluid which has responded to therapy. The duration of treatment is five days, after which time a follow-up lumbar puncture should show a clear spinal fluid, few cells, negative smear, sterile culture, and normal sugar. The child should be acting well.

We have mentioned the Waterhouse-Friderichsen syndrome, which occurs as part of a severe meningococcemia. It is presumably due to the severe infection (toxemia) and results in adrenal insufficiency. Usually there is hemorrhage or necrosis of the adrenal gland, although at the Kings County Hospital we have had a number of instances in which this was not apparent at necropsy. When treating the shock syndrome not only hydrocortisone and norephinephrine should be given but also infusions of 5% glucose in saline intravenously, and plasma or blood. Recently the use of adrenal steroids has been questioned. See the article by Koch and Carson.

In addition to specific therapy, the child with meningitis should receive sedation like phenobarbital, for undue pain, restlessness, or convulsion, and get good nursing care. Supportive therapy as indicated above should be given as needed. Care should be exercised in administering fluids. An excess may produce symptomatic hyponatremia with seizures. Evaluation of the sodium content in the serum will establish the presence of a low level. This can be corrected by injecting saline.

COMPLICATIONS: The most serious and frequent complication is hydrocephalus. In infants this is suspected if there is an increase in the size of the head. Other diagnostic aids are undue vomiting, convulsions, or an increase in the opisthotonic position suggesting a chronic basilar meningitis. The flow of spinal fluid through the lumbar puncture needle may be slowed and a rise in pressure is noted. At the same time fluid is freely obtained from the ventricle. Fortunately, this complication is becoming rare today, occurring usually in infancy and when early diagnosis is not made. Drug and antibiotic therapy should be intensive. Varidase may be administered into the lateral ventricle. If necessary, craniotomy should be performed to reestablish the flow of fluid through some circumventing procedure. The problem is treated more fully under Hydrocephalus.

Subdural collections of fluid are treated by aspiration.

A serious complication is eighth nerve deafness which is bilateral and permanent due to involvement of the cochlear division of the eighth nerve. This type of deafness should be distinguished from that due to otitis media which is temporary and ends in recovery of hearing. Ocular palsies such as external strabismus usually disappear. In recent times, coincident with the reduction of the mortality rate, there has been noted, especially in infancy, an increase in mental impairment, hemiplegia, convulsions, and occasionally peripheral neuritis.

Other complications include arthritis, which usually clears spontaneously and infections of the eyes such as conjunctivitis, panophthalmitis, and choroiditis with blindness resulting occasionally. Pericarditis and endocarditis may also occur.

PREVENTION FOR THOSE EXPOSED: Give one gram sodium sulfadiazine orally, daily for three days.

PROGNOSIS: The outlook is excellent. The general recovery rate is 90-95 per cent, usually with few sequelae, except as previously mentioned in infancy.

H. Influenzal Meningitis. This is the most frequent type amongst the purulent meningitides in children, except during epidemic periods, as in war times, when the meningococcus form takes precedence. It is not usually seen before two months of age since antiobodies derived from the mother appear to protect the newborn for this period, but is common in the first to third years. It is due to H. influenzae type B, a gram-negative bacillus. The clinical picture is similar to the description given in the preceding discussion of meningococcus meningitis in its acute onset, symptoms and signs of meningeal involvement, and complications. The spinal fluid findings are also similar except for the presence of H. influenzae. Several points however should be stressed. Influenzal meningitis may be preceded by an ear infection (acute otitis media). To avoid the complication of meningitis, it should be emphasized that the use of penicillin alone for the treatment of ear infections is not sufficient, as this antibiotic will not destroy H. influenzae. Therefore, some other agent such as sulfadiazine or chloramphenicol which is effective against gram-negative organisms should always be used in addition. A second factor is that in influenzal meningitis obstruction of the cerebrospinal pathways occurs rapidly; therefore, it is imperative to recognize and actively treat this disease early so as to avoid hydrocephalus. Finally, there is a great tendency for subdural collections of purulent fluid to develop when H. influenzae is the infecting organism. Therefore, if the child is not responding well and has persistent fever, convulsions, and focal neurological signs, this complication should be seriously considered and subdural punctures performed.

TREATMENT: Specific therapy consists of 100 mg./kg. of chloramphenicol initially, the total dose to be administered intravenously with saline over a period of thirty minutes or intramuscularly. Following this injection a calculated dose of 100 mg./kg. per day should be given intravenously or intramuscularly in eight to twelve hour periods or by continuous drip intravenously; or 200 mg./kg. per day orally q. 8 hours or in four periods. Sodium sulfadiazine 50 mg./kg. should also be given initially intravenously as a 5% solution in saline. This should be followed by the administration of 200 mg./kg. per day, divided into two doses, q. 12 h., and injected subcutaneously or intramuscularly. If there is no vomiting, it may then be given orally on the second day. This should give a blood level of 10-15 mg. per 100 ml. Lumbar puncture should be repeated in forty-eight hours, following the diagnostic tap on admission. If the spinal fluid indices (rise in sugar, lowered cell count, negative smear, and subsequent negative culture) are favorable, therapy without change is continued. Lumbar puncture should be repeated in about seven days. If all is favorable the chloramphenicol is discontinued, but the sulfadiazine, 100 mg./kg. per day, orally, should be administered for one more week. In very severe cases or in young infants, 20 cc. of type specific rabbit serum may be given intramuscularly. This should be preceded by an eye or skin test for sensitivity.

PROGNOSIS: The prospects are favorable as there is about 90 per cent recovery. The complications and sequelae are similar to those which have been discussed under meningococcus meningitis.

Pneumococcus Meningitis. This type, similar to influenzal meningitis, does not usually occur the first few weeks following birth because of antibody protection received from the mother. However, this immunity is soon lost and pneumococcus meningitis is very often seen in early infancy. One of the difficulties in this disease is that it is most often associated with other areas of infection, such as pneumonia, otitis media, or acute sinusitis. These foci may precede or appear together with the onset of meningitis. This means that therapy must correct a multiplicity of foci, rather than just meningitis. Trauma to the head with skull fracture is an occasional factor in older children. Any type of pneumococcus may be found as the causative agent.

The pathology in this disease occurs more extensively over the convexity of the brain and anteriorly rather than in the base, as in meningococcus or influenzal meningitis.

The clinical picture is similar to the description under meningococcus meningitis. The spinal fluid is likewise the same, except for the presence of the gram-positive pneumococcus in smear and culture.

TREATMENT: The treatment depends on massive doses of penicillin and sulfadiazine. Aqueous penicillin, 2,000,000 units, is injected intravenously stat. Then a total of 6,000,000 to 12,000,000 units per day should be given in four divided doses q. 6h., intravenously for three days. This is followed by 3,000,000 units of procaine penicillin per day intramuscularly, divided into two doses q. 12h. With this, sodium sulfadiazine 50 mg./kg. is given stat, either intravenously or subcutaneously. This should be followed by a total of 200 mg./kg. per day, including the first day, administered q. 12h., or in two injections intravenously or subcutaneously. A continuous drip including the drugs may be used. If there is no vomiting after the second day, the sulfadiazine may be offered orally. Chloramphenicol may be added for infants, 50 mg./kg. per day intramuscularly, twice daily. Chloramphenicol and penicillin should be discontinued at the end of a week if the spinal fluid at that time is clear, with few cells, negative smear and culture, and normal sugar. Sulfadiazine, 100 mg./kg. per day, should be continued for one more week.

The problem of treating the associated areas of infection is also present. In most instances the intensive treatment of the meningitis will also correct the accompanying pneumonia or sinusitis. However, if there is a collection of pus in the sinus, e.g., ethmoid, or evidence of mastoiditis in an older child, this may be corrected surgically, but only after the fulminating meningitis is under control. This same procedure is to be followed if the organism is H. influenzae or streptococcus.

The complications are similar to those following meningococcus and influenzal meningitis.

PROGNOSIS: The outlook is more serious than in meningitis caused by the meningococcus or H. influenzae. However, great progress has been made, for there is now about 80 per cent recovery.

ORGANISM UNKNOWN: When the organisms causing meningitis are unknown, we have already referred to the combined use of penicillin, sulfadiazine, and chloramphenicol. The dosage and procedure should follow the amounts prescribed for meningococcus infection in the case of penicillin and sulfadiazine, and for influenzal meningitis in the use of chloramphenicol.

Streptococcus Meningitis. The beta hemolytic streptococcus has decreased in importance as a factor in meningitis since the advent of chemotherapy. It is always to be considered in children when either otitis media or mastoiditis or acute ethmoid sinusitis is present, or there is a recent history of such infection. Meningitis may follow by direct extension from these foci, in which case there may also be lateral sinus thrombosis or epidural abscess, or develop by way of a bacteremia. Meningitis may also follow head trauma. In the newborn period and in early infancy streptococcus meningitis may follow secondary infection of a meningocele with direct invasion of the cerebrospinal fluid pathway, or may be the result of blood stream infection secondary to inflammation of the umbilicus. Streptococcus meningitis may also occur with no visible focus, but this is uncommon.

As in the other meningitides there is a purulent exudate, particularly over the superior surface of the brain.

The spinal fluid is similar to the other purulent types, except that direct smear shows gram-positive cocci and culture confirms the diagnosis of streptococcus.

TREATMENT: Treatment consists of aqueous crystalline penicillin, 4 to 12 million units, injected intravenously in 5% glucose daily for the first three days, then 2 to 3 million units daily intramuscularly, divided into two doses. Sodium sulfadiazine should be given, 50 mg./kg. initially intramuscularly or intravenously, followed by 200 mg./kg. per day, either subcutaneously in two doses or orally three times a day. Treatment should be continued for a total of two weeks from the onset. The associated focus, such as the infected mastoid or lateral sinus, may require surgery after the acute meningeal picture is under control. Penicillin should be discontinued after a week if the spinal fluid at that time is clear, contains few cells, is negative on smear and culture, and there is a normal sugar. Sulfadiazine, 100 mg./kg. per day should be continued for one more week.

PROGNOSIS: There is about 90 per cent recovery. Sequelae are similar to meningococcus.

Staphylococcus Meningitis. This form of meningitis is occasionally seen in infancy secondary to skin infections or following an injury with infection of the wound. The organism also enters the meninges through infection of a meningocele, especially the occipital type. As with staphylococcus elsewhere in the body there is a tendency to abscess formation (epidural and cerebral). The clinical picture resembles the other meningitides. The spinal fluid is similar except for the presence of the gram-positive staphylococcus in smear and culture.

TREATMENT: Treatment consists of aqueous penicillin 500,000 to 1,000,000 units/kg./day, chloramphenicol as previously outlined under H. influenzae therapy, and erythromycin 100 mg./kg. per day. All three may be given intravenously at the onset. Subsequently erythromycin and chloramphenicol may be given orally q. 6 h. and penicillin intramuscularly.

PROGNOSIS: There are more recoveries taking place in infancy, but at the same time, there is an increasing number with sequelae, both mental and neurological, due to brain damage.

Alexander, H. E.: Guide to Optimal Therapy in Bacterial Meningitis. J.A.M.A. 152:662, 1953.

———: Treatment of Pyogenic Meningitis. A. Res. Publ. Ass. Nerv. Ment. Dis. Proc. 34:3, 1954.

———: The Treatment of Purulent Meningitis. Advances in Pediatrics, New York, Interscience Publishers, Inc. Vol. II, P. 121, 1947.

Davies, J. A. V., Meyer, E. and Hyde, H.: Follow-up Studies of Patients Who Have Recovered from Meningitis. Am. J. Dis. Child. 79:958, 1950.

Gardner, L. I.: Adrenocortical Metabolism of the Fetus, Infant and Child. Pediat. 17:897, 1956.

Hodes, H. L., Moloshok, R. E. and Markowitz, M.: Fulminating Meningococcemia Treated with Cortisone; Use of Blood Eosinophil Count as a Guide to Prognosis and Treatment. Pediat. 13:138, 1952.

Horner, F. A., Webb, Jr., N. C., Welch, K.: Diagnosis of Collection of Subdural Fluid by Transillumination. American Pediatric Society Program and Abstracts, May 8 and 9, 1958.

Koch, R. and Carson, M. J.: Meningococcal Infections in Children. New England J. Med. 258:639, 1958.

Matson, D. D. and Ingraham, F. D.: Intracranial Complications of Congenital Dermal Sinuses. Pediat. 8:463, 1951.

Nyhan, W. L. and Cooke, R. E.: Symptomatic Hyponatremia in Acute Infections of the Central Nervous System. Pediat. 18:604, 1956.

Smith, M. H. D.: Acute Bacterial Meningitis. Pediat. 17:258, 1956.

Watson, D. G.: Purulent Neonatal Meningitis: A Study of Forty-five Cases. J. Pediat. 50:352, 1957.

OTHER LESS FREQUENT TYPES OF ACUTE BACTERIAL MENINGITIS

Salmonella Meningitis. Infection with the Salmonella group takes the form of gastroenteritis in some children, while in others there is evidence of severe septicemia. In the latter group, particularly, there may be localization in the meninges.

Henderson reported three cases of salmonella meningitis and reviewed 144 more in the literature. He noted that salmonella meningitis in the newborn occurred in epidemic form in nurseries. He also stressed a decrease in resistance as a factor, citing five cases which followed meningococcic meningitis.

In the newborn diarrhea is an outstanding and presenting symptom. The course of the illness is very rapid. In infancy and childhood there are more classical signs of meningeal irritation present.

LABORATORY: The spinal fluid is turbid and under increased pressure. There are increased numbers of cells, polymorphonucleated in type. The smear of the sediment shows gram-negative rods. Culture of the spinal fluid is positive for Salmonella.

TREATMENT: Chloramphenicol and other drugs such as sulfadiazine may be used depending on the response to sensitivity tests. These shoud be administered as described under the previous group of meningitides (meningococcus, etc.). If the tetracyclines are used, the dosage by mouth is 20-25 mg./kg./day. If injected intravenously or intramuscularly, 15 mg./kg./day should be administered.

PROGNOSIS: In the newborn and in those under one month the mortality is almost 100 per cent. Over one month of age the mortality is about 80 per cent.

COLON GROUP

E. Coli Meningitis and Klebsiella Pneumoniae (Friedlander Group) and other Gram-negative Bacilli. This type of meningitis is seen mainly in the newborn period and infancy. The onset is often insidious and there is no characteristic clinical picture. In any newborn who is not doing well, especially prematures, or where there has been obstetrical difficulty, meningitis should be suspected and a lumbar puncture done. The diagnosis is based on recovering the organism in the spinal fluid culture, together with fermentation tests. Treatment consists of chloramphenicol, with either sulfadiazine or streptomycin. Similar forms of therapy may be tried with pseudomonas aeruginosa and the proteus group. If polymyxin B is used, especially in pseudomonas aeruginosa, it is injected intramuscularly, 2-5 mg./kg./day for seven days and intrathecally 2.5 mg. once a day for one to four days.

PROGNOSIS: The outlook is poor. In one series there was only 15 per cent recovery. As with other meningitides of infancy, while recoveries are increasing, mental and neurological sequelae are also rising.

Listeria. Listeria meningitis is caused by Listeria monocytogenes, a gram-positive rod, which may be cultured from the spinal fluid. It is seen especially in infancy, where the major symptoms are poor feeding, diarrhea, cyanosis, drowsiness, and convulsions.

The spinal fluid may appear clear or cloudy. The organism must be differentiated from the beta-hemolytic streptococcus and diphtheroids, both in the blood and in the spinal fluid.

The treatment consists of chloramphenicol or penicillin, depending upon the response to sensitivity tests.

SALMONELLA

Beene, M. L., Hansen, A. E. and Fulton, McD.: Salmonella Meningitis: Recovery from Meningitis due to Salmonella Tp. (type Montevideo), with consideration of the problem of Salmonella Meningitis. Am. J. Dis. Child. 82:567, 1951.

Henderson, L. L.: Salmonella Meningitis: Report of three cases and review of 144 cases from the literature. Am. J. Dis. Child. 75:351, 1948.

Powell, S. M.: Typhoid with Meningitis (Salmonella Typhosa). Report of Case in Infant with Recovery. A.M.A. J. Dis. Child. 91:380, 1956.

COLON GROUP AND OTHER GRAM NEGATIVE ORGANISMS

Biehl, J. P. and Hamburger, M.: Polymyxin B Therapy of Meningitis following procedures on Central Nervous System. Beneficial Therapeutic Effect of Polymyxin B in Meningitis due to Organisms of the Colon Group. A.M.A. Arch. Int. Med. 93:367, 1954.

David, J. K. and Owens, J. W.: Tularemia Meningitis. Am. J. Dis. Child. 67:44, 1944.

Freedman, R. H., Love, J. G. and Hallberg, O. E.: Otitic Proteus Meningitis with Recovery; Report of Case. Proc. Mayo Clin. 27:390, 1952.

Gordon, H. S. and Aronow, J.: Escherichia Coli Meningitis in Five Day Old Infant. Report of a Case with Complete Recovery. J.A.M.A. 159:1288, 1955.

Trice, P. A. and Townsend, T. E.: Meningitis due to Klebsiella Pneumoniae. J.A.M.A. 149:1471, 1952.

Watson, D. G.: Purulent Neonatal Meningitis. A Study of Forty-five Cases. J. Pediat. 50:352, 1957.

LISTERIA

Line, F. G. and Appleton, F. C.: Listeria Meningitis in a Premature Infant. J. Pediat. 41:97, 1952.

Mathieu, Jr., P. L., Young, R. M., Mennillo, E. P. and Sherwood, E. S.: Listeria Meningitis. Pediat. 48:349, 1956.

TUBERCULOUS MENINGITIS. Tuberculous meningitis occurs as a secondary manifestation of primary tuberculosis. The latter is usually noted in the lungs and bronchial lymph nodes but may be seen elsewhere. The development of meningitis may be associated with generalized miliary spread, or it may be the only manifestation of

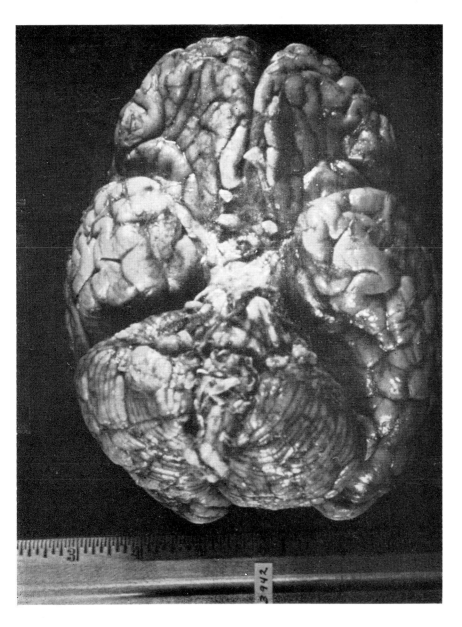

11. Tuberculous meningitis showing typical opaque leptomeningeal exudate at the base of the brain.

159

tuberculous infection. It is essentially a disease of the first two years of life. The organism is the Mycobacterium tuberculosis.

PATHOLOGY: As a result of the investigations of Rich and Mc-Cordock, it has been shown that tuberculous meningitis generally develops through the discharge of bacilli from caseous foci in the brain into the spinal fluid pathways. The tubercles rupture into the meninges or the ventricles from adjacent areas in the cortex. The base of the brain may be studded with tubercles along the paths of the blood vessels. There is a thickened exudate of fibrin and mononuclear cells which blocks the subarachnoid channels. The brain is edematous and the ventricles distended. The blood vessels show evidence of arteritis and phlebitis, leading to thrombosis and rarely infarction.

CLINICAL PICTURE: The onset is insidious as a rule, with irritability and change in personality. The child is not as friendly as formerly and may be somewhat drowsy at odd times. There may be occasional headache, vomiting, and a slight rise of fever. These continue for a week or so.

Soon the picture changes as the meningeal phase sets in. There are now present neck stiffness, convulsions, intense drowsiness leading to stupor, and cranial nerve paralyses. If the condition continues untreated, there is coma. The child is disoriented and exhibits irregular respiration, reflexes are absent, and choked discs are seen. Choroidal tubercles may be noted.

In infants the onset and course are usually more rapid. There are apt to be convulsions, a bulging fontanel, and stupor; there may be marked diarrhea.

In other instances there is a picture of the first stage with irritability and change of personality from which the child may recover completely instead of progressing to the meningeal phase immediately. However, after a few weeks, he develops the meningeal picture suddenly and rapidly.

LABORATORY: The spinal fluid is clear or opalescent and contains several hundred cells per cu. mm. Early in the disease there may be a number of polymorphonucleated cells, but later the characteristic mononuclear type predominates. The spinal fluid sugar is decreased, protein elevated, and chlorides decreased. If the fluid is allowed to stand for twenty-four hours in a test tube, a web or pellicle may form, which when stained by the Ziehl-Neelsen method will reveal tubercle bacilli. The culture of the spinal fluid is carried out on Frobisher media (a modification of Petragnani) and on Dubos' agar or liquid media. Various strains of tubercle bacilli may grow on one and not on the other. Culture should be done, if possible, before the onset of therapy.

DIAGNOSIS: When carefully inquired into, there will almost always be a history of exposure to an adult with tuberculosis, usually a parent or close relative. The tuberculin skin test, using tuberculin PPD first strength, is usually positive. If this strength is negative and tuberculous meningitis is suspected, the intermediate strength should be used. Where the child is extremely ill, or has recently had a severe case of measles or pertussis, there may be failure to obtain a positive skin test even though tuberculous meningitis is present. But allowing for these exceptions, the tuberculin skin test is usually positive, generally indicating active infection, especially in infancy and early childhood. There is commonly evidence of primary tuberculosis elsewhere, as in the lungs (X-ray).

Thus, a history of exposure, positive intradermal skin test, evidence of tuberculosis in the lungs, lymph nodes, or bones, characteristic spinal fluid findings, and above all the demonstration of tubercle bacilli in smear and culture of the spinal fluid establish the diagnosis. The presence of a clear or opalescent spinal fluid usually eliminates purulent meningitis. Smear and culture will establish the diagnosis here. Encephalitic and poliomyelitic spinal fluid on the other hand appear similar to that of tuberculous meningitis. However, the low spinal fluid sugar suggests that encephalitis or poliomyelitis is not present. In our discussion of cryptococcosis we have stressed the necessity of considering fungus infection where tuberculous meningitis is suspected but not proven and have described the techniques of demonstrating C. neoformans by smear and culture. In lead encephalopathy there are usually a history of chewing paint peelings, elevated blood level of lead, and increased excretion in the urine associated with raised coproporphyrin level. The long bones may also show changes. Brain abscess is usually associated with a focus in the ear or paranasal sinuses. If the abscess is localized, the spinal fluid does not show lowered sugar or any real degree of cellular reaction. Brain tumor is usually associated with a different clinical course, nor are there the changes in the spinal fluid as a rule.

The meningomyelitis associated with Behcet's syndrome may be differentiated by the associated ocular and cutaneous manifestations in the latter.

Neurological lesions occur occasionally in sarcoidosis. These in children consist mainly of facial paralysis associated with "uveoparotid fever" and more infrequently meningoencephalitis or hydrocephalus. The confirmation of the diagnosis of tuberculous meningitis will eliminate the question of sarcoidosis.

In all of these conditions, when the tubercle bacillus can be demonstrated, there is no problem. However, when it cannot be found, then the use of the other differential features should be resorted to. When in doubt, the condition should be treated as a case of tuberculous meningitis.

TREATMENT: Specific therapy consists in the use of isoniazid (INH), para-aminosalicylic acid (PAS), and streptomycin.

The isoniazid is calculated on the basis of 15-25 mg./kg. body weight per day. This should be given orally in two to four doses a day or injected intramuscularly. Pyridoxine to combat the neurotoxicity of isoniazid may be added, 10-15 mg. per day.

Streptomycin 50 mg./kg. per day should be injected intramuscularly. In the average case the total daily dose of streptomycin is one gram. It is divided into two injections daily.

Para-aminosalicylic acid (PAS) 0.3 gm/kg per day should be given orally in one or two divided doses.

In addition to specific drug therapy general measures should be taken to help the child, such as seeing that adequate food is taken. Electrolytes may be needed, such as potassium and sodium; this can be verified by chemical determinations of the serum.

While these measures have considerably improved the outlook in tuberculous meningitis, they may at times fail to correct one feature of the disease. This is the tendency to develop sequelae, such as hydrocephalus and spinal cord block. Because steroids, such as cortisone, are known to suppress the usual effects of inflammation in tissues including the development of fibrous adhesions, they have been added to the treatment of tuberculous meningitis. Cortisone may be injected intramuscularly daily, from 25 to 100 mg. depending on the weight of the child. Therapy with the steroids is continued for about one month, reducing the dosage gradually.

The isoniazid, PAS, and streptomycin are continued regularly for about a year, with the amounts gradually reduced during this time. Too early cessation of therapy may bring about a relapse. Penicillin or tetracycline may be used while the cortisone is being given to counteract the loss of inflammatory reaction or leucocytic response. In a recent report Ratner and his associates suggested that isoniazid alone is effective in the treatment of tuberculous meningitis, without the added streptomycin. However, until more evidence is available, streptomycin should also be used, at least during the hospital period.

COMPLICATIONS: The complications in tuberculous meningitis consist of mental impairment, hydrocephalus, blindness, deafness, cranial nerve palsies, and paralysis of the extremities. There have also been some cases in which primary spinal cord infection was present with spinal canal block.

In the group showing beginning hydrocephalus, or in the less common cases with spinal block, craniotomy may be done. The purpose is to relieve the increased pressure. With the present use of cortizone intramuscularly and hydrocortisone intraventricularly, it is evident that a good number of these complications will be prevented, or if the diagnosis is not made in time and a block has already occurred, the use of cortisone may overcome the obstructive effects.

PROGNOSIS: The outlook in this once universally fatal disease is steadily improving. The mortality is now about fifteen per cent, and the complications and sequelae previously discussed are occurring less often. However, the mortality and sequelae are greater in infants under two years. There is a return to normal, clinically, as well as in the chemistry and EEG, about two months after the onset of therapy.

PROPHYLAXIS: Prevention is the big goal and need in tuberculosis. This means isolation of the child from any individual with tuberculosis. Secondly, BCG vaccine may be used for the potentially exposed patient. The question of giving isoniazid to children who live in contact with tuberculosis but are tuberculin negative is still open. Lastly, isoniazid 10 mg./kg. per day should be given for about a year to any infant who is tuberculin-positive and to every child who has active primary tuberculosis to prevent the spread toward meningitis. In conjunction with this, these children should receive 200 mg./kg. per day of para-aminosalicylic acid, or a maximum of 12 grams per day, to avoid drug resistance, and finally multiple vitamins including 1 to 2 mg. of pyridoxine daily.

Applebaum, E. and Anderson, T. A.: Treatment of Tuberculous Meningitis with Isonicotinic Acid Hydrazides. J.A.M.A. 156:673, 1954.
Boyd, G.: Tuberculous Meningitis in Children. A.M.A. J. Dis. Child. 91:477, 1956.

Choremis, C., Papadatos, C., Gargoulas, A. and Drosos, C.: Intrathecal Hydrocortisone in the Treatment of Tuberculous Meningitis. J. Pediat. 50:138, 1957.

Choremis, C., Papadatos, C., Arzimanoglon, A., and Drosos, C.: Spontaneous Fractures in Tuberculous Meningitis. A.M.A. J. Dis. Child. 94:17, 1957.

Colover, J.: Sarcoidosis with Involvement of the Nervous System. Brain. 71:451, 1948.

Hsu, K. H. K.: Diagnosis and Antimicrobial Therapy of Primary Tuberculosis in Children. J.A.M.A. 164:1204, 1957.

Pennell, W. H.: Boeck's Sarcoid with Involvement of the Central Nervous System. Arch. Neurol. and Psychiat. 66:728, 1951.

Ratner, B., Klimkiewicz, G. R., Ellis, W. C., Rialone, H. J. and Dolgin, J.: The Relative Merits of Isoniazid and Other Therapeutic Agents in the Treatment of Tuberculous Meningitis in Children. Pediat. 20:676, 1957.

Rich, A. T. and McCordock, H. A.: The Pathogenesis of Tubercular Meningitis. Bull. Johns Hopkins, 52:5, 1933.

Sweetnam, W. P. and Sykes, C. G. W.: The Treatment of Tuberculous Meningitis without Injections. A.M.A. J. Dis. Child. 92:2, 1956.

Szabo, G., Sterk, V. V. and Berman, S.: Tuberculous Meningitis Treated with Hydrocortisone and Cortisone. Pediat. 19:580, 1957.

Wadia, N. and Williams, E.: Behcet's Syndrome with Neurological Complications. Brain. 80:59, 1957.

FUNGI

Cryptococcus or Torula Meningitis.

ETIOLOGY: Torulosis is caused by the Cryptococcus neoformans (Torula histolytica), a yeast-like fungus which has a gelatinous capsule, thus differentiating it from other yeasts. It is found in nature, plants, canned milk, animals and pigeons.

PATHOLOGY: Meningitis develops usually secondary to some other focus in the body. It is a chronic type with a gelatinous exudate similar to that seen in tuberculous meningitis. There is also involvement of the brain substance in the form of perivascular invasion, with giant and epithelioid cells simulating tubercule formation. There is little cellular reaction.

The disease may be generalized with involvement of the skin, lymph nodes, lungs, and pancreas, but is primarily noted in the central nervous system.

CLINICAL PICTURE: The mode of infection and method of spread to the meninges are not known, but it is suspected that the lungs may be the primary focus. The usual symptoms of meningitis, headache, vomiting, fever, neck stiffness, and drowsiness are noted. The disease progresses slowly after the initial onset with signs of increasing intracranial pressure developing, including papilledema and hydrocephalus in infants. Cranial nerve palsies are also noted. While infection of the meninges is the only manifestation in most instances, there may be associated pathology in the lungs and skin in some cases. With generalized cryptococcosis, there is involvement of the lymph nodes, spleen, and liver, so that the disease simulates Hodgkin's disease or tuberculosis.

LABORATORY: The spinal fluid is under increased pressure, opalescent to cloudy in appearance. The cell count is usually over 100, but may be normal or be elevated to 1,000 per cu. mm. The cells are usually lymphocytic and mononuclear. The protein is elevated, whereas the sugar and chlorides are usually reduced.

Centrifuged spinal fluid forms a gelatinous sediment. When the sediment is mixed with India ink under a cover glass, the fungus is seen as a thick walled, budding cell, 5 to 15 micra in diameter, spherical in shape, and surrounded by a wide gelatinous capsule.

Culture on Sabouraud's glucose agar at room temperature and blood agar at 37° C. is positive in two to four days for Cryptococcus neoformans.

DIAGNOSIS: The disease may be mistaken for tuberculous meningitis, brain abscess, brain tumor, encephalitis, central nervous system syphilis, or lymphocytic choriomeningitis.

The diagnosis of C. neoformans can only be made with certainty by finding the yeast fungus in culture or injecting the spinal fluid intracerebrally into mice and recovering the fungus. Therefore when a child has a long continued course of fever with evidence of meningitis or encephalitis and a definite diagnosis of tuberculosis cannot be made, C. neoformans should be looked for. Furthermore if there is evidence of block of the flow of the cerebrospinal fluid, and tumor or abscess of the brain are being considered because of signs of increased intracranial pressure, the presence of this fungus should be kept in mind.

PROGNOSIS: The outlook is poor. There is about 90% mortality.

TREATMENT: At present, Amphotericin B, given intravenously in 5% glucose over a period of six to eight hours, 0.25 mg./kg./

day, appears to be the best therapeutic agent. The drug should be administered every other day.

Other fungi have invaded the nervous system occasionally to produce meningitis in children. They include Candida albicans, the actinomyces group, Blastomyces, Coccidioides immitis and Histoplasma capsulatum.

Recently several reports have been published concerning a relatively new fungus disease, cerebral mucormycosis. It is carried by either Rhizopus or Mucor. While adults are mainly infected, two cases have occurred in male infants of 2½ and 5 months of age, and one in a five year old girl. There was a preceding diarrhea in one and nephritis in the other two. The disease appears to follow diabetes, cortisone intake, debilitating illnesses, and the use of antibiotics which suppress bacterial growth and favor the invasion of the fungus. The portal of entry is often the paranasal sinuses or orbit. The fungus permeates the walls of the arteries and veins, causing cerebral and meningeal vascular thrombosis. This is followed by mycotic encephalitis and meningitis. Diagnosis may be made by spinal fluid culture. The disease is usually fatal in about ten days. There is as yet no effective treatment.

Baker, R. D.: Mucormycosis—A New Disease? J.A.M.A. 163:805, 1957.

Carton, C. A. and Liebig, C. S.: Treatment of Central Nervous System Cryptococcosis. A.M.A. Arch. Int. Med. 91:773, 1953.

Dubos, R. J.: Bacterial and Mycotic Infections of Man. Philadelphia, J. B. Lippincott, 1948.

Harris, J. S.: Mucormycosis. Pediat. 16:857, 1955.

Lepow, H., Rubinstein, L., Chu Foo, Shandra, J.: A Case of Cryptococcus Neoformans Meningoencephalitis complicating Boeck's Sarcoid. Pediat. 19:377, 1957.

Merriam, Jr., J. C. and Tedeschi, C. G.: Cerebral Mucormycosis; a Fatal Fungus Infection complicating other Diseases. Neurology, 7:510, 1957.

Nanda, S. P., Kass, I., Cohn, M. and Dressler, S. H.: Coexistence of Tuberculosis and Cryptococcal Meningitis. Pediat. 20:45, 1957.

Rubin, H. and Furcolow.: Promising Results in Cryptococcal Meningitis. Neurology 8:590, 1958.

Schulz, D. M.: Histoplasmosis of the Central Nervous System. J.A.M.A. 151:549, 1953.

Sprofkin, B. E., Shapiro, J. C. and Lux, J. J.: Histoplasmosis of Central Nervous System; Case Report of Histoplasma Meningitis. J. Neuropath. and Exper. Neurol. 14:288, 1955.

Whitehill, M. R. and Rawson, A. J.: Treatment of Generalized Cryptococcosis with 2-Hydroxystilbamidine. Virg. Med. Monthly 81:591, 1954.

Wilson, H. M. and Duryea, A. W.: Cryptococcus Meningitis (Torulosis) Treated with a New Antibiotic, Actidione. Arch. Neurol. & Psychiat. 66:470, 1951.

Meningism

Meningism may be associated with the onset of an acute infection such as tonsillitis or pneumonia. There is neck stiffness, which is the main and often only manifestation. Kernig's sign, Brudzinski's sign, and opisthotonos may also be present. The spinal fluid is normal. Apparently there is cerebral irritation without any meningeal inflammatory reaction. The picture of meningism disappears after the first day, as the major disease becomes clarified.

Meningism must be differentiated from the onset of an acute bacterial meningitis.

Brain Abscess

This condition was a frequent and serious problem prior to the advent of chemotherapy and antibiotics. Today, it is infrequently seen in children.

Abscess of the brain in children usually results from extension of an original focus, such as otitis media or mastoid infection, especially the chronic type. The route is either direct extension into the brain or by way of the venous channels. This usually results in a single temporal or cerebellar lobe abscess. The organism is apt to be the streptococcus, pneumococcus, or staphylococcus, but any other may occasionally be seen. There may be direct extension into the frontal lobe from an ethmoid or frontal sinusitis, or the brain abscess may be the result of an orbital infection which has extended to the frontal lobe either through venous channels or via an osteomyelitis. Epidural or subdural abscess may precede the brain abscess.

Brain abscess also results from hematogenous spread from infected foci elsewhere, such as lung abscess, endocarditis, empyema, or erysipelas. In these cases there are usually multiple brain abscesses.

Trauma to the skull with compound fracture may introduce the organism directly into the brain.

A form of brain abscess which is receiving increasing attention, particularly with the decrease in other causes, is that associated with congenital heart disease. More cases of this type are being reported, especially as increasing surgery is being done for the correction of congenital cardiac defects. The brain abscess is referred to as a paradoxic type. It occurs in those congenital heart defects where the venous blood is shunted directly into the systemic circulation without passing through the lungs. The children are cyanotic, and the condition is referred to as right-to-left shunt. The most common types are the tetralogy of Fallot, i.v. septal defect, and patent ductus. The pathogenesis is not clear. There is assumed to be a bacteremia. However, the organisms escape the normal filtering action of the lung capillaries because of the right-to-left shunt, thus reaching the brain directly. Blood culture is usually sterile. Paradoxical embolus precedes the infection, aided in its formation by polycythemia with secondary slowing of the blood stream. The brain abscess is usually single. The children are usually well prior to the onset of symptoms. Occasionally there is a history of preceding tonsillectomy. The major symptoms are headache, lethargy, seizures, and weakness of the extremities. Cases have been reported prior to surgery. In other instances brain abscess followed several years after cardiac surgery, during which time the children appeared well.

PATHOLOGY: There are an accumulation of polymorphonucleated cells, necrotic brain tissue, and organisms. The purulent encephalitis is then limited by a wall of connective tissue and fibroblasts if the infection comes under control. Surrounding this area the brain is edematous. As the abscess becomes more chronic, the capsule is thicker and the cells change to lymphocytes. The abscess may break through into the ventricle or subarachnoid space and cause meningitis if it is not brought under control.

CLINICAL PICTURE: The initial picture is that of the preceding cause of the brain abscess. There are fever, headache, and pain in the area of the ear or sinus, which are found to be due to an acute upper respiratory infection with otitis media or acute sinusitis. In some cases there has been a tonsillectomy followed by persistent low grade fever. In others the original infection had been so slight as to have been forgotten. In still other instances there is a history of direct trauma, or of erysipelas, furunculosis, empyema, lung abscess, or congenital heart disease which may or may not have had surgery.

Most children will have received some form of chemotherapy or antibiotics in the initial stages for their ear or other infection. The latter may have appeared to heal, or low grade fever and lack of well-being may continue. In other instances the ear may drain pus. In view of the modification of the clinical picture by therapy, it is rare now to see a clearly defined picture of the invasive stage of the onset of brain abscess. However, within a few weeks after the onset of the original infection, the child complains of headache, drowsiness, vomiting, and fever. Convulsions are noted, especially in infancy.

Examination may reveal focal signs. In temporal lobe abscess there are changes in the visual fields, with homonymous hemianopia, facial paralysis, and hemiparesis. If on the left side of the brain, there is aphasia, especially anomia, or inability to name an object, although the child knows what it is. These points are, however, difficult to bring out in children. Cerebellar signs are more apparent. There are ataxia, hypotonia, and incoordination on the same side as the lesion, and nystagmus, more marked when the head is turned to the side of the lesion. In cerebellar abscess there is more obvious evidence of increased intracranial pressure, with choked discs and occipital headache. Frontal lobe abscess may lead to changes of personality, confusion, seizures, and aphasia.

SPINAL FLUID: If the clinical picture is obvious and there is evidence of marked increase in intracranial pressure, lumbar puncture may be avoided. If necessary, as little fluid as needed for study may be withdrawn, especially in cerebellar abscess.

The character of the fluid depends on the stage of the abscess. In most instances the fluid is under increased pressure, clear, sterile, and contains about 25 to 500 cells/cu. mm., mostly lymphocytes; the protein is slightly elevated at 50-75 mg./100 ml. Sugar and chlorides are normal.

If the abscess is near the surface of the brain or not as yet encapsulated, there will be more cells with a polymorphonuclear preponderance.

Finally, if there is rupture into the ventricles or invasion of the meninges, the fluid takes on the aspects of meningitis. It is turbid with thousands of cells/cu. mm., polymorphonuclears predominating, sugar is reduced, and organisms are demonstrated by Gram-stain and culture.

X-ray of the mastoids, paranasal sinuses, and chest may show evidence of infection. The skull may show suture separation in infants. The ventriculogram may indicate the area of the abscess. Ventriculography, however, should only be done when the diagnosis is not clear and should be followed by surgery if an abnormality is demonstrated. EEG may show a focal source for abnormal discharges.

DIAGNOSIS: Brain abscess should be suspected in any child when there is a known history of ear infection or sinusitis. It should also be considered if there is a preceding infection in the lungs or a history of trauma. Finally it should be kept in mind in cases of congenital heart disease, before and after surgery. The symptoms and signs of increased intracranial pressure, focal neurological signs, fever, and spinal fluid changes all help to make the diagnosis. The EEG aids in localizing a supratentorial brain abscess. Where there is no definite history obtainable or the clinical picture is confused, one should resort to ventriculography.

To be differentiated are brain tumor, encephalitis, meningitis, dermal sinus with secondary meningitis, and otitic hydrocephalus. Subdural and epidural abscess as well as septic sinus thrombosis may accompany abscess or may need differentiating. If surgery is indicated, the association or differential will be made at the time of operation. Acute labyrinthitis following ear infection or without antecedent history may require consideration. There are vertigo, nausea, vomiting, disturbed equilibrium, and nystagmus. Cerebellar abscess shows papilledema and ataxia on the same side.

TREATMENT: The abscess should be removed by surgical drainage. The child should receive appropriate chemotherapy and antibiotics. If there is a preceding focus elsewhere which requires surgical correction, this should be done later. In infants where there is a tendency to cerebrospinal fluid block, varidase may be injected into the lateral ventricle.

PROGNOSIS: This depends on whether the brain abscess is single or multiple and on its location. The advent of antibiotics makes use of older mortality figures valueless. In a recent report on cerebral abscess following cardiac surgery, the results of neurosurgery were excellent.

Campbell, M.: Cerebral Abscess in Cyanotic Congenital Heart Disease. Lancet 1:111, 1957.
Cohen, I., Bergman, P. S. and Malis, L.: Paradoxic Brain Abscess in Congenital Heart Disease. J. Neurosurg. 8:225, 1951.
Eagleton, W. P.: Brain Abscess. New York. Macmillan Co., 1922.
Gluck, R., Hall, J. W. and Stevenson, L. D.: Brain Abscess Associated with Congenital Heart Disease. Pediat. 9:192, 1952.
Loeser, Jr., E. and Scheinberg, L.: Brain Abscesses: A Review of Ninety-nine Cases. Neurology 7:601, 1957.
Matson, D. D. and Ingraham, F. D.: Neurosurgery of Infancy and Childhood. Springfield, Ill. Chas. C. Thomas, 1954.
Munslow, R. A., Stovall, V. S., Price, R. D. and Kohler, C. M.: Brain Abscess in Infants. J. Pediat. 51:74, 1957.

Wishingrad, L., Rosenthal, I. M. and Cascino, J. P.: Brain Abscess Seven Years after a Potts Anastomosis in Case of Tetralogy of Fallot. J.A.M.A. 164:1465, 1957.
Ziegler, D. K. and Hoeffer, P. F. A.: Electroencephalographic and Clinical Findings in Twenty-eight Verified Cases of Brain Abscess. EEG Clin. Neurophysiol. 1:41, 1952.

ABSCESS OF SPINAL CORD

This is extremely rare in childhood. It is generally apt to be part of a systemic infection or meningitis. Other factors include local trauma, osteomyelitis, furuncles, or extension of infection from adjacent foci, such as a perinephritic abscess. A congenital dermal sinus may be present.

The most common organism is the Staphylococcus aureus, but a variety of others such as streptococcus, salmonella, and E. coli have been reported. If the spinal cord is involved, there is a picture of transverse myelitis with pain in the back, weakness and flaccid paralysis of the legs, absent deep tendon reflexes, sensory loss below the level of the lesion, and urinary retention. In those instances where there is an abscess of the epidural space, the infection is usually posterior and in the upper thoracic region. The pus and granulation tissue spread longitudinally along the dorsal part of the dura. The clinical picture develops within a few days to weeks after onset of the infection. There are fever and pain in the back of the spine and root pains along the affected trunks. Impairment of cord function with flaccid paralysis and loss of deep tendon reflexes may develop if there is compression of the cord. When extension into the subarachnoid space occurs, meningitis develops.

LABORATORY: The spinal fluid shows increased numbers of cells and excess protein; there may be xanthochromia. Organisms may be present on direct smear and culture if meningitis is present. The diagnosis of epidural abscess is made on the history and spinal puncture. The latter must be done carefully so as not to carry infection into the subarachnoid space by puncturing the dura. If spinal puncture does not reveal pus, a space higher may be tried. In the case of Mincks and Pulaski this procedure made the diagnosis possible. Confirmation and localization may be aided by myelography.

TREATMENT: This consists of laminectomy for drainage of the epidural space and antibiotic therapy. Reference may be made to the chapter on meningitis for the use of the proper drugs.

PROGNOSIS: Occasional cases of recovery are now reported. Prior to the advent of antibiotics, the outlook was almost universally fatal.

Hulme, A. and Dott, N.: Spinal Epidural Abscess. Brit. M. J. 1:64, 1954.
Mincks, J. R. and Pulaski, E. J.: Acute Lumbar Epidural Abscess in a Thirty Months Old Child; Complete Recovery Following Surgery and Antibiotic Therapy. Antibiotic Medicine and Clinical Therapy 3:202, 1956.

CEREBRAL SINUSES

Thrombosis of the dural sinuses was of common occurrence in infants and children in the early period of pediatrics when a widespread knowledge of proper nutrition was not available and there were no chemotherapeutic or antibiotic agents. Today it is rarely seen.

The two major factors are undernutrition associated with dehydration, and infection, especially otitis media with secondary spread to the dural sinuses.

SUPERIOR LONGITUDINAL SINUS

This venous sinus is involved most frequently in infancy, secondary to infantile diarrheas with subsequent marasmus or athrepsia. Thrombosis is also seen in chronic diseases with marked anemia. Infection from the nasal cavities or dura is a rare cause. I have seen cases with congenital heart disease, and occasional instances in the past from the use of the longitudinal sinus for taking and administering blood. Thrombosis has also followed blood transfusions in dehydrated infants.

The mechanism producing thrombosis is a combination of increased viscosity and stagnation of the blood flow due to dehydration, and possibly cardiac weakness.

At times no clinical signs are evident; the marantic infant may be found dead in its crib. Postmortem examination reveals the sinus occluded with non-septic thrombi. In other instances there are no symptoms until there is a spread into the cerebral veins. There is then evidence of increased intracranial pressure with a bulging anterior fontanel, or edema of the forehead with distension of the superficial veins. Convulsions of the Jacksonian type and hemiplegia may follow.

LABORATORY: The spinal fluid is under increased pressure, usually clear, but it may be xanthochromic or bloody. Protein is increased. The cell count is normal, culture sterile.

DIAGNOSIS: This condition should be suspected when convulsions or paralysis suddenly occur in an infant who is undernourished, or has diarrhea or severe anemia. Subdural hematoma should be ruled out by bilateral punctures. Angiography may be helpful by locating the area of block.

PROGNOSIS: The outcome is usually fatal.

TREATMENT: Prophylactic therapy should be used to improve hydration. Electrolytes and glucose are administered first. Transfusion should not be done until good circulation is established.

LATERAL SINUS

Lateral sinus thrombosis usually follows otitis media, or acute and especially chronic mastoiditis. The mastoid cells overlying the sinus wall are infected and there is direct extension into the lateral sinus, first involving the wall, followed by the development of a septic thrombus.

CLINICAL PICTURE: Involvement of the lateral sinus usually occurs in the course of an acute upper respiratory infection associated with purulent otitis media. Mastoiditis may develop first, followed by direct extension of the infection into the sinus with the development of clinical signs. Occasionally the venous sinus is infected at the beginning of the respiratory and otitic infection without intervening chronic mastoiditis. In either case the symptoms and signs are those of bacteremia and increased intracranial pressure. The child has chills and a marked rise of fever of septic type. Whereas the temperature may have been ranging between 100°-102° F, it now spikes between 99° and 105° F, indicating that infection has spread to the venous sinuses. In addition there may be signs of increased intracranial pressure, headache, vomiting, papilledema, and rarely convulsions. When the last occur, they usually indicate extension to the cerebral veins over the lateral aspect of the cortex, or posteriorly toward the midline (torcular Herophili).

In view of the use of chemotherapy and antibiotics, the picture today may not show the classical temperature spikes or chills. There may not be a marked rise of fever. It is therefore necessary to keep in mind that any child with a continuous draining ear should be checked for symptoms and objective signs of mastoid infection (tenderness over the bone, edema). Use should be made of X-rays of the mastoid and blood cultures, to be sure there is no extension of the process.

LABORATORY: The blood shows leucocytosis and severe anemia when bacteremia develops. Blood culture is positive, usually for hemolytic streptococcus, but occasionally for H. influenzae or pneumococcus. X-ray of the mastoid shows evidence of infection and sclerosis. The spinal fluid is clear and under increased pressure. There is a slight cellular increase. The sugar is normal, unless meningitis complicates the venous sinus infection. Bacteriological culture is sterile.

DIAGNOSIS: The diagnosis is based on the sudden rise of temperature, with marked spikes and associated chills, in a patient who has otitis media or mastoiditis. This may occur before or after operation on the mastoid. Blood culture is usually positive. Following diagnostic lumbar puncture, while the needle is still in the subarachnoid space, if pressure is made with the fingers over the jugular veins in the neck there is recorded a rise of spinal fluid pressure. Sudden release of the neck pressure should normally produce a fall of the spinal fluid pressure. Failure of the release of neck pressure on either side to be followed by reduction of spinal fluid pressure suggests lateral sinus thrombosis on that side (Ayer).

Meningitis is ruled out by the spinal fluid findings. In meningitis the spinal fluid contains thousands of cells per cu. mm., positive culture for organisms, and low sugar.

Brain abscess may be associated with lateral sinus thrombosis or it may have to be differentiated from it. With abscess there are more apt to be localizing signs, choked discs, and hemiplegia; however, at times, ventriculography or needle aspiration at operation may be needed to make the differential.

PROGNOSIS: In the period prior to chemotherapy and antibiotics, there was serious possibility of death because of bacteremia with secondary infection of the lungs, pleura, joints, meninges, and brain. There was also extension into the cavernous sinus or petrous bone. Today, we rarely see any of these complications.

TREATMENT: The primary aim in therapy is to bring the infection under control with chemotherapy and antibiotics. It is stressed here, as in the discussion of meningitis, that penicillin alone is insufficient in the treatment of otitis, as the organism may not be responsive, e.g., influenza B. Therefore a broad spectrum antibiotic should be used so that all types of organisms are covered. This procedure is both prophylactic and therapeutic. It has not only almost eliminated lateral sinus thrombosis in childhood, but when the complication has occurred, the use of combined therapy, such as penicillin, sulfadiazine, and chloramphenicol, has lessened the need for surgery. If the latter must subsequently be performed, a mastoidectomy with exposure of the lateral sinus is done. The wall is incised and the infected clot drained. The internal jugular vein may need ligation. Transfusions are used for supportive therapy.

CAVERNOUS SINUS THROMBOSIS

This results from infections of the orbit, paranasal sinuses, or face. We have seen it in association with lateral sinus thrombosis. From the lateral sinus there may be extension to the cavernous. Involvement of one cavernous sinus may spread to the other by way of the circular sinus.

CLINICAL PICTURE: As in lateral sinus thrombosis there are signs of bacteremia including septic temperature and chills. Outstanding, however, is the pain in the region of the eyes, edema of the tissues of the orbit, and proptosis of the eyeball (exophthalmos). There may be papilledema. Vision is affected. Neurological signs include ptosis of the lid, strabismus, diplopia, and dilation of the pupils.

LABORATORY: Since cavernous sinus thrombosis may be an extension of lateral sinus thrombosis of otitic origin, the laboratory data may be that of the latter, previously described. If directly produced, from a furuncle of the face, orbital abscess, or an infected paranasal sinus, the spinal fluid will be clear, with few cells and normal sugar. With spread to the meninges, the spinal fluid would take on the features of meningitis.

DIAGNOSIS: This is based on the presence of exophthalmos, coming on acutely, in association with a clinical picture of sepsis and a positive blood culture. There may be a history of ear infection with signs of lateral sinus thrombosis, or a preceding infection of the face or orbital tissues. Cavernous sinus thrombosis must be differentiated from abscess of the orbit or sinusitis. These latter conditions are more often unilateral and are usually associated with a negative blood culture and different history (no otitis). Hemorrhage into the orbit following injury may require differential. Finally, tumors of the orbit, exophthalmic goiter, and traumatic internal carotid-cavernous sinus fistula should be considered.

TREATMENT: This condition was invariably fatal in the past. As previously remarked, chemotherapy and the use of broad spectrum antibiotics have not only diminished the incidence of cranial venous sinus thrombosis, but have improved the chances for recovery.

Byers, R. K. and Haas, G. M.: Thrombosis of the Dural Venous Sinuses in Infancy and in Childhood. Am. J. Dis. Child. 45:1161, 1933.
Eagleton, W.: Cavernous Sinus Thrombophlebitis. New York, Macmillan, Co. 1926.
Tobey, G. L. and Ayer, J. B.: Dynamic Studies on the Cerebrospinal Fluid in the Differential Diagnosis of Lateral Sinus Thrombosis. Arch. Otolaryng. 2:50, 1925.

ENCEPHALITIS

Encephalitis in children is produced by a variety of factors. While the term should be restricted to indicate inflammation of the brain, it is actually broadened to include reactions resulting from chemical and physical agents as well. The child who is ill with encephalitis presents so many of the early symptoms and signs associated with meningitis or poliomyelitis that one can only make a presumptive diagnosis on clinical impression and send the patient to the hospital for lumbar puncture and further study. As in meningitis there may be sudden onset with fever, headache, vomiting, irritability, drowsiness, and neck stiffness. The clinical picture in encephalitis depends also on the areas involved, irrespective of the type of virus. With brain stem pathology there are often cranial nerve palsies. Therefore, in addition to meningitis and poliomyelitis, other conditions which affect cranial nerve nuclei and their pathways, such as brain tumor and abscess, must be ruled out.

Lumbar puncture (following the procedure previously outlined for meningitis) usually reveals a clear or slightly opalescent fluid, under normal or increased pressure. This will tentatively eliminate acute purulent meningitis where the fluid in an untreated case is turbid. In tuberculous meningitis or poliomyelitis the appearance of the fluid is similar to that in acute encephalitis. If, however, the spinal fluid sugar and chlorides are normal, which is characteristic in encephalitis and poliomyelitis, tuberculous meningitis is less likely. The season of the year, if other than summer or early autumn, and the absence of spinal cord signs, as indicated by flaccid paralysis of muscle groups in the legs or arms, will tend to eliminate paralytic poliomyelitis. The acute onset, normal optic discs and skull X-rays, and absence of a history of previous ear or acute sinus infection should help rule out either brain tumor or abscess; in the latter the spinal fluid may be similar to encephalitic fluid. Of course, a complete study of the spinal fluid must be carried out, including immediate Gram stain for organisms, culture, and cell count. The last, in a patient with encephalitis, may range between 10 to 200 per cu./mm., usually lymphocytes. Smears are negative and cultures are sterile.

In considering an outline of the types of encephalitis, one must include infectious agents and their toxins: viruses, bacteria, protozoa, fungi, spirochetes, and rickettsiae, as well as chemical and physical causes.

If the brain and cord are involved, we refer to the condition as encephalomyelitis. Some viruses attack the brain directly; they are referred to as neurotropic. In other types of encephalitis the brain is indirectly attacked, no virus being demonstrable. In other words, the brain is secondarily involved, perhaps through an allergic reaction.

Where there is a virus present, the cells of the brain including their fibres may be destroyed. There is also evidence of inflammatory reaction with cellular infiltration in the sheaths of the small blood vessels (adventitial reaction). The gray matter of the brain stem, including the basal ganglia and cerebellum, is often primarily attacked in some forms (polioclastic), as in the original acute epidemic type, but the cortex and subcortical white matter (leucoclastic) as well as the gray and white matter of the spinal cord are also involved in other types. In the postinfectious and post-vaccination types there is noted a marked diffuse, demyelinizing process, presumably due to an allergic response.

Ideally the diagnosis of viral encephalitis should be based on isolating the virus, but this is impractical because it is time-consuming and expensive. Therefore, serological methods, such as neutralization and complement fixation tests are utilized. Similar methods are used for the postinfectious and other demyelinizing types where no virus has been demonstrated. When the child is first seen, a blood serum specimen is drawn. After the acute stage is over, in about ten days to two weeks, a second blood specimen is drawn and together with the original tested to see whether there has been a significant rise of antibody titer. This is very diagnostic, especially when there is a sharp rise, about four times the original. If the increase in titer is not present or is inconclusive and encephalitis is strongly suspected on clinical grounds, the blood serum test for rise in antibody titer should be repeated a third time, about three or four weeks later.

Regardless of whether antibody is present or not in the original sample, a marked rise in titer on the second specimen is diagnostic of virus or rickettsial disease.

Encephalitis Lethargica (Von Economo) Type A

This disease occurred in epidemic form throughout the world from 1916 on. It was described by von Economo in 1917 and is now essentially of historical interest since no epidemics have been observed in several decades. In many of the patients there were prolonged periods of lethargy, hence the name "lethargic encephalitis" or "sleeping sickness."

Clinical Picture: The onset was gradual in the vast majority, but in about 10 per cent, it was acute with chills, fever, vomiting, convulsions, and sudden paralysis. The most frequent combination of symptoms was headache, lethargy, vomiting, diplopia, and changes in character. The disease was especially prevalent in the winter and spring months. As it progressed, a variety of clinical types were noted: the somnolent-ophthalmoplegic, with emphasis on the pronounced lethargy and the presence of extraocular palsies; a hyperkinetic form in which there was a stage of excitement rather than lethargy together with myoclonias and choreiform movements. Still other patients showed paralytic manifestations or akinetic features along with tremors or rigidity; finally there was a group who showed marked psychotic manifestations.

It is of no value to attempt a separate description of these and other types, since they were never so clearly demarcated clinically.

Laboratory: The spinal fluid is usually clear, under normal or slightly increased pressure. The cell count averages about 10 to 100 per cu./mm., mostly lymphocytes. The sugar is normal. Bacterial culture is sterile. The blood shows a leucocytosis of about 15,000.

PATHOLOGY: Every part of the nervous system is involved, but especially the basal ganglia, midbrain, and pons. Microscopically there are many areas of small hemorrhages. There is evidence of inflammatory reaction about the blood vessels of the brain and cord, with degeneration of the neurons. The perivascular lymphocytic infiltration is seen especially in the gray matter but not exclusively so. In the chronic stage there is a loss of cells with gliosis, especially in the substantia nigra and periaqueductal nuclei.

ETIOLOGY: This is unknown. It was believed to be due to a virus, although none has ever been isolated.

PROGNOSIS: The mortality in the epidemic form was estimated at 20 per cent.

TREATMENT: There was no specific therapy. Hypertonic glucose (10-20 per cent) given intravenously was used in the acute cases where there was evidence of increased intracranial pressure with cerebral edema. For the specific late features or sequelae such as tremor or rigidity appropriate drugs may be used. (See chapter on cerebral palsy for drugs and surgery.)

DISCUSSION: The significance of this disease lies in the development of residual features during the acute stage and the later occurrence of profound sequelae. It was estimated that only about 12 per cent of the patients recovered completely. The remainder developed some residual or late feature.

The residual features remained as an aftermath of the acute stage, and included paralysis of the eye muscles with disturbance in accommodation, pupillary inequalities, nystagmus, and ptosis. Facial paralysis occurred in some. In infants where the disease was often ushered in acutely with convulsions, delirium, coma, neck stiffness, and high fever the residuals were more severe, consisting of marked mental deterioration and various forms of paralysis of the extremities.

The late features or sequelae most often occurred after an interval of months or years following the acute stage. In children of adolescent age the "Parkinson" picture developed with mask-like facies, tremors, rigidity, and flexion deformities of the trunk. Some showed reversal of their sleep mechanism, being awake all night and sleeping by day. In others, myoclonias and myorhythmias, choreiform and athetoid movements, facial tics, torticollis, grimaces, and torsion spasms were noted. Oculogyric crises, consisting of a fixed stare with the eyes rolled upward while there is cessation of all activity, occurred alone or in association with the Parkinson syndrome. In some, a peculiar type of respiration similar to the panting of a dog was observed. An endocrine change took place in a few children evidenced by polyuria, obesity, or genital hypoplasia. Finally, and perhaps most important, was the marked amount of psychic disturbance which developed.

As previously stated, this disease has not recurred epidemically. It appears today only in sporadic form. Diagnosis becomes therefore a matter of eliminating all known causes. When this has been carefully done, a diagnosis of acute encephalitis may be made, probably viral, but etiology not determined. If the child shows residual damage, especially severe in infancy, with mental impairment, blindness, or paralysis, or subsequently shows sequelae similar to those of epidemic encephalitis, e.g., oculogyric crises or sleep perversion, we are apt to feel this is a sporadic case of the latter form. This is obviously an unsatisfactory diagnosis, which will disappear as more causal agents are discovered.

Perhaps of greater importance today is the fact that a child may be brought to the physician because of personality alteration with behavior difficulties. There may be no definite history of any previous acute illness. The problem is to determine whether the abnormal pattern of behavior is due to any form of encephalitis such as lethargic, viral, or postinfections, since all types may result in distortion of personality, or whether we are dealing with a purely emotional problem in an otherwise structurally normal child. The usual complaints vary from incorrigibility or truancy to more serious types of improper behavior such as sexual assault, attempted arson, and other delinquencies. When these children are carefully observed they show little or no self-control and exhibit a marked lack of judgment and inability to concentrate, even though their I.Q. may be normal. At times there may be associated neurological signs, and the electroencephalogram may show some cerebral dysrhythmia. The postencephalitic syndrome should be suspected in any child who is extremely hyperactive, lacks ability to concentrate for any period of time, is easily distractible, and has lack of self-control (brain-injured syndrome). The intellectual level may be normal or superior in these children. Psychomotor epilepsy and post traumatic behavior are discussed in their respective chapters. They also require differential from postencephalitic behavior.

Social psychotherapy is not successful in children with posten-

PROGNOSIS: The mortality in the Massachusetts epidemic was 90 per cent. Follow-up of the 10 per cent who survived revealed that only one child had recovered completely without sequelae. The others had severe brain damage with mental impairment and hemiplegia.

TREATMENT: There is no specific therapy.

WESTERN EQUINE ENCEPHALOMYELITIS

ETIOLOGY: Western equine encephalomyelitis is primarily found in the western parts of the United States and Canada. The natural reservoir for the virus is horses, chickens, and birds. Vectors are the Aedes and Culicine mosquitoes and tics. The disease occurs in the early summer, especially where there has been intermittent flooding of the land for irrigation, which causes an influx of mosquitoes.

CLINICAL PICTURE: The onset is marked by headache, vomiting, drowsiness, and fever, after an incubation period of five to ten days. Neck stiffness, convulsions, cranial nerve palsies, and occasional paralysis of the extremities follow. The whole course of the disease is milder than the Eastern equine type and lasts only about seven to ten days. In an epidemic in California 370 cases confirmed by laboratory testing were studied. In eighty per cent of the infants under one year fever and convulsions of brief duration occurred. Fifty per cent of the older children had fever, vomiting, drowsiness, irritability, and convulsions. Few cases went beyond this point in their clinical picture as recovery set in.

LABORATORY: The spinal fluid is clear with 50 to 500 cells per cu. mm., mononuclear mainly. The protein is increased, the sugar normal. The blood shows a moderate leucocytosis.

PATHOLOGY: There is infiltration of the meninges, though not as marked as in the eastern type. There are also perivascular infiltration in the gray matter and demyelination of the fibres with areas of softening or necrosis in the white matter. Moderate nerve cell destruction is present. Changes are noted in some of the blood vessel walls.

DIAGNOSIS: This is suggested by the seasonal incidence and geographical location. Clinically, one must rule out meningitis by examination of the spinal fluid, especially tuberculous and coccidioidal. Paralytic poliomyelitis is recognized by the presence of flaccid paralysis of the extremities. A history of previous mumps should be considered. The laboratory tests will identify the western type of equine encephalitis and differentiate it from the St. Louis encephalitis, with which it is clinically similar. The diagnosis is confirmed serologically, primarily by complement fixation tests showing a rising antibody titer on the second specimen of blood. Neutralization tests and isolation of the virus from brain tissue in fatal cases may also be done to identify the disease.

PROGNOSIS: The outlook is good. The mortality is about 10 per cent. All but 13 per cent of those who have recovered did so without residuals or sequelae. Infants experience a higher attack rate than others and 54 per cent of all major sequelae have been reported in those under one year. These consist of cerebral palsy, seizures, and mental retardation. In older children Parkinsonism may develop.

ST. LOUIS ENCEPHALITIS

ETIOLOGY: St. Louis virus is the cause of this disease. It was isolated during an epidemic of encephalitis in 1933, in which there were 1,130 cases. Chickens and birds are the natural reservoir for the virus. Vectors are mosquitoes, tics, and chicken mites. The disease occurs in the late summer and early fall.

CLINICAL PICTURE: The incubation period is four to twenty-one days. In infants the disease is violent, with high fever, convulsion and severe paralysis. Where death does not occur, there is marked residual disturbance.

In the epidemic of 1933 various forms of the disease were described. In some children there occurred an abortive type with mild headache and fever and slight gastrointestinal upset. Lumbar puncture was done only because there was an epidemic. In others, a more severe illness developed, with one to four days of systemic infection manifested by prodromal symptoms including fever, chills, sore throat, headache, and generalized muscular pains. This was followed by invasion of the central nervous system evidenced by neck stiffness, Kernig's sign, tremors, ataxia, variable reflexes, and mental confusion. Finally, in the most common form there were encephalitic manifestations from the onset, with marked headache, vomiting, high fever, neck stiffness, delirium, and convulsion. Reflexes were variable, the abdominals being absent at first, but returning with convalescence. Speech was disturbed. There were tremors of the hands, lips, and tongue. Fourteen per cent of the cases had blurred vision.

LABORATORY: The spinal fluid is clear, under increased pressure, with 50 to 250 cells per cu. mm., mononuclears mainly. There are increased protein and normal sugar. The blood count shows a moderate leucocytosis.

PATHOLOGY: The meninges exhibit inflammatory reaction. The brain shows edema and petechial hemorrhages. There is marked destruction of the neurons. All areas of the brain and cord are involved with perivascular and glial proliferation. The pathological changes are most marked in the brain stem.

DIAGNOSIS: The clinical picture is similar to Western equine encephalitis. It must be differentiated from tuberculous meningitis, other encephalitides, and poliomyelitis. Neutralization and complement fixation tests, two specimens of serum, will show rising titer, which is diagnostic.

PROGNOSIS: The course is favorable except in infancy. In the St. Louis epidemic there was a 20 per cent mortality. Residual damage is not as common as in the Eastern or Western equine encephalitis. The incidence of major sequelae in different series is one to 7.7 per cent.

JAPANESE B ENCEPHALITIS

Japanese B encephalitis has occurred in epidemic form during the summer months and early fall. The vector for transmission of the virus is the mosquito. Animals are the natural reservoirs. Its clinical picture and spinal fluid findings are similar to the equine encephalitides.

While the virus may be obtained from the blood and spinal fluid, the diagnosis is usually made by serological tests, complement fixation and neutralization, as in the other viral encephalitides. The mortality in children is about 50 per cent. In those surviving there may be mental defect and severe neurologic disturbance.

The Australian X disease is considered to be caused by a virus which is either the same as Japanese B or similar to it.

Ayres, J. C. and Feemster, R. F.: The Sequelae of Eastern Equine Encephalomyelitis. New England J. Med., 240:960, 1949.

Dent, J. H.: Pathological Changes in the Brains of Children Infected with the Virus of Eastern Equine Encephalomyelitis. Bull. Tulane Univ. Med. Faculty 14:85, 1955.

Dickerson, R. B., Newton, J. R. and Hansen, J. E.: Diagnosis and Immediate Prognosis of Japanese Encephalitis. Observations based on more than 200 patients with detailed analysis of 65 serologically confirmed cases. Am. J. Med. 12:277, 1952.

Finley, K. H., Longshore, Jr. W. A., Palmer, R. J., Cook, R. E. and Riggs, N.: Western Equine and St. Louis Encephalitis. Preliminary report of a Clinical Follow-up study in California. Neurology 5:223, 1955.

Fothergill, L. D., Dingle, J. H., Forbes, S. and Connerley, M. L.: Human Encephalitis Caused by the Virus of the Eastern Variety of Equine Encephalomyelitis. New England J. Med. 219:411, 1938.

Hammon, W. McD.: Encephalitis:—Eastern and Western Equine and St. Louis Types, as observed in 1941 in Washington, Arizona, New Mexico and Texas. J.A.M.A. 121:560, 1943.

Hempleman, T. C.: The Symptoms and Diagnosis of Encephalitis (1933 St. Louis Epidemic). J.A.M.A. 103:733, 1934.

Herzon, H., Shelton, J. T., and Bruyn, H. B.: Sequelae of Western Equine and other Anthropod-Borne Encephalitides. Neurology 7:535, 1957.

Pond, W. L., Russ, S. B., and Warre, J.: The Russian-Spring-Summer Encephalitis and Louping Ill Group of Viruses; Relationship of European and Asiatic strains of Russian Spring-Summer Encephalitis Viruses and Louping Ill Virus. J. Infect. Dis. 93:294, 1953.

LYMPHOCYTIC CHORIOMENINGITIS

ETIOLOGY: Lymphocytic choriomeningitis is caused by a specific virus which produces an acute, benign form of meningeal irritation. It may be transmitted to humans by the household mouse in whom the disease is endemic. Since the virus is present in the urine, feces, and nasal secretions of the mouse, inhalation of contaminated dirt or ingestion of infected food may produce the disease. One case of probable transplacental transmission has been reported.

CLINICAL PICTURE: The incubation period is about eight to twenty-one days. As with other viral infections, there is a clinical form of the disease in which the etiology is rarely recognized. This is the type in which there is a systemic infection with symptoms of "grippe" but without central nervous system manifestations. The patients may have fever, chills, and generalized aches and pains. The virus is recoverable from the blood stream. In a few days these patients are well. Armstrong found that eleven per cent of 2,000 blood sera, collected as random specimens from various parts of the United States, contained antibody for the virus of lymphocytic choriomeningitis despite lack of knowledge on the part of the donors of ever having had any central nervous system infection. This data would be explained by such "influenza types" of infections previously described.

The picture of meningitis or meningoencephalitis is the usual one presented when the child is admitted to the hospital. This occurs in those children whose preceding "grippe" has not cleared. There are fever, headache, vomiting, and neck stiffness. Kernig's sign is present. In those in whom encephalitis is more marked there are present profound lethargy, hyperactive deep tendon reflexes, and paralysis both of the extremities and cranial nerves.

LABORATORY: The spinal fluid is clear, pressure increased. There is a marked increase in cells, 1,000-3,000 per cu. mm., mostly all lymphocytic. Protein is increased, sugar normal. Culture is sterile for bacterial organisms.

PATHOLOGY: The meninges are markedly infiltrated with lymphocytes. There is also lymphocytic infiltration of the choroid plexus, the latter appearing necrotic.

DIAGNOSIS: Since the clinical picture is that of meningitis or encephalitis, it must be differentiated from other causes for these conditions. It may be suspected when the spinal fluid is clear, under increased pressure, and there are a great number of cells mostly all lymphocytes, and a normal sugar.

Absolute diagnosis is made by isolating the virus from the blood or spinal fluid, but as previously indicated this procedure is not practical. The usual method is the demonstration of complement fixing antibodies in the second blood specimen about three weeks after the original blood was taken, or of neutralizing antibodies in six to eight weeks. The latter persist for years.

PROGNOSIS: Recovery is the usual outcome in one to two weeks, without complications or sequelae. A case of arachnoiditis leading to a non-communicating hydrocephalus was recently reported in a fifteen-year-old girl.

TREATMENT: There are no specific drugs for this disease.

Armstrong, C. and Lillie, R. D.: Experimental Lymphocytic Chorio-meningitis of monkeys and mice produced by a virus encountered in studies of the 1933 St. Louis Encephalitis epidemic. Pub. Health, Rep. 49:1019, 1934.

————: Studies on Choriomeningitis and Poliomyelitis. Harvey Lectures, 36:39, 1940-41.

Haas, V. H.: Some Relationships between Lymphocytic Choriomeningitis (LCM). J. Infec. Dis. 94:187, 1954.

Komrower, G. M., Williams, B. L., and Stones, P. B.: Lymphocytic Choriomeningitis in newborn: Probable Transplacental Infection. Lancet 1:697, 1955.

Miles, J. A. R.: Benign Lymphocytic Meningitis. Med. J. Australia, 41:659, 1954.

Rivers, T. M. and Scott, T. F. M.: Meningitis in Man Caused by a Filterable Virus. Science 81:439, 1935.

Tindall, G. T. and Gladstone, L. A.: Hydrocephalus as a Sequel to Lymphocytic Choriomeningitis. Neurology 7:516, 1957.

POSTINFECTIOUS ENCEPHALITIS

This group includes the exanthemata such as measles, chicken pox, rubella, scarlet fever, and smallpox. Encephalitis may also follow influenza or upper respiratory infection, and vaccination against smallpox or rabies.

The primary pathological picture is a disseminated encephalomyelitis. The reason for the development of encephalitis during the course of these diseases is unknown. A hypothetical neurotropic virus suddenly activated by the illness or vaccination has been postulated, but none has been demonstrated. The virus of the overt disease itself has been suggested, but rarely found. Recently Ferraro and Roizin designated this group of encephalomyelitides as "hyperergic," meaning that there is either a constitutional predisposition due to allergy, an inadequate hemato-encephalic barrier, a central nervous system susceptibility due to the previous exanthem, or that the infectious agent, such as a virus, combines with antigen to form an anti-neural antigen.

The pathology is diffuse and involves the cortex, brain stem, and spinal cord. Both the white and gray matter are affected, but especially the white. There are perivascular infiltration and vascular engorgement. About these areas many cells accumulate, both microglial and lymphocytic. The nerve cells in these areas show degenerative changes, and there is a destruction of the myelin sheath. The axis cylinder, however, is not as greatly affected.

Ferraro, A. and Roizin, C.: Hyperergic Encephalomyelitides Following Exanthematic Diseases, Infectious Diseases and Vaccination. J. Neuropath. and Exper. Neurol. 16:423, 1957.

Kabat, E. A., Wolf, A. and Bezer, A. E.: Rapid Production of Acute Disseminated Encephalomyelitis in Rhesus Monkeys by Injection of Brain Tissue with Adjuvants. Science 104:362, 1947.

MEASLES ENCEPHALOMYELITIS

Encephalomyelitis as a complication of measles occurs about once in every 1,000 cases, or 0.1 per cent.

CLINICAL PICTURE: The appearance of encephalitic manifestations in measles takes place most frequently about the third to sixth day after the onset of the rash, but there are variations, including an onset a day before or with the beginning of the rash; and some cases have been reported in which symptoms began eight to fourteen days after the first day of the eruption.

Usually the mode of onset is acute with coma and convulsion. There is a marked change in sensorium and the child shows increasing lethargy or stupor. The fever rises sharply, whereas in the usual case of uncomplicated measles the fever and rash are declining at this time. In conjunction with coma, convulsions, changes in sensorium, and rise of fever, there are noted on examination a stiff neck, Kernig's sign, and twitching of the extremities.

There are varied clinical types of measles encephalomyelitis. In some instances the onset is gradual. Swanson reports a child who showed a Parkinson type of clinical picture with mask-like facies. Other cases have shown cranial nerve palsies, especially facial and oculomotor. Still others have profound brain stem pathology which results in difficulty in swallowing, respiratory disturbance, and death. There may be cerebellar symptoms with ataxia and in others hemiplegia (vascular). Paraplegia, urinary retention, and loss of deep tendon reflexes suggest myelitis or cord involvement.

LABORATORY: The spinal fluid is clear, under normal or increased pressure. The cell count is increased to about 100 cells per cu. mm., with lymphocytes mainly. The sugar is normal, but quite often increased. The protein is also increased. There is no bacterial growth on culture.

The electroencephalogram is abnormal with high voltage and slow waves, with or without focal evidence. With clinical improvement there is a slow return of the electroencephalogram to normal. In four of thirty-three cases of measles encephalitis the electroencephalogram remained abnormal paralleling clinical evidence of residual damage to the central nervous system. Grossman et al., correlated this date with their electroencephalographic studies of other children who had measles without clinical evidence of involvement of the central nervous system. In the latter there were 74 of 189 who had an abnormal electroencephalogram. They concluded that the electroencephalogram may be of help in detecting minor as well as major involvement of the central nervous system.

PATHOLOGY: This consists primarily of a diffuse perivascular demyelination. There are also glial proliferation and a slight meningeal reaction. In some instances there may be thrombosis of the major arterial channels or acute cerebral edema.

DIAGNOSIS: The presence of measles complicated by the onset of symptoms and signs of encephalitis or myelitis is diagnostic. When the child is admitted to the hospital with signs of encephalitis and no rash is obvious, or the history of preceding measles doubtful, other encephalitides, purulent meningitis, brain tumor, tuberculous meningitis, and poliomyelitis must be considered.

PROGNOSIS: In some cases the symptoms and signs spontaneously abate after several days and the child recovers completely in two to four days. In about twenty per cent a variety of complications occur, including personality and behavior disorders, mental impairment, convulsions or paralysis. The behavior disorders are typical of the brain injured child and include lack of concentration and disturbed memory. The mortality ranges from ten to thirty per cent in different series.

TREATMENT: Previous experimental work has suggested that damage to the nervous system with resultant demyelinization may be of an allergic nature. Corticotropin and cortisone have therefore been used in measles encephalitis. In a series of seventeen cases reported by Applebaum and Abler, fifteen of sixteen who were followed for periods of seven months to three years and nine months showed no sequelae. Swanson, comparing seven cortisone treated cases with seventeen non-cortisone treated cases, felt that the clinical course was not altered but that the sequelae in the cortisone treated cases were much milder. Further information will be needed to assess the value of steroid therapy but it appears promising at this time.

Applebaum, E., Dolgopol, V. B. and Dolgin, J.: Measles Encephalitis. Am. J. Dis. Child. 77:25, 1949.
———, E. and Abler, C.: Treatment of Measles Encephalitis with Corticotropin. A.M.A.J. Dis. Child. 92:147, 1956.
Grossman, H. J. Gibbs, E. L. and Spies, H. W.: Electroencephalographic Studies on Children having Measles with no Clinical Evidence of Involvement of the Central Nervous System. Pediat. 18:556, 1956.

Hoyne, A. L. and Slotkowski, E. L.: Frequency of Encephalitis as a complication of measles. Am. J. Dis. Child. 73:554, 1947.
Riley, Jr., H. D.: Encephalitis Complicating Attenuated Rubeola. A.M.A.J. Dis. Child. 95:270, 1958.
Spragins, M., Shinners, B. M. and Rochester, B.: Measles Encephalitis, Clinical and Electroencephalographic Study. Pediat. 5:599, 1950.
Swanson, B. E.: Measles Meningoencephalitis: A Summary of Twenty-four Cases Treated at Grasslands Over A Ten Year Period. A.M.A.J. Dis. Child. 92:272, 1956.
Tyler, H. R.: Neurological Complications of Rubeola (Measles). Medicine 36:147, 1957.

CHICKEN POX ENCEPHALOMYELITIS

Encephalomyelitis following chicken pox is caused by the varicella virus which has characteristics allied to the virus of herpes zoster.

CLINICAL PICTURE: The onset of encephalitic symptoms occurs about four to fourteen days after the beginning of the rash. There are present mild fever, delirium or stupor, vomiting, and occasionally convulsion. With recovery from the stupor, evidence of muscular weakness or paralysis, especially in the lower extremities is noted. Cranial nerve palsies, tremors, or ataxia may be seen.

LABORATORY: The spinal fluid is clear, with a pleocytosis, mostly lymphocytes. Culture is sterile. Sugar is normal.

PATHOLOGY: There is a widespread, nonspecific degenerative lesion in the ganglion cells of the brain and cord. There is also perivascular demyelinization throughout the brain and spinal cord, but especially noted in the frontal and occipital lobes.

PROGNOSIS: The outlook has been considered good for complete recovery. The encephalomyelitis following chicken pox is usually of a mild type. However, in three recent admissions to Kings County Hospital (State University Division) the children were left with devastating residuals.

TREATMENT: There is no specific therapy.

Zimmerman, H. M. and Yannet, H.: Non-suppurative Encephalomyelitis accompanying Chicken Pox. Arch. Neurol. & Psychiat. 26:322, 1931.
Underwood, E. A.: The neurological complications of varicella: a clinical and epidemiological study. Brit. J. Child. Dis. 32:83, 1935.

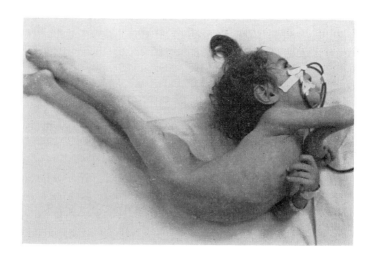

12. Opisthotonus following attack of chicken pox encephalomyelitis.

ENCEPHALOMYELITIS FOLLOWING GERMAN MEASLES
(RUBELLA)

This complication occurs in about 1:6,000 cases of German Measles. In a series reported by Davison and Friedfeld it was noted that the age range was from fourteen to forty-three years with the majority of the series during puberty, an age level above the usual for viral attacks.

CLINICAL PICTURE: The onset takes place about four to six days after the appearance of the rash and is explosive in type. There are symptoms of headache, irritability, vomiting, and pain in the extremities. In severe cases convulsions occur. Examination reveals a stiff neck, Kernig's sign, strabismus, diplopia, or nystagmus. The pupils are dilated and may be unequal. The optic discs are blurred. The superficial reflexes are diminished, abdominals absent. There may be paraplegia or ataxia. The fever is only slightly elevated.

LABORATORY: The spinal fluid is clear with normal or slightly increased pressure. There is an average of forty to ninety lymphocytes per cu. mm., with variations of no cells to five hundred. The sugar is normal, protein slightly elevated. Bacterial culture is sterile. In the blood a leucocytosis replaces the leucopenia when encephalitis develops.

PATHOLOGY: There are edema and hyperemia of the brain. The nerve cells are damaged. A perivascular infiltration of the gray and white matter of the cortex, cerebellum, and brain stem is noted. Meningeal reaction is mild. There is no demyelination as in measles encephalitis.

PROGNOSIS: Chances for recovery are good, although the mortality is twenty per cent. Neurological sequelae such as ataxia and tremors, when present, usually disappear in a few months.

TREATMENT: There is no specific therapy.

Davison, C. and Friedfeld, L.: Acute Encephalomyelitis following German Measles. Am. J. Dis. Child. 55:496, 1938.
Margolis, F. J., Wilson, J. L. and Top, F. H.: Postrubella Encephalomyelitis. Pediat. 23:158, 1943.

Mumps Encephalomyelitis

Mumps is a viral disease which affects the salivary glands, the mature gonads, pancreas, and breasts. The central nervous system is involved in about thirty per cent of all cases of mumps. It takes the form of a meningoencephalitis, usually following salivary gland involvement, but may precede the swelling or develop without the latter being noted. The encephalitis following mumps is the most common type of viral encephalitis we see and is classified as a primary neurotropic infection because the virus is recovered from the brain and spinal fluid in an acute attack. In this form there is evidence of meningeal irritation. It is also listed under postinfectious meningoencephalitis, which is the form it takes less often, and the pathology is then similar to others of this group, namely, a diffuse perivascular demyelination.

CLINICAL PICTURE: The onset is acute with headache, vomiting, neck stiffness, and marked rise of fever, which represents the meningitic phase. The brain involvement (encephalitic) usually affects the 8th nerve producing deafness, which very often is unilateral and permanent. Seventh or facial nerve paralysis also occurs. These symptoms and signs usually follow the appearance of the parotitis, but may be present without swelling of the gland. If the spinal cord is affected, transverse myelitis may follow.

LABORATORY: Lumbar puncture usually reveals a clear fluid under increased pressure; the number of cells ranges from ten to nine hundred per cu. mm., but in most instances averages about fifty to five hundred. The differential is lymphocytic. Protein is increased. Sugar and chlorides are normal.

DIAGNOSIS: The diagnosis is suggested clinically by the history of preceding or associated mumps. It is confirmed by serological tests. Complement fixing antibodies against mumps virus are present at the end of the first or second week. A blood serum specimen taken at this time and compared with one taken at the onset should show a four-fold increase in antibody titer. In suspected cases of viral encephalomyelitis due to mumps, where an original sample of blood serum was not taken because of the absence of parotitis, a titer over 1:128 may be considered indicative of recent mumps.

PROGNOSIS: The outlook is good, both for survival and recovery from most sequelae, except for the nerve deafness which is usually permanent.

TREATMENT: There is no specific therapy.

Holden, E. M., Eagles, A. Y. and Stevens, Jr., J. E.: Mumps involvement of the Central Nervous System. J.A.M.A. 131:382, 1946.
Macrae, J. and Campbell, A. M. G.: Neurological Complications of Mumps. Brit. M. J. 2:259, 1949.

ENCEPHALITIS FOLLOWING SMALLPOX (VARIOLA)

CLINICAL PICTURE: The most common nervous system complication following smallpox is an encephalomyelitis. This takes place about a week after the onset of the rash. There are present fever, headache, vomiting, and neck stiffness. Drowsiness may be marked. Tremors, occipital sweating, and intense salivation are also noted. Cranial nerve palsies including bulbar involvement with disturbed speech and swallowing may occur. There may also be spinal cord infection with paraplegia.

LABORATORY: The spinal fluid is clear, with several hundred cells per cu. mm., either lymphocytic or polymorphonuclear early in the disease, later changing to mononuclears. The sugar and protein are normal. Culture is sterile.

PATHOLOGY: This is similar to measles and vaccination encephalomyelitis with the development of perivascular demyelinization.

PROGNOSIS: In the eleven cases of Marsden and Hurst there were four deaths.

TREATMENT: There is no specific therapy.

Marsden, J. P. and Hurst, E. W.: Acute Perivascular Myelinoclasis (Acute disseminated encephalomyelitis) in Smallpox. Brain 55:181, 1932.

PERTUSSIS ENCEPHALOPATHY

Encephalopathy following pertussis occurs especially in infants under two years of age. Various theories have been offered to explain the cause. The presence of petechial hemorrhages in the brain together with the marked anoxemia produced by the spasms of coughing has suggested a vascular basis. In other instances, a meningoencephalitis or inflammatory reaction has been given as the factor.

CLINICAL PICTURE: The cerebral complications of pertussis usually appear at the peak of the paroxysmal stage, or at about the third and fourth weeks of the disease. The onset is marked by a rise of fever and convulsions. The child goes into a stupor or coma. Neurological signs develop including hemiplegia or spastic paraplegia, and sensory changes such as aphasia, deafness or blindness. Meningeal signs include neck stiffness, Kernig's, and Brudzinki's. The pupils are unequal and there may be evidence of hemorrhages in the optic discs. Bulbar symptoms with disturbance in speech and swallowing may appear. Mental changes are marked.

LABORATORY: The spinal fluid is clear. There are about 10 to 100 cells per cu. mm., mostly lymphocytes. The sugar and protein are normal or slightly increased. Culture is sterile.

PATHOLOGY: There are edema and congestion of the brain. Microscopically there are punctate hemorrhages, including areas of small hemorrhages in the subarachnoid space. In some cases there are marked degeneration of the nerve cells and cortical atrophy. In general neither massive hemorrhages are noted, nor are there marked areas of thrombosis. The lesions have been considered vascular with the circulatory disturbances related to toxemia or anoxemia.

PROGNOSIS: The outcome of pertussis encephalopathy is poor. There is about forty per cent mortality but under two years the mortality rate rises to sixty per cent. Of those who survive about half are left with sequelae such as complete blindness or deafness, mental retardation, permanent paralysis, recurrent convulsions, or alteration of behavior.

TREATMENT: There is no specific treatment of the encephalopathy. Attempts to prevent its occurrence should be made, especially in early childhood, by treating the onset of the pertussis itself with hyperimmune gamma globulin, injected intramuscularly.

Dolgopol, V. B.: Changes in the Brain in Pertussis with Convulsion. Arch. Neurol. & Psychiat. 46:477, 1941.
Litvak, A. M., Gibel, H., Rosenthal, S. E., Rosenblatt, P.: Cerebral Complications in Pertussis. J. Pediat. 32:357, 1948.
Nelson, R. L.: Neurological Complications of Whooping Cough: Review of Literature with Reports of Two Cases of Pertussis Encephalitis. J. Pediat. 14:39, 1939.
Powers, G. F.: Tetany as a Cause of Convulsions in Whooping Cough. Am. J. Dis. Child. 30:632, 1925.

POST-VACCINAL ENCEPHALOMYELITIS

Encephalomyelitis following vaccination against smallpox occurs about 1:100,000 vaccinations. It usually follows the primary or original vaccination but occasionally occurs on revaccination. It is not common in the United States, for in 1938 there were only about seventy-five cases reported in the literature. On the other hand, it has been noted quite frequently in England, Holland, and Germany. There is no explanation for this difference, although vaccination in the United States has been carried out in the first year of life, whereas on the continent it has been performed most often at school age.

CLINICAL PICTURE: After an incubation period of about seven to twelve days following vaccination, the disease is usually ushered in with acute manifestations of a meningoencephalitic character, including headache, fever, vomiting, drowsiness, neck stiffness, and convulsion. In some the signs are primarily those of an encephalitis, including stupor, seizures, and hemiplegia. Cranial nerve palsies such as ophthalmoplegia and ptosis may occur with involvement of the brain stem, and death may supervene with medullary extension. In other cases there are indications of spinal cord involvement with an ascending type of paralysis or transverse myelitis. In these there are sensory disturbances, retention of urine, and flaccid paralysis.

LABORATORY: The spinal fluid is clear with few cells, which are usually lymphocytic. The protein is slightly elevated, sugar normal. Bacterial culture is sterile.

PATHOLOGY: There is a diffuse encephalomyelitis involving especially the brain stem and spinal cord, but in other instances the cortex or cerebellum may be affected. The process is most intense in the white matter. There are areas showing marked perivascular demyelination. The blood vessels are engorged and there is cellular infiltration around the vessels. The nerve cells and axones are not as markedly affected.

DIAGNOSIS: This is based on a history of vaccination against smallpox within two weeks of the onset of symptoms. The disease develops irrespective of whether or not there was a vaccination "take."

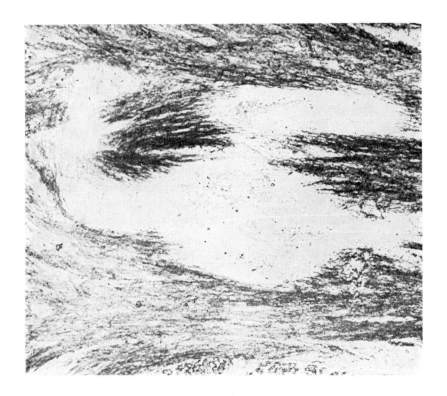

13. Demyelinization of medullated fibers in the pons. In the center of the field the lumen of a small vessel is seen. The originally continuous transverse band of black-stained medullated fibers is interrupted in the area about the vessel. Spielmeyer stain. Magnification 200.

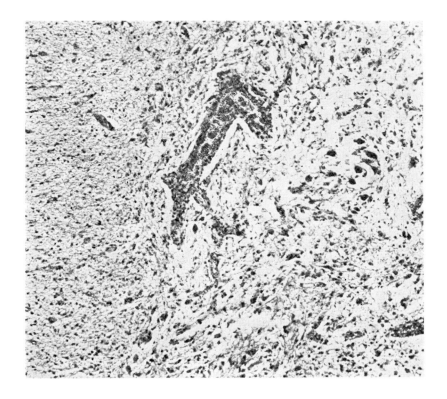

14. Cellular infiltration and extensive disintegration of the gray substance about a vessel in the lumbar portion of the cord. Note the persisting ganglion cells to the right of the vessel. To the left of the vessel the white substance of the cord is well preserved. Magnification 200.

PROGNOSIS: The mortality is about forty per cent. In those who survive, recovery is usually complete in about two weeks with few sequelae. The latter, when present, consist of hemiplegia or seizures.

TREATMENT: There is no specific therapy once the disease has set in. The best way to avoid this condition is to vaccinate early in infancy, around the third month and certainly within the first year, for it is extremely rare to see encephalomyelitis follow vaccination at this age. The only contraindication to this rule would be the presence of severe eczema in the infant or chickenpox in the siblings.

Greenberg, M. and Applebaum, E.: Post-vaccinal Encephalitis: Report of 45 cases in New York City. Am. J. Med. Sc. 216:565, 1948.
Lamm, S. S.: Post-vaccinal Encephalomyelitis. Am. J. Dis. Child. 56:824, 1938.
Miller, H. G.: Prognosis of Neurologic Illness Following Vaccination Against Smallpox. Arch. Neurol. & Psychiat. 69:695, 1953.
Stuart, G.: Memorandum on Post-vaccinal Encephalitis. World Health Org. 1:36, 1947.

ENCEPHALITIS FOLLOWING ANTIRABIES VACCINE INJECTION

The use of antirabies vaccine is followed by an encephalomyelitis in about 1:2,000 injected cases.

CLINICAL PICTURE: The onset occurs from eight to twenty-one days following beginning of injections. The symptoms are of various types, depending on the area of the central nervous system involved. They may be those of an encephalitis, radiculitis involving the nerve roots and trunk, polyneuritis, or myelitis, especially in the dorsolumbar area, resulting in paraplegia or an ascending Landry type of paralysis.

LABORATORY: With encephalitic manifestations the spinal fluid is clear and under increased pressure. There are about 200 cells per cu. mm., lymphocytes predominating, slightly elevated protein, and normal sugar. Bacterial culture is sterile.

PATHOLOGY: There is a diffuse perivascular demyelination, especially in the white matter, with glial proliferation.

PROGNOSIS: The prospects are good for complete recovery in most instances. However, in one report, death in some cases and permanent paralysis in three others were noted.

TREATMENT: Cortisone may be of value in treatment since the central nervous system manifestations are considered to be secondary to the development of hypersensitivity to the brain tissue in the vaccine.

Since embryonated duck eggs are now being used to make the antirabies vaccine, we may expect a subsidence of central nervous system reactions to antirabies vaccine injection. (Refer to the section on Rabies.)

Applebaum, E., Greenberg, M. and Nelson, J.: Neurological Complications Following Anti-rabies Vaccination. J.A.M.A. 151:188, 1953.

CAT SCRATCH ENCEPHALITIS

Cat scratch disease is characterized by generalized involvement of the lymph glands. In a few instances there are nervous system complications, of which encephalitis is the most frequent manifestation.

CLINICAL PICTURE: The incubation period is variable, from ten to thirty days. There may be evidence of a healing lesion in the skin, presumably the scratch of a cat. In addition to a cat scratch, slivers, thorns, and porcupine quills have been implicated.

The onset is marked by fever and enlargement of the regional glands. Evidence of encephalopathy occurs most frequently about the second week after the onset of adenopathy and is marked by convulsions and coma in addition to the fever. In Stevens' case, a thirteen-year-old boy, there was a papule on the right forearm with enlargement of the right epitrochlear and axillary nodes. A week later convulsions occurred, together with nuchal rigidity. In Thompson and Miller's case of a sixteen-year-old boy, coma appeared six weeks after the onset of the illness. There may be facial palsy, muscle weakness, a Babinski sign and sensory changes. Paxon and McKay, Jr. in a review of the literature found twelve cases of neurologic complication in cat scratch disease and added two of their own. Of the fourteen, ten had encephalopathy (the authors prefer this term to encephalitis because of the lack of cellu-

lar response and an elevated spinal fluid protein), two encephalomyelitis, one myelitis, and one radiculitis.

LABORATORY: The spinal fluid is usually normal, but in some
cases there may be a slight increase in cells with elevated protein.
Culture is sterile. The electroencephalogram shows a generalized
dysrhythmic pattern. Biopsy of a gland reveals numerous granulomata with central necrosis. Culture is sterile.

ETIOLOGY: No virus has been isolated. Paxon and McKay, Jr.
favor an immunologic reaction related to the infective agent or
to an associted toxin. However, there is no evidence, as yet, as to
the etiologic factor.

DIAGNOSIS: The diagnosis is based upon a history of exposure
to a cat scratch or of contact with a cat, the presence of regional
adenopathy, biopsy of a lymph node, and a clinical picture of
encephalitis which develops within six weeks of the onset of
adenopathy. It may be confirmed by an intradermal test using cat
scratch antigen. A positive test consists of persisting erythema and
induration of the skin within twenty-four to forty-eight hours.

A differential diagnosis should be made from other causes of
lymphadenitis including tuberculosis, Hodgkin's, bacterial infection, and infectious mononucleosis. Viral studies should be carried
out to be certain the encephalopathy is not due to a specific type
complicating cat scratch disease.

PROGNOSIS: The outlook is good for complete recovery.

TREATMENT: There is no specific therapy.

Paxon, E. M. and McKay, Jr., R. J.: Neurologic Symptoms Associated with
    Cat Scratch Disease. Pediat. 20:13, 1957.
Stevens, H. Cat Scratch Fever Encephalitis. Am. J. Dis. Child. 84:218,
    1952.
Thompson, Jr., T. E. and Miller, K. F.: Cat Scratch Encephalitis. Ann. Int.
    Med. 39:146, 1953.

RABIES

Rabies is an acute viral disease producing an infection of the
central nervous system of an encephalomyelitic character. It is
usually transmitted through the bite of a dog or wild animal,
such as a wolf, suffering from the disease, or an insectivorous bat.

Following the bite there is an incubation period of about one to three months. Occasionally shorter incubation periods of seven days are noted, especially when the wound is about the face and head. Longer intervals of seven months have also been reported. The virus of rabies passes to the central nervous system by way of the peripheral nerves. From here it spreads by way of the neural route to the salivary glands, where it again multiplies and is excreted in the saliva. There is no significant viremia.

PATHOLOGY: The virus of rabies is neurotropic and in response to its presence the characteristic inclusion body (Negri body) is found in the nerve cell. The neurons show degeneration and there is diffuse perivascular infiltration of the brain and cord, especially the brain stem, akin to acute epidemic encephalitis. Occasionally cases of acute myelitis without encephalitis have been noted.

CLINICAL PICTURE: At the onset of the disease there may be generalized pain and a feeling of numbness, followed by irritability and drowsiness. There are also a rise of fever, vomiting, and sore throat. This stage soon passes into a phase of excitation. Convulsions, twitchings, neck stiffness, and high fever occur, followed by spasms of the pharyngeal and laryngeal muscles, especially when an attempt is made to eat or drink. There is a fear of food or water (hydrophobia) because the sight of these, or efforts to take any, intensify the spasms. The excitatory period is followed by coma and death, the total illness lasting about four or five days.

LABORATORY: The spinal fluid is clear, pressure normal or increased. There are several hundred cells per cu. mm. of the polymorphonucleated type. The protein is increased, sugar and chlorides are normal. Culture is sterile.

DIAGNOSIS: The differential diagnosis is based on the history of a bite by a dog. In the case of tetanus, the spasm takes the form of trismus (lock-jaw). The history of the wound is different, there are no spasms of the pharynx and the larynx, and the spinal fluid is normal. Hysteria may occasionally simulate true rabies. Acute encephalitis, lead encephalopathy, and tuberculous meningitis must also be ruled out.

TREATMENT: Attempts at sedation with barbiturates or anesthesia may be made, especially for the seizures. However, once the disease has set in there is no specific therapy and death follows.

Therefore, prophylactic treatment is the major therapeutic goal. Children who are bitten should have their wounds washed thoroughly with soap and water. In addition a tetanus toxoid booster should be administered and an antibiotic prescribed to prevent secondary infection. The dog should be impounded by notifying the authorities and carefully observed for about ten to twelve days for any signs of rabies.

Since the incidence of rabies is not great in the United States, the decision to give vaccine routinely to those who are bitten by dogs or other animals depends on the risk involved from the reaction to the vaccine itself. The risk of encephalitis or myelitis varies between 1:600 to 1:2,000 of treated cases. (The mortality in this group lies between 10 to 25 per cent.) The reaction from the vaccine has been due to the brain tissue of rabbits, especially the myelin in it. The new duck-embryo rabies vaccine is free of neurological reactions. Therefore the vaccine may now be given more freely.

However, there is still a risk involved since foreign protein is being injected, so that a careful history concerning the presence of allergy, especially to egg, must be ascertained and proper precautions exerted.

Where the animal is unknown and there is a deep wound about the face, head, or neck, antirabies hyperimmune serum followed by antirabies vaccine should be given immediately. The serum should be injected intramuscularly, but only after careful testing for horse serum sensitivity has been carried out. The dose of serum given should be based on a ratio of 0.5 ml./kg. of body weight of the child. The vaccine should be administered subcutaneously, 0.5 ml. of a 20 per cent emulsion, daily, for fourteen days. In severe cases, the injections should be continued for twenty-one days.

If the biting animal is known and appears to have signs of rabies, serum should be given followed by vaccine as outlined above. If, however, by the fifth day of observation, the animal acts normally, vaccine injections should be stopped.

Where there is a severe wound and the animal acts healthy, serum should be given and the animal observed. If it develops rabies, vaccine therapy should be added. In the case of a bat, however, vaccine as well as serum should be given immediately without any observation period.

This brings us to those cases where the skin has just been licked, or there is a slight simple bite or abrasion. If the skin has not been broken, no therapy is necessary. If there is a slight wound, the animal should be observed. Treatment with vaccine is begun if rabies develops. If there is any doubt, one might use serum while waiting. When the animal is unknown, give vaccine treatment immediately. For complete details, one may consult the article by Habel, which includes a report on the indications for specific treatment after exposure to rabies, as prepared by the "Expert Committee on Rabies, World Health Organization."

The outlook for prevention of rabies is good, provided serum and vaccine are used at the proper time.

Applebaum, E., Greenberg, M., and Nelson, J.: Neurological Complications following Antirabies Vaccination. J.A.M.A. 151:188, 1953.
Blatt, N. H. and Lepper, M. H.: Reactions Following Antirabies Prophylaxis. A.M.J. Dis. Child. 86:395, 1953.
Habel, K. and Koprowski, H.: Laboratory data supporting the Clinical Trial of Antirabies Serum in persons bitten by a rabid wolf. Bull. World Health Org., 13:773, 1955.
————: Rabies Prophylaxis in Man. Pediat. 19:923, 1957.
Knutti, R. E.: Acute Ascending Paralysis and Myelitis Due to the Virus of Rabies. J.A.M.A. 93:754, 1929.
Peck Jr., F. B., Powell, H. M., and Culbertson, C. G.: Duck-Embryo Rabies Vaccine. Study of Fixed Virus Vaccine Grown in Embryonated Duck Eggs and Killed with Beta-proprolactone (BPL). J.A.M.A. 162:1368, 1956.

HERPES SIMPLEX MENINGOENCEPHALITIS

Acute encephalitis due to herpes simplex virus has been occasionally reported in children. In most instances the outcome was fatal both in children and adults.

CLINICAL PICTURE: The onset is acute, with fever, delirium, and coma. Convulsions have occurred in some. Encephalitic manifestations develop, such as ocular and facial palsies, and paralysis of the extremities. There are signs of meningeal irritation in others, with headache and neck stiffness. In one instance, the mother was subject to recurrent herpes labialis; although no evidence of external herpes was noted in the infant, the latter developed herpes simplex viral encephalitis. In the newborn the clinical picture is similar to that of cytomegalic disease.

LABORATORY: The spinal fluid is clear, under increased pressure. It contains from 90 to 800 cells per cu. mm., mostly lymphocytes, increased protein, and normal sugar. Bacterial culture is sterile. The virus can be isolated from the spinal fluid.

PATHOLOGY: The pathology consists of extensive necrosis of the cortex. There is perivascular infiltration with mononuclear cells. Acidophilic intranuclear inclusion bodies are found in the oligodendroglia and ganglion cells. The virus may be isolated from brain tissue.

DIAGNOSIS: The diagnosis is based on the development of neutralizing antibodies in the patient's serum following recovery and isolation of the virus from the spinal fluid during the acute stage. In fatal cases the virus is isolated from the brain tissue. There may also be evidence of herpes on the skin, on the mucous membrane as a gingivostomatitis, or in the eye, as a keratoconjunctivitis. In the newborn period, cytomegalic inclusion disease and toxoplasmosis should be ruled out.

PROGNOSIS: The disease lasts about four to twelve days, usually ending in death.

TREATMENT: There is no specific therapy.

Ginder, D. R., and Wharton, C. M.: Herpes Simplex Encephalitis. J. Pediat. 39:298, 1951.
Haymaker, W.: Herpes Simplex Encephalitis in Man. Report of three cases. J. Neuropath. and Exp. Neurol. 8:132, 1949.

LYMPHOGRANULOMA VENEREUM

A meningoencephalitis may be produced by the virus of lymphogranuloma venereum with or without the presence of enlarged lymph nodes. Fever, headache, delirium, and neck stiffness are present. In this type, contrary to the other viral forms, there are a low spinal fluid sugar and decreased spinal fluid chlorides. The spinal fluid appears turbid with thousands of cells per cu. mm., mostly lymphocytes, and some increase in protein. Bacterial culture is sterile.

The diagnosis is made through isolation of the virus from the spinal fluid, complement-fixation with the antigen of lymphogranuloma venereum, and the Frei test (intradermal skin test).

Sabin, A. R. and Aring, C. D.: Meningoencephalitis in Man Caused by the Virus of Lymphogranuloma. J.A.M.A. 120:1376, 1942.

ASEPTIC MENINGITIS

The three types of Poliomyelitis viruses, Coxsackie A and B and the ECHO strains form a group of enteroviruses belonging to a similar biologic family which may produce a viral meningitis (aseptic meningitis). Some of the members of the Coxsackie and ECHO groups have also produced a flaccid paralysis similar to the clinical picture of Poliomyelitis.

COXSACKIE VIRUSES

This group of viruses (A and B) may produce a benign lymphocytic meningitis (aseptic meningitis). Illnesses similar to poliomyelitis and epidemic myalgia or pleurodynia have also been described. In the meningitic form there may be an acute onset with high fever, vomiting, headache, abdominal pain, and later, neck stiffness. In others the development of meningitis follows a prodromal period of malaise, lack of appetite, abdominal discomfort and elevated fever of 3 to 10 days. The cerebrospinal fluid is clear, under moderate pressure, contains 50 to 500 cells per cu. mm., early polymorphonuclears, later mostly lymphocytes, with normal sugar and slight protein increase. Bacteriological culture is sterile. The diagnosis is made by isolating the Coxsackie virus from the stools. A differential from other viral diseases may also be made by serological tests demonstrating increasing titer of neutralizing antibodies for Coxsackie virus in the serum. Recovery is complete.

ECHO VIRUSES (ENTERIC CYTOPATHOGENIC HUMAN ORPHANS)

This group of viruses may also produce an aseptic meningitis. The symptoms include fever, frontal headache, nausea, vomiting, and pains in the chest, abdomen, and extremities. Examination reveals evidence of meningeal irritation such as stiff neck and back, and spasm of the hamstring muscles. Some patients have a pinkish red rash, especially on the face. The cerebrospinal fluid is clear, containing about 30 to 200 cells per cu. mm., mostly lymphocytes, but in one group of cases there were from 300 to 2,400 cells per cu. mm.; the protein is slightly increased or normal, and the sugar is normal. The virus may be cultured from the spinal fluid.

The diagnosis is made by isolation of the ECHO virus from the stool, pharynx, and spinal fluid. Neutralizing antibody can be demonstrated during the course of the illness. A differential diagnosis should be made from poliomyelitis, Coxsackie, and other infections which may produce an aseptic meningitis syndrome.

Barron, A. L., Karzon, D. T. and Pollock, B. F.: Isolation of ECHO Virus Type Two from the Cerebrospinal Fluid in Aseptic Meningitis. A.M.A.J. Dis. Child. 95:235, 1958.

Curnen, E. C.: Human Disease associated with the Coxsackie Viruses. Bull. N. Y. Acad. Med. 26:335, 1950.

Dalldorf, G.: The Coxackie Viruses: Isolation and Properties, Second International Poliomyelitis Conference, Copenhagen, Denmark, 1951. Philadelphia, J. B. Lippincott Company, 1953.

Heubner, R. J., Beeman, E. A., Cole, R. M., Biegelman, P. M., and Bell, J. A.: The Importance of Coxsackie Viruses in Human Disease Particularly Herpangina and Epidemic Pleurodynia. New England J. Med. 247:249 and 285, 1952.

Miles, J. A. R.: Benign Lymphocytic Meningitis. Med. J. Australia, 1:659, 1954.

Rivadeneira, J. C., Robbins, F. C., Crea, M., and Eiben, R. M.: The distribution of Group B Coxsackie Viruses in a children's institution. Pediat. 20:468, 1957.

Sabin, A. B., Krumbiegel, E. R. and Wigand, R.: Echo Type 9 Virus Disease. A.M.A.J. Dis. Child. 96:197, 1958.

Syverton, J. T., McLean, D. M., Martins da Silva, M., Doany, H. B., Cooney, M., Kleinman, H., and Bauer, H.: Outbreak of Aseptic Meningitis caused by Coxsackie B5, Virus. Laboratory, Clinical and Epidemiologic Study. J.A.M.A. 164:2015, 1957.

ACUTE HEMORRHAGIC ENCEPHALITIS

Acute hemorrhagic encephalitis may occur secondary to infectious diseases such as pneumonia, influenza, septicemia, typhoid, malaria, scarlet fever, and drugs like the sulfa compounds.

CLINICAL PICTURE: The onset is sudden and acute, with vomiting, headache, convulsion, and high fever. Paralysis, coma, and death may follow in two to three days. If the patient survives, the paralysis persists, and the mental level is impaired. These children comprise a portion of the spastic hemiplegias, postnatal type, who are treated in cerebral palsy clinics. Rarely they recover completely. The spinal fluid is clear and usually normal as to cells and chemistry. Occasionally the fluid may contain a few red blood cells. Bacteriological culture is sterile.

PATHOLOGY: There are widespread lesions of a necrotizing type in the brain and cord, with perivascular hemorrhages noted in the cortex, mid-brain, pons, and medulla. The white matter is particularly affected. The pathology may be due to sensitivity to the toxin or infective agent.

DIFFERENTIAL DIAGNOSIS: These cases have also been called acute superior polioencephalitis hemorrhagica (Wernicke), brain purpura, or Strümpell encephalitis. One must rule out meningitis, viral encephalitis, poliomyelitis, thrombosis of the basilar artery, or pontine hemorrhage.

Adams, R. D.: Acute Necrotizing Hemorrhagic Encephalopathy. J. Neuropath. and Exper. Neurol. 8:1, 1949.
Alpers, B. J.: So-called "Brain Purpura" or "Hemorrhagic Encephalitis." Arch. Neurol. and Psychiat. 20:497, 1928.

INCLUSION BODY ENCEPHALITIS (DAWSON)

This disease is marked by progressive mental deterioration associated with variable neurological signs due to a diffuse involvement of the central nervous system. It was first described by Dawson, who noted intranuclear inclusion bodies in the brain in fatal cases of encephalitis.

CLINICAL PICTURE: The disease is limited to the first two decades of life. The onset is insidious, the course slowly progressive. Mental deterioration appears early. There are also optic atrophy with blindness, convulsions, and motor disturbances due to involvement of the pyramidal, extrapyramidal, and lower motor pathways. Usually fever sets in near the end of the disease.

LABORATORY: The spinal fluid is normal except for a strong first zone colloidal gold curve. The electroencephalogram shows paroxysms of atypical spike wave patterns.

PATHOLOGY: There is a diffuse involvement of the white and gray matter of the central nervous system, with perivascular infiltration, demyelinization, and gliosis. There is also a meningeal reaction. Intranuclear inclusion bodies are seen in the brain.

ETIOLOGY: The cause of Dawson inclusion body encephalitis is unknown.

DIAGNOSIS: The disease must be differentiated from herpes simplex virus encephalitis where the inclusion bodies are of a similar type morphologically. Another condition, subacute sclerosing leucoencephalitis (Van Bogaert), simulates the Dawson type of encephalitis, but inclusion bodies are only rarely noted. The two appear to be closely related and may be similar.

PROGNOSIS: Death comes anywhere from a year to as long as seven and one-half years after the onset of symptoms.

TREATMENT: There is no specific therapy.

Dawson, J. R.: Cellular Inclusion in Cerebral Lesions of Lethargic Encephalitis. Am. J. Path. 9:7, 1933.
————: Cellular Inclusions in Cerebral Lesions of Epidemic Encephalitis. Arch. Neurol, and Psychiat. 31:685, 1934.
Greenfield, J. G.: Encephalitis and Encephalomyelitis in England and Wales During the Last Decade. Brain 73:141, 1950.
Malamud, N., Haymaker, W., and Pinkerton, H.: Inclusion Encephalitis, with a Clinico-pathologic Report of Three Cases. J. Path. 26:133, 1950.

SUBACUTE SCLEROSING LEUCOENCEPHALITIS
(VAN BOGAERT TYPE)

This condition is marked clinically by the onset of intellectual deterioration in a young child or adolescent who has previously been well. Along with the mental disturbance, seizures and motor disabilities appear. These include dyskinesias and hyperkinesias. Finally bilateral spasticity with decerebrate rigidity and complete dementia precede death.

LABORATORY: The blood and spinal fluid are normal. The EEG is characteristic: the first portion begins with a few spike discharges; then there follow rhythmic discharge complexes associated clinically with myoclonic jerks. The complexes are of high voltage, slow waves, and regular rhythms, followed by waves of decreasing amplitude.

PATHOLOGY: The main process is a fibrillary gliosis, especially noted in the subcortical white matter, but also seen with less intensity in the basal ganglia, thalamus, brain stem, and cord. There is a subacute inflammatory reaction, but very little or no demyelinization. Inclusion bodies are occasionally found.

ETIOLOGY: The cause is unknown. No virus has been isolated. There is no familial pattern. Birth and early development are normal.

DIAGNOSIS: This is based on early intellectual deterioration, dyskinesias, bilateral spasticity with decerebrate rigidity, and the electroencephalographic patterns. Poser and Radermecker, who reported twenty cases diagnosed antemortem, state that these cases are not Schilder's or diffuse sclerosis, but are closely related to Dawson's subacute inclusion body encephalitis and Pette-Döring's nodular panencephalitis.

Lesse, S., Hoefer, P. F. A. and Austin, J. H.: The Electroencephalogram in Diffuse Encephalopathies. A.M.A. Arch. Neurol. and Psychiat. 79:359, 1958.
Poser, C. M. and Radermecker, J.: Subacute Sclerosing Leukoencephalitis, Van Bogaert Type. J. Pediat. 50:408, 1957.

INFECTIOUS MONONUCLEOSIS

Infectious mononucleosis is an acute illness of unknown origin possibly due to a virus, with protean systemic manifestations which include enlarged cervical glands and spleen, and changes in the blood.

CLINICAL PICTURE: At times, in children, the nervous system is involved (one per cent). Evidence of the latter may antedate the usual symptoms and signs of infectious mononucleosis by a few days or may appear at the onset of the disease. At other times neurological complications may appear after the usual signs of the disease have disappeared.

Silver and his associates have classified six groups of cases showing nervous system involvement in addition to the usual features of infectious mononucleosis:

1. Serous meningitis with headache and nuchal rigidity in which there is increased pressure in the cerebrospinal fluid.

2. Meningitis, similar to the above, plus abnormal reflexes. The spinal fluid shows increase in cells and protein as well as pressure.

3. Encephalitis with the presence usually of fever, lethargy, delirium and convulsion. The spinal fluid protein and pressure are elevated, but there is no increase in cells.

4. Acute polyneuronitis (Guillain-Barré syndrome). Symmetrical flaccid paralysis of the extremities and loss of deep tendon reflexes. There is increased protein in the spinal fluid with absence of cells (albumino-cytologic dissociation).

5. Peripheral neuritis with flaccid paralysis limited to isolated groups of muscles, associated with a normal spinal fluid.

6. Optic neuritis with papilloretinal edema and hemorrhages. In all of these the spinal fluid sugar is normal and culture of the fluid is sterile.

These forms of nervous system involvement in infectious mononucleosis may thus be said to take on the manifestations of meningitis with or without increase of cells in the spinal fluid (Groups I and II of Silver's classification), encephalitis, pure or combined with meningeal or myelitic symptoms (Group III), and peripheral neuritis (Groups IV, V, and VI), with VI being the ocular form.

LABORATORY: The spinal fluid findings are as described above. The diagnosis of infectious mononucleosis is made on the basis of the atypical lymphocytes in the peripheral blood smear and the heterophile antigen reaction. An agglutination titer of 1:64 or higher is diagnostic.

DIAGNOSIS: The differential diagnosis must be made from bacterial meningitis, acute encephalitis, poliomyelitis, acute infectious lymphocytosis, and the various types of neuritis. If jaundice is present, viral hepatitis associated with meningitic or encephalitic manifestations must be considered. The heterophile test and blood smear examination will establish the presence of infectious mononucleosis.

PROGNOSIS: The outlook is good with complete recovery from the neurological signs in most cases. Occasionally permanent brain damage may occur, and even death, if the brain stem is involved. Leibowitz, in seventy-one cases of infectious mononucleosis with neurological involvement collected from the literature, reported a mortality of eleven per cent.

TREATMENT: Recently steroids have been used with apparent success in the treatment of the neurological complications.

Beloff, J. S. and Goug, K. M.: Acute Poliomyelitis and Acute Infectious Lymphocytosis. J. Pediat. 26:586, 1945.

Doran, J. K. and Weisberger, A. S.: Use of ACTH in Infectious Mononucleosis. Ann. Int. Med. 38:1058, 1953.

Friedlander, W. J.: Neurologic Signs and Symptoms as a Prodrome to Virus Hepatitis. Neurology 6:574, 1956.

Frenkel, E. P., Shiver, Jr., C. B., Berg, P. and Caris, T. N.: Meningoencephalitis in Infectious Mononucleosis. Report of a case treated with cortisone. J.A.M.A. 162:885, 1956.

Lazar, H. P., Manfredi, R. and Hammond, J. H.: Seizures in Infectious Mononucleosis: With a review of the Literature. Amer. J. Med. 21:990, 1956.

Leibowitz, S.: Infectious Mononucleosis. Modern Medical Monographs, New York, Grune & Stratton, Inc. 1953.

Silver, H. K., Robertson, W. O., Wray, J. D. and Gruskay, F. L.: Involvement of the Central Nervous System in Infectious Mononucleosis in Childhood. A.M.A.J. Dis. Child. 91:490, 1956.

Stokes, J. F., Owen, J. R., and Holmes, E. G.: Neurological Complications of Infective Hepatitis. Brit. Med. J. 2:642, 1945.

Tiese, M. J., Chen, S. and Radding, J.: Guillain-Barre Syndrome in Infectious Mononucleosis: Report of case with recovery following Administration of Cortisone. A.M.A. Arch. Int. Med. 92:438, 1953.

Walsh, F. C., Poser, C. M. and Carter, S.: Infectious Mononucleosis Encephalitis. Pediat. 13:536, 1954.

POLIOMYELITIS

Poliomyelitis is a viral disease with general manifestations which include upper respiratory or gastrointestinal symptoms. On occasion the disease involves the central nervous system, especially the spinal cord and brain stem, producing flaccid paralysis of various muscle groups.

CLINICAL PICTURE: After an incubation period of seven to fourteen days the disease is ushered in with sore throat, headache, nausea, vomiting, and fever. Constipation and some general abdominal pain may be present. The picture is one of an upper respiratory or gastrointestinal upset during the summer or fall season. In most instances the child returns to normal. This form has been classified as abortive. On the basis of epidimological studies such as isolation of the virus and demonstration of high antibody titer in the blood, it is felt that numerous instances of inapparent infection or abortive forms must take place to account for the immunity to poliomyelitis present in so much of the population.

Instead of recovery as in the abortive form, the clinical picture may become more extensive and involve the nervous system. There is then noted stiffness of the neck and rigidity of the back "poker spine," due to muscle spasm. This is brought out even more by asking the child to sit up from a supine position and attempt to kiss his knees while they are being held down. He will be unable to do this because of muscle spasm of the back muscles. The child maintains a sitting posture by putting his hands on the bed behind him for support. There is also spasm of the hamstring muscles. Kernig's sign is present; also Brudzinski's. A lumbar puncture done at this stage shows a clear fluid under increased pressure and some increase in cells, 50-200 per cu./mm., with a lymphocytic differential. If the fluid is examined very early at the onset of the disease, there may be a polymorphonuclear preponderance. The sugar is normal, protein increased. Culture is bacteriologically sterile. This stage is referred to as non-paralytic poliomyelitis. Many children go on to resolution as in the abortive forms without paralysis setting in.

Finally, we have the paralytic form of poliomyelitis. This most often occurs immediately following the development of the symptoms and signs of the non-paralytic stage, but instead of resolution, paralysis sets in. In other instances, after the abortive form has ended, following an interval of about three days, there is a recrudescence of symptoms and signs with the development of paralysis. This is called the dromedary type.

In the course of the development of paralysis there are present marked hyperesthesia, increased muscle tenderness, and spasm. Two major types of paralysis are seen, spinal and bulbar. The spinal type is associated with flaccid paralysis since the major pathology is present in the ventral horn cells. The greatest number of children have combinations of paralysis of the legs and some other part of the body. Involvement of the legs alone occurs in about fifty per cent of cases. The arms or trunk muscles are rarely solely involved. The paralysis of muscles is usually not symmetrical. It is selective rather than involving an entire extremity. Thus, the muscles of the hip or shoulder girdle may show paralysis and not other parts of the leg or arm. At the onset of the attack the reflexes may be present, but soon the superficial reflexes, especially the abdominals, are lost, and finally the deep tendon reflexes are also abolished. There is no sensory loss.

In the bulbar form the various cranial nerve nuclei are affected, especially V, IX, X, and XI. There may be combined bulbar and spinal cord involvement (bulbospinal type). The muscles used for swallowing, normally the palatal and pharyngeal, are frequently involved. There is a nasal tone to the voice, and regurgitation of fluid through the nose is observed. The facial muscles may become paralyzed. Paralysis of respiration may be due to bulbar involvement, or to intercostal or diaphragmatic paralysis. Occasionally encephalitic manifestations of drowsiness, irritation and lack of orientation may develop in association with the bulbospinal type.

The paralysis sets in in most all cases within five days of the appearance of central nervous system involvement. It increases or spreads for about one to two days. At this time fever begins to abate or subside completely. When fever continues, there is apt to be a greater amount of paralysis.

In the course of the illness marked constipation and excessive sweating occur. Bladder function may be disturbed with urinary retention. Hypertension may develop. Electrocardiographic changes are present in about twelve per cent, and include high grade sinus tachycardia, T-wave alterations, and AV conduction variations. These disappear with recovery.

LABORATORY: The spinal fluid is clear, under increased pressure, with an average of about 50-200 cells per cu. mm., highest in the pre-paralytic stage. The majority of the cells are lymphocytes. The protein is slightly elevated, about 50-60 mg. per 100 ml, but in the second and third weeks it becomes markedly elevated to 200 mg. or higher. At this time the cell count returns to normal. The sugar and chlorides are normal. On rare occasions the virus of poliomyelitis may be isolated on culture. Serological tests demonstrate a rising titer of neutralizing antibodies for the poliomyelitis virus.

PATHOGENESIS: The virus of poliomyelitis resides primarily in the alimentary tract. It is present in the oropharynx where it enters the body and much of it has passed from the alimentary canal by way of the feces. The virus multiplies in the alimentary tract and in the regional lymph nodes. If the latter absorb and neutralize it, there is no viremia, so that the major antibody resistance is in the nodes. However, when this does not occur, the excess virus spills into the blood, whence, the principal invasion of the nervous system takes place. Sabin postulates that from the various sites of multiplication in the alimentary tract and extraneural tissues the virus invades the corresponding ganglia and then spreads to the corresponding areas of the central nervous system.

There is also some axonal spread of the virus along nerve pathways. This is seen in the bulbar type which follows tonsillectomy and in the poliomyelitis which develops in an extremity after an inoculation. Newborns rarely are affected by poliomyelitis probably because maternal antibodies are transferred to the baby in utero, or because of a placental barrier. Elliot and McAllister believe this is due to the inactivity of the fetal muscles and associated inactivity of the motor cells in the cortex and spinal cord. When the mother has paralytic poliomyelitis during pregnancy prior to delivery, the newborn baby may become infected with poliomyelitis virus, but does not develop congenital poliomyelitis. If, however, the mother is in the preparalytic state at the time of labor, there is a greater chance of paralytic poliomyelitis in the baby after birth because the transfer of protective antibody may not as yet have occurred. The mechanism of infection may be viremia, ingestion of virus during passage through the birth canal, or squeezing of placental virus into the infant's circulation during labor.

PATHOLOGY: The major change is a selective destruction of the neuron since mainly the motor neurons of the ventral horns and cranial nuclei are involved. In the area of necrosis there are perivascular infiltration of cells as well as infiltration of the adventitia of the arterioles with lymphocytes (perivascular cuffing). Glial proliferation is noted. The large motor cells of the ventral horns of the spinal cord are mostly involved. They show chromotolysis, disappearance of Nissl bodies, and eccentric nuclei. In the neurons which recover from attack there may be acidophilic intranuclear inclusion bodies, but these are not diagnostic. There is little edema or meningeal reaction.

The loss of function of the peripheral nerves and muscles is secondary to the motor cell destruction. Other areas are involved such as the medulla, especially the motor nuclei for the cranial nerves, and reticular formation. The spinal cord and medulla are the chief areas of pathology. However, the cerebellum, brain stem, and cortex (motor areas) are also damaged. To a much lesser extent the posterior ganglia (sensory) are likewise affected.

ETIOLOGY: There are three types of virus immunologically separated, I or Brunhilde, II or Lansing, and III or Leon. Type I has been responsible for most of the cases. One may have had poliomyelitis with Type I and be susceptible to another attack from the other strains.

EPIDEMIOLOGY: In the United States outbreaks occur sporadically throughout the year, but the greatest incidence is from May through September.

The virus is present in the mucosa of the oropharynx, alimentary tract, and blood. It has been demonstrated in the feces for weeks after an acute illness. It is also found in the spinal cord and brain of humans. The method of spread is not completely known, but it is thought to be by way of the feces and pharyngeal secretions. Insects such as flies and mosquitoes, and food such as contaminated milk, may play a secondary role. Fatigue and chilling make for greater susceptibility. Pregnancy, especially in the second and third trimesters, exposes a woman to greater risk. Potential danger to the embryo for the development of congenital pathology is greatest in the first trimester.

DIAGNOSIS: In the non-paralytic stage of poliomyelitis quite a number of clinical entities must be differentiated. The bacterial meningitides have turbid instead of clear fluid, organisms are found on smear and culture, and there is a low spinal fluid sugar. Tuberculous spinal fluid, while similar in many respects to that of poliomyelitis, has a low spinal fluid sugar and chloride; organisms are found on smear and culture. There are usually other evidences of tuberculous infection, a positive tuberculin skin test, and a history of exposure. The aseptic meningitis syndrome due to Coxsackie A & B group and ECHO viruses has similar spinal fluid findings, but the three agents can be differentiated by serology (rising titer neutralizing antibodies) and isolation of the virus. The postinfectious encephalitic group can be differentiated by the associated disease (e.g., measles or mumps) and serologic techniques; infectious mononucleosis by the presence of atypical cells in the blood smear and the heterophile test. Epidemic pleurodynia (Coxsackie-Group B) is separated by isolation of the virus and rise in antibody titer in the patient's serum. Other viral encephalitides may be tested for by two stage serology study. Other conditions such as osteomyelitis and acute rheumatic fever must be thought of under certain conditions.

When the paralytic stage has been reached, the diagnosis is readily made. Infectious neuronitis (Guillain-Barré) produces an albuminocytologic dissociation (few or no cells in the spinal fluid with very high protein); this may be confusing in the later stages of poliomyelitis. However, in infectious neuronitis the paralysis is more symmetrical and sensory symptoms more prominent. Peripheral neuritis may be associated with a history of an injection or chewing of paint flakes, for example. In diphtheria there may be peripheral neuritis or palatal palsy, but there are usually ocular palsies with loss of accommodation, which are lacking in poliomyelitis. Together with diphtheria, both tetanus and rabies may be ruled out by the history. Bulbar palsy due to food poisoning (botulism) is recognized by the history of eating contaminated food and marked involvement of the ocular muscles. Paralysis due to brain abscess or encephalitis is apt to be associated with pyramidal tract signs, e.g., spasticity and Babinski. Paralysis following vaccination against smallpox or injections for rabies or pertussis can be diagnosed by the history of inoculation. Transverse myelitis is characterized by sensory and motor paralyses, a definite cord level, and spastic paralysis subsequently. Occasionally a child is brought for examination because of sudden "paralysis" of a limb. The child cannot stand on one leg, or limps. This may be due to unnoticed injury, producing sprain or epiphyseal separation. Undue use of the limb may produce pseudoparalysis, as in excessive bicycle riding. There may be a toxic synovitis producing a limp due to involvement of the hip. In infants, scurvy, osteomyelitis, congenital syphilis, and bone complications secondary to salmonella infection also should be differentiated.

TREATMENT: The patient should lie on a good, firm mattress or bedboard. When paralysis is present, a padded footboard is used for the legs. This will prevent pressure from the bedclothes and keep the ankles flexed, avoiding ankle drop. The patient's position should be changed frequently to prevent bed sores. In the acute stage, warm, moist packs may be applied to the painful areas for twenty minutes, several times a day if possible. Furmethide® may be used subcutaneously to empty the bladder; otherwise catheterization is employed. When the pain in the extremities has subsided, passive motion may be used for the paralyzed parts. When bulbar symptoms are present, a nasal tube for feedings is necessary. Parenteral fluids and antibiotics should be given if needed. Sedation should be administered for marked anxiety.

In intercostal and diaphragmatic paralysis with resulting respiratory difficulty there are first noted an increased rate of breathing and asymmetry of the thorax, a staccato type of speech, and anxiety and restlessness with inability to sleep. For therapy, a tank respirator is best to supply oxygen and get rid of CO_2. Later this can be replaced by a cuirass-type respirator and rocking bed for the purpose of weaning the child away from the tank respirator.

In bulbar poliomyelitis with pharyngeal paralysis the patient requires postural drainage and aspiration of the throat (tube in pharynx) to eliminate secretions in order to avoid block of the airway. If not successful, tracheotomy should be done. It is important to watch the blood pressure, for a fall may mean medullary involvement and death.

Fluid should be carefully administered to avoid edema, and electrolytes should be controlled, observing especially the potassium and CO_2 levels in the blood.

With convalescence, various therapies may be instituted to restore function. These include hydrotherapy after the pain is gone, electrical stimulation of the muscles, physical and occupational therapy, and muscle reeducation. The orthopedist should be brought in to help in preventing deformity and crippling. In this way the child may be rehabilitated, so that he can get the maximum use of what muscle function he has left.

PROGNOSIS: The prognosis for life in poliomyelitis is good. The mortality is about five per cent. It is highest in bulbar poliomyelitis, in which it reaches thirty per cent. If recovery occurs in the bulbar form there are usually no residuals. However, in a recent report of an epidemic in Israel, there were quite a number of facial palsies which persisted, especially where there had been severe bulbar palsy. In the spinal form recovery begins about a week after the onset of paralysis and may be marked for two or three months, particularly if there is an active therapeutic program for muscle training. Beyond this time there is apt to be a residual difficulty which will require a long term program of rehabilitation. Bennett has listed the factors determining recovery. These include the site and extent of central nervous system involvement. Lesions in the cervical region will produce greater loss of functional capacity than those in the thoracolumbar region. When a muscle has innervation from more than one cord level, it may not be as severely affected as a muscle receiving its supply from only one level. Community resources are another factor. The age of the patient is important, for in the young child who has not yet learned to walk prior to his attack, there are more apt to be disturbances of growth and the development of abnormal muscular patterns with deformity. The attitude of the patient and his family also plays a great role.

PROPHYLAXIS: There is no specific drug therapy once the disease has set in. Therefore, the prevention of poliomyelitis has always been the goal. This appears to have been accomplished through the use of the Salk vaccine. All children and adults should receive the vaccine, even if they have had poliomyelitis, for having had the disease with Type 1, for example, does not protect against Types 2 and 3. The vaccine, containing as it does all three types, will protect against all three strains. The Salk vaccine is administered subcutaneously in 1 cc. doses. Three injections are given, the first two, four to six weeks apart, the third seven months after the second injection.

Tonsillectomy should not be performed during the poliomyelitis season. The weight of evidence suggests that there is a greater susceptibility to the bulbar type if the child does contract poliomyelitis in the few weeks following tonsillectomy.

A Symposium on Poliomyelitis. Pediat. Clin. N. A. Philadelphia, W. B. Saunders Co. Vol. I, No. 1A, 1952.
Bodian, D.: Pathology and Immunity in Poliomyelitis, p. 5.
Steigman, A. J.: Diagnosis and general care of acute poliomyelitis, p. 12.
Wilson, J. L.: Treatment of Acute Respiratory Difficulty, p. 20.
Wright, J.: Physical therapy in Poliomyelitis, p. 26.
Bennett, R. L.: Evaluation of End Results of Acute Anterior Poliomyelitis. J.A.M.A. 162:851, 1956.
Bradford, H. A. and Anderson, L. L.: Electrocardiographic observations during a poliomyelitis epidemic. Ann. Int. Med. 32:270, 1950.
Coryllos, E.: Etiology and Occurrence of Arterial Hypertension in Poliomyelitis. A Review of Literature. Arch. Pediat. 70:122, 1953.
Enders, J. F., Weller, T. H., and Robbins, F. C.: Cultivation of the Lansing Strain of Poliomyelitis Virus in Cultures of various Human Embryonic Tissues. Science 109:85, 1949.
Galloway, T. C.: Relation of Tonsillectomy and Adenoidectomy to Poliomyelitis. J.A.M.A. 163:519, 1957.
Godenne, M. O., and Riordan, J. T.: Tissue culture diagnosis of Poliomyelitis and Aseptic Meningitis. J.A.M.A. 158:707, 1955.
McCrea, M. G.: Isolation of the Type I Poliomyelitis Virus from Human Cerebrospinal Fluid. Pediat. 19:869, 1957.
Neva, F. A.: Poliomyelitis in a family with occurrence of localized paralysis after inoculation with combined Diphtheria, Pertussis, Tetanus Vaccine. Pediat. 18:59, 1956.
Rosen, L. and Thoaris, G.: Poliomyelitis following injection. A.M.J. Hyg. 57:237, 1953.
Sabin, A. B.: Pathogenesis of Poliomyelitis. Science 123:1151, 1956.
Salk, J. E.: Studies in human subjects on active immunization against poliomyelitis. 1. A Preliminary report of experiments in progress. J.A.M.A. 151:1081, 1953.

Siegel, M. and Greenberg, M. J.: Poliomyelitis in Pregnancy: Effect on fetus and newborn infant. Pediat. 49:280, 1956.
Winsser, J., Pfaff, M. L., and Seanor, H. E.: Poliomyelitis Viremia in a Newborn Infant. Pediat. 20:458, 1957.
Winter, S. T.: Facial paralysis in Poliomyelitis. Pediat. 19:876, 1957.

HERPES ZOSTER

Known also as "shingles," this disease is an acute viral infection which attacks primarily the posterior root ganglia. It may be accompanied by vesicular eruptions on the skin which occupy the same dermatome as the affected ganglion. There is marked pain.

ETIOLOGY: Herpes zoster is due to a virus. The elementary bodies may be seen under the electron-microscope in vesicular fluid taken in the first forty-eight hours of the attack. The viruses of herpes zoster and chicken pox are similar, and inoculation of the zoster vesicular fluid will produce chicken pox lesions in children who have not had the disease, but not in those who already have been afflicted. Cross fixation of complement and cross agglutination of elementary bodies occur between the two diseases.

The incubation period is seven to fourteen days, as determined by human inoculation experiments. The disease occurs only occasionally in childhood. At times it develops secondary to irritation from trauma to the spine, lumbar puncture, or osseous tuberculosis. Pressure on the ganglia from malignancy such as Hodgkin's disease may produce the symptomatology of herpes zoster. X-ray therapy and intramuscular injections have also been mentioned as secondary causes. Two cases of herpes zoster were reported following the use of cortisone or ACTH for other illnesses.

Involvement of the nervous system most often occurs in the lower thoracic and upper lumbar areas in children. Rarely, the maxillary and cervical regions are affected.

PATHOLOGY: In the acute stage hemorrhages may be found in the ganglia, along with mononuclear infiltration in the form of perivascular cuffs and degenerative changes in the nerve cells. The inflammatory reaction extends to the meninges.

CLINICAL PICTURE: In children the attacks are usually milder than in adults. There is pain, followed by the vesicular eruption on the skin in about four days. The vesicles appear in clusters and may produce a burning sensation. This takes place in the same dermatome as the affected nerve and is usually unilateral. One or more dermatomes may be affected. Encephalitic symptoms are not common but may occasionally be seen. The skin lesions dry up and scab and disappear in one to two weeks.

Various types of zoster in the nervous system have been described, such as ophthalmic zoster from the first division of the gasserian ganglion (ophthalmic division of the 5th nerve), which may cause conjunctivitis, keratitis, iritis, scarring of the cornea, or secondary glaucoma. In geniculate zoster there may be facial paralysis with loss of taste in the anterior two-thirds of the tongue. There may be spread of the inflammation from the posterior (sensory) to the anterior (motor) horn, which may lead to wasting of the muscles.

LABORATORY: In the meningoencephalitic form there is a lymphocytosis in the spinal fluid. The protein is normal or slightly increased, sugar and chlorides are normal. Bacterial culture is sterile. Elementary bodies are usually not seen in the spinal fluid.

DIAGNOSIS: A diagnosis is made by the presence of the characteristic skin lesions.

PROGNOSIS: In children the course is generally favorable.

TREATMENT: Soothing lotions may be used for the skin lesions and sedation for the pain. X-ray therapy may be given to the affected segments in Hodgkin's disease. Steroids may be tried, but their value is questionable.

Brain, W. R.: Zoster Varicella and Encephalitis. Brit. Med. Journal 1:81, 1931.
Burgoon, Jr., C. F., Burgoon, J. S., and Baldridge, G. D.: The Natural History of Herpes Zoster. J.A.M.A. 164:265, 1957.
Good, R. A., Vernier, R. L. and Smith, R. T.: Cortisone and Adrenocorticotropin in Pediatric Practice (Part I). Pediat. 19:95, 1957.
Schmidt, R. P., Roseman, E. and Steigman, A. J.: Cranial Nerve Paralysis in Herpes Zoster Encephalitis of Childhood. J. Pediat. 46:215, 1955.
Shev, E. E.: Ramsay Hunt Syndrome (Geniculate Zoster): Pediat. Clin. N. A. Philadelphia, W. B. Saunders Co. Feb. 1955.

RICKETTSIAL DISEASES

Tick Typhus or Rocky Mountain Spotted Fever

This is an acute, febrile, self-limited, infectious disease. It is caused by Rickettsia rickettsii, an obligate, intracellular parasite of ticks and rodents. The latter are the probable reservoir. The disease is transmitted to man by the bite of the adult tick. In the western U.S.A. the wood tick, Dermacentor andersoni, and in the eastern U.S.A. the dog tick, Dermacentor variabilis, are the principal vectors.

The western disease affects mainly adults over forty. It occurs in the spring and early summer and has a higher mortality than the eastern. The latter occurs chiefly in the summer, and almost half the cases are in children under fifteen years. The seasonal incidence is in keeping with the prevalence of the wood and dog ticks.

CLINICAL PICTURE: After an incubation period of four to eight days there is an abrupt onset with headache, chills, and sharp rise of fever. On the second or third day of the illness a characteristic rash appears, beginning in the extremities, particularly the ankles and wrists, then extending to the trunk. It is macular at first, then petechial. Toward the end of the first week neck stiffness and cloudy sensorium appear due to acute meningoencephalitis. The illness lasts about two to three weeks.

LABORATORY: The spinal fluid shows a pleocytosis of a few cells to one hundred eighty per cu. mm., mostly lymphocytes, increased protein, and normal sugar. At the onset the blood picture may show a leucopenia, later leucocytosis. Complement fixation is positive and diagnostic during the second week of the illness. Agglutinins against Proteus ox19 are present in rising titer, seven to fifteen days after the onset (Weil-Felix Reaction).

PATHOLOGY: Changes are especially noted in the skin, central nervous system, and testis in the form of an acute arteritis, although all tissues are somewhat involved. There is endothelial proliferation leading ultimately to occlusion, thrombosis, or necrosis of the small arterioles. There is also a generalized capillary injury, which is a major feature of the disease. Rickettsia organisms are found in the vessels. The brain shows petechial hemorrhages as well as arteriole thrombosis, and perivascular inflammation. Glial nodules are noted. The vessels of the brain stem are particularly involved.

DIAGNOSIS: The diagnosis should be made on the history, rash, and Proteus agglutination and complement fixation tests showing rising antibody titers in the second week of the disease.

The differential diagnosis is made from meningococcemia by the history of tick bite and characteristic skin rash. Often ticks are still to be found on the child's clothing. Furthermore, spinal fluid and blood cultures should identify meningococcus. In murine typhus the rash is much milder and mostly on the trunk. Typhoid fever and measles should also be ruled out.

PROGNOSIS: There is a fifteen per cent mortality in children. Various central nervous system sequelae may occur, including mental deterioration and disturbances of speech, vision, and hearing.

TREATMENT: Prophylaxis can be accomplished by preventative vaccination, but this would be required yearly; therefore, it is not practical as a general measure. Ticks should be looked for through daily inspection and carefully removed from the clothing and scalp. They should be picked up with tweezers and gloves, not crushed. Once the disease has set in, chloramphenicol or terramycin should be used. Electrolytes and blood transfusion are also helpful in severe cases.

ENDEMIC (MURINE) TYPHUS

Murine typhus is caused by the parasite Rickettsia mooseri, which is transmitted to children by the bite of the rat flea. It occurs mostly in the summer and fall.

CLINICAL PICTURE: There is an abrupt onset with fever, headache, chills, and a rash which usually appears on the trunk on the third day. The rash then extends to the remainder of the body, especially the extremities. The illness terminates by lysis in about two weeks. In some patients there are meningeal signs, including neck stiffness and Kernig's sign.

The European type (Epidemic Typhus), due to Rickettsia prowazeki and transmitted by the body louse, does not usually affect children. When it does, the attack is generally mild. The clinical picture is somewhat similar to the above.

PATHOLOGY: As in tick fever, the lesions are primarily vascular, especially in the skin and brain. In the brain there is arteriole thrombosis and endothelial proliferation. Glial nodules are also present.

DIAGNOSIS: The Weil-Felix reaction is positive in at least 1:320 dilution, and also complement fixation. These positive tests are obtained at the end of the first week.

TREATMENT: Chrolamphenicol and Terramycin should be used for therapy. For prophylaxis, typhus vaccine should be administered. In addition, measures such as delousing and D.D.T. should be applied.

Cawley, E. P. and Wheeler, C. E.: Rocky Mountain Spotted Fever. J.A.M.A. 163:1003, 1957.
Peterson, J. C., Overall, J. C., and Shapiro, J. L.: Rickettsial Diseases of Childhood. J. Pediat. 30:495, 1947.
Smadell, J. E.: Present Status of Antibiotic Therapy in Viral and Rickettsial Disease. Bull. N. Y. Acad. Med., 26:221, 1951.
Thomas, M. H., and Berlin, L.: Neurologic Sequelae of Rocky Mountain Spotted Fever. Arch. Neurol. and Psychiat. 60:574, 1948.

BEHCET'S SYNDROME

Behcet's syndrome consists primarily of lesions in the eyes, and ulceration in the mouth and genitalia.

CLINICAL PICTURE: The patient is most often a young adult. The presenting complaint is usually ulceration in the mouth or genitalia or a painful infected eye. Ulcers also appear on the skin and are recurrent and painful. The commonest eye lesion is hypopyon. Other ocular lesions include uveitis, iridocyclitis and conjunctivitis. There is low grade fever. Thrombophlebitis may be present.

When the central nervous system is affected there is evidence of meningoencephalitis with neck stiffness, Kernig and Babinski sign, and active deep tendon reflexes. Ophthalmoplegia may be present. In some cases, there is marked mental confusion with progressive deterioration. Wadia and Williams reported thirteen cases of Behcet's syndrome with neurological complications and stated that these involved the brain stem or were meningomyelitic. They stressed the development of progressive dementia.

LABORATORY: The spinal fluid shows a slight cellular increase, occasionally marked, otherwise it is normal.

PATHOLOGY: There is a diffuse involvement of the meninges, cortex and brain stem particularly. This consists of small softenings in relation to smaller blood vessels. The inflammatory reaction is mild. Myelin loss is secondary.

ETIOLOGY: The cause of this disease is unknown. A viral basis has been postulated (see reference of Evans, Pallis and Spillane).

DIAGNOSIS: The diagnosis is based upon the presence of ocular and cutaneous manifestations, complicated by the development of meningoencephalitis. Other etiological factors, bacterial and viral must be eliminated, especially syphilis, tuberculosis and sarcoidosis. Multiple sclerosis must also be considered.

PROGNOSIS: The outlook for recovery is promising after a protracted course, including remissions and exacerbations. If the nervous system is involved, the prospects are more grave.

TREATMENT: Cortisone appears to be of some value.

Evans, A. D., Pallis, C. A. and Spillane, J. D.: Involvement of the Nervous System in Behcet's Syndrome. Lancet 273:349, 1957.
McMenemey, W. H. and Lawrence, B. J.: Encephalomyelopathy in Behcet's disease. Lancet 273:353, 1957.
Wadia, N. and Williams, E.: Behcet's Syndrome with Neurological Complications. Brain 80:59, 1957.
Whitty, C. W. M.: Neurologic Implications of Behcet's Syndrome. Neurology 8:369, 1958.

PARASITIC INFECTIONS OF THE CENTRAL NERVOUS SYSTEM

CYSTICERCOSIS CEREBRI

Invasion of the brain is caused by the Cysticercus cellulosae, the larval stage of the cestode, Taenia solium. This is usually due to eating uncooked pork. The larvae are encysted in the skeletal muscles of the pig and so ingested. Man is also infected by eating food contaminated with the feces of an individual who harbors the adult tapeworm. The eggs are hatched in the small intestine, and the organisms penetrate the wall, enter the blood stream, and encyst wherever they localize, mainly in the skeletal muscles, chambers of the eye, and especially in the brain.

PATHOLOGY: In the nervous system the cysticerci are usually present in the leptomeninges or brain tissue. They become encapsulated and calcify. They are usually multiple, each about one cm. in size. A cyst may project from the meninges into the brain tissue, especially in the cerebellum and brain stem (racemose cysts). With death of the larvae there is marked granulomatous inflammatory reaction in the leptomeninges with giant cells and fibrosis. The cysts may be seen in the cortex, ventricles, basal ganglia, and base of the brain.

CLINICAL PICTURE: The clinical picture may be similar to that of a tumor with block of the flow of cerebrospinal fluid, headache, and papilledema. The symptoms and signs are those of the area involved. If cerebellar, there is ataxia and hypotonia. If cortical, there may be focal epilepsy. Cysts at the base of the brain produce arachnoiditis. There may be involvement of the cisterna magna with resulting hydrocephalus.

In children the course of the disease may be more rapid with fever, headache, and convulsion. There are signs of increased intracranial pressure, papilledema, and mental impairment, but the impression is often one of generalized infection rather than of localized tumor.

Usually, however, the course is slow and insidious with symptoms from infection of the brain developing years after the original entry of the larvae.

LABORATORY: The spinal fluid shows an elevated protein and a pleocytosis of 15 to 100 cells, per cu. mm., either neutrophiles, lymphocytes, or eosinophiles in the early stages. Occasionally there is a low sugar.

X-RAY: The skull may show evidence of increased pressure with an enlarged sella and erosion of the clinoid processes. Extremely diagnostic is the presence of multiple, small, diffuse areas of intracranial calcification. Ventriculography may show dilatation of the ventricles and diffuse cortical atrophy.

Complement fixation (serum) and skin tests may be positive.

DIAGNOSIS: Cysticercosis cerebri should be suspected when brain tumor is being considered. The diagnosis may be made by identifying the ova or segments of the worm passed in the stools. Scolices from the material removed at operation may be diagnostic.

Cysticercosis should be differentiated from infection by Echinococcus granulosis which forms hydatid cysts. Humans are infected in the latter by the accidental ingestion of dog feces. The differential is made by identification of the hooklets or scolices if a cyst is removed. Otherwise the Casoni test may be used to establish the presence of echinococcus disease. One-quarter cc. of antigen obtained from hydatid fluid is injected intradermally. A positive reaction (infiltration and edema of at least 4 cm. in diameter) at the end of twenty-four hours indicates present or past infection and in association with the hydatid cysts is diagnostic.

PROGNOSIS: If there is a solitary cerebral cyst, this may be completely removed. Otherwise the outlook is grave.

TREATMENT: Surgery should be used to evacuate the cysts.

Dent, J. H.: Cysticercosis Cerebri-Cestode Infestation of Human Brain. J.A.M.A. 164:401, 1957.
Griponissiotis, B.: Hydatid Cyst of the Brain and Its Treatment. Neurology 7:789, 1957.
Obrador, S.: Clinical Aspects of Cerebral Cysticercosis. Arch. Neurol. & Psychiat. 59:457, 1948.
White, J. C., Sweet, W. H., and Richardson, Jr., E. P.: Cysticercosis Cerebri: A Diagnostic and Therapeutic Problem of Increasing Importance. New England J. Med. 256:479, 1957.

TRICHINOSIS

This is probably the most common parasitic infection in the United States. Autopsy data suggest that twenty per cent of the population is infected. The disease is caused by the ingestion of uncooked meat, usually pork. The larvae migrate through the intestinal walls and localize especially in the diaphragm, intercostal muscles, and muscles of the eyes. When the myocardium or central nervous system is invaded the outlook is most serious.

CLINICAL PICTURE: There are usually three clinical stages in trichinosis. In the first there are gastrointestinal symptoms of nausea, vomiting, diarrhea, and abdominal cramps. This probably corresponds to the period when the encysted larvae are liberated from the ingested meat and develop into adult worms (T. spiralis). The ova of the female worms are deposited in the duodenal mucosa where they mature into larvae. During the second stage, about a week after the onset, when the larvae are migrating by way of the systemic circulation to the various tissues, there is marked pain in the skeletal muscles, urticaria, periorbital edema, and fever. This stage lasts three to six weeks. During this period the central nervous system may be invaded. Those whose course is fatal usually die at this time. Recovery, however, is the rule, and the final stage is one of slow convalescence with encystment of the larvae.

With involvement of the nervous system there may be general features including headache, neck stiffness, mental confusion, and stupor. There is also a loss of deep tendon reflexes in about ten per cent. This type has a good outlook. A more severe form occurs with the development of focal cerebral pathology. There may be cerebellar signs or hemiplegia with a Babinski sign. Convulsion is not a frequent feature here as it is in cysticercosis.

LABORATORY:
> The blood shows a leucocytosis and eosinophilia.
> The precipitin test (blood) and intradermal skin test are positive in the third week.
> Muscle biopsy shows the encysted larvae.
> The spinal fluid may be normal or contain a few cells including eosinophiles. Larvae are occasionally seen in the spinal fluid.

PATHOLOGY: The neurological symptoms appear to be due to mechanical obstruction of the end-arteries and capillaries by the larvae, or to a toxic or allergic reaction. The latter consists of an antibody-antigen reaction with altered permeability of the capillaries and edema of the nerve cells. In the brain there are microscopic changes in the form of granulomata containing lymphocytes, plasma cells, giant cells, and microglia. Larvae may be seen in the nodules. There are also perivascular infiltration and endothelial proliferation.

PROGNOSIS: Recovery with few if any residuals is the rule since the advent of steroid therapy.

TREATMENT: Cortisone should be used in adequate doses.

Greenstein, N. M. and Steinberg, D.: The Prompt and Effective Response of Trichinosis to Corticotropin. A.M.A.J. Dis. Child. 95:261, 1958.
Hurd, R. W.: Focal Cerebral Injury Due to Trichinella Spiralis. J. Nerv. and Ment. Dis. 117:526, 1953.

Meltzer, L. E. and Bockman, A. A.: Trichinosis Involving the Central Nervous System. Treatment with Corticotropin (ACTH) and Cortisone. J.A.M.A. 164:1566, 1957.

Merritt, H. H. and Rosenbaum, M.: Involvement of Nervous System in Trichinosis. J.A.M.A. 106:1646, 1936.

Most, H. and Abeles, M. M.: Trichinosis Involving Nervous System: Clinical and Neuropathologic Review, with Report of Two Cases. Arch. Neurol. and Psychiat. 37:589, 1937.

CHOREA

Chorea is characterized by a series of movements of the muscles of the face, extremities, and trunk, which are sudden, rapid, purposeless, and involuntary. The basis for the disturbance lies primarily in the cortex and extrapyramidal system. It is noted as a congenital form, in pregnancy (chorea gravidarum), as a chronic progressive adult disease (Huntington's), and as a childhood type (Sydenham's) with which we are primarily concerned.

SYDENHAM'S CHOREA (CHOREA MINOR, ST. VITUS DANCE)

CLINICAL PICTURE: Chorea minor occurs most often between the ages of seven to twelve years. There have been occasional case reports of an onset before four years or over twenty, but for clinical purposes it is a disease which appears in the prepuberty and puberty age primarily. Chorea is seen more often in girls, the ratio being 2:1. Its onset is most frequent in the winter and spring. The beginning of the attack may be gradual or sudden, often being attributed to some experience which has frightened or shocked the child. The mother may note that her daughter is frequently dropping a spoon while eating, or a pencil while writing. Facial grimaces and a change in disposition may be observed. There are increased fatigue and a tendency to emotional upsets. Purposeless movements of the face, extremities, and trunk are noted. The tongue is uncontrollable. Speech is thick, slurred, and indistinct. The gait is poor and the child stumbles or falls. The muscles are weak and hypotonic. The movements are jerky, aimless, incoordinated, and lack control, but cease during sleep.

Examination brings out the main features of the disease. When the child is asked to hold the arms and hands extended forward, there is inability to keep the hands in this position; instead, there are jerky movements resulting in marked flexion of the wrists and hyperextension of the fingers. When the arms are held upward there is pronation of the forearms, so that the backs of the hands face each other. The tongue when protruded cannot be held in one position; it is extended quickly, or rapidly pulled into the mouth. If an extreme effort is made to hold it out, it may be bitten by the uncontrollable action of the jaw muscles. Speech is indistinct because the tongue wobbles about the mouth. When the child is offered a pencil and asked to write her name, the scrawl is obvious and incoordination is demonstrated. Hand grasp may begin with firmness due to spasmodic contraction of the muscles, but soon becomes weak and gradually limp. This is due to inability of the muscles to sustain any effort. When the child is asked to walk, she displays unsteadiness, incoordination, and jerky movements of the head and trunk which interfere with the steadiness of the gait. At rest all movements are diminished. At times there may be involvement of only one side of the body (hemichorea). The cranial nerves are not affected.

There are no sensory disturbances. The reflexes are normal but may vary. At times, when the knee (patella tendon) is tapped, the leg remains extended for a few seconds, then relaxes slowly (hung-up or caught-up reflex). At other times the knee jerk is diminished and may be pendular, relaxing in a series of slow, jerky movements.

There are apt to be mental and emotional changes. The children vary in their moods. They are unstable, easily provoked to tears or laughter. There is marked hyperexcitability in the presence of visitors. Occasionally there are bad dreams or mania, the children thrashing in their beds violently.

LABORATORY: The blood count and sedimentation rate are generally normal. The spinal fluid is also negative. The electroencephalogram is not significant.

PATHOLOGY: Since chorea minor is a disease in which complete recovery usually occurs, there is no clear evidence as to the nature of the pathology. In the older literature changes of a degenerative, vascular, and inflammatory nature have been observed in the cortex, basal ganglia, and cerebellum. Colony and Malamud refer to Sydenham's chorea as a syndrome of rheumatic fever, disseminated lupus, encephalitis, and toxi-degenerative conditions of undetermined etiology.

ETIOLOGY: Chorea is discussed in the pediatric literature as one of the forms of rheumatic fever, which is regarded as related to Group A streptococcus infection. The mechanism whereby rheumatic fever occurs is not as yet clear. The evidence favoring the idea that chorea minor is a major manifestation of rheumatic fever rests on the development of chorea in about 50 per cent of rheumatic fever patients at some time in the course of their illness. Chorea developed as an initial manifestation, with or without carditis, in 127 of 689 children with rheumatic fever. The recurrence rate of carditis and the nature and severity of the recurrent carditis are the same in those with an onset of chorea alone as in those with some other rheumatic manifestation (Jacobsson). Elevation of antistreptolysin titer occurs in "pure chorea" as well as in chorea associated with obvious rheumatic fever. On the other hand, instances of so called "pure chorea" are seen in which there is no evidence of preceding streptococcal infection in the form of sore throat or scarlet fever, and in which there are no manifestations of rheumatic fever either major or minor. In uncomplicated chorea there is no fever, leucocytosis, or increased sedimentation rate. Obviously psychological factors and personality disorders play an important role in the onset and recurrences.

Summarizing the data, the author feels that there is a definite relationship between chorea and rheumatism in most instances but that there are many unexplained cases in which the association cannot be demonstrated. Long-term follow-up studies of "pure chorea" do reveal the development of carditis or other rheumatic manifestations in 50 to 75 per cent.

DIAGNOSIS: The diagnosis of chorea minor depends upon recognition of the abnormal choreiform movements. They must be differentiated from tics or habit spasms. In the latter the involuntary movements affect only a particular group of muscles at one time. While the movements are spasmodic, they can be controlled. There may be repeated winking of the eye, or jerking of the head, or constant sniffling. When the child is asked to look at the examiner or at a pencil, or is otherwise distracted, the tic may cease for a short period. This is not so in chorea. Furthermore, there is no incoordination of movements in the child with habit spasm. He can walk or speak freely. In tic there is apt to be a spread from one localized muscle group to another, cephalad to caudad. The presence of rheumatic manifestations will help in the differential. Tics may follow encephalitis or chorea. In both groups the children are highly emotional and neurotic. The treatment of tic is through psychotherapy.

When the chorea has developed insidiously, or in cases of hemichorea, there may be some difficulty in diagnosis. The athetoid group in cerebral palsy is easily differentiated by the earlier onset and different character of the movements (see Cerebral Palsy). In hemiparesis with pyramidal tract involvement there are increased tendon reflexes, Babinski sign, and spasticity. Chorea secondary to acute encephalitis has spinal fluid changes and cranial nerve palsies diagnostic of the latter. The age of onset rules out congenital chorea. Huntington's disease is usually observed in adult life. In the occasional instance when its onset occurs in childhood, it may be differentiated from Sydenham's chorea by the following characteristics: it is inherited as a Mendelian dominant, strongly familial; the chorea is progressive and associated with mental deterioration; psychotic manifestations are common; and the course of the disease ends in death.

PROGNOSIS: The outlook in chorea is good. Uncomplicated, the average course runs from six to twelve weeks ending in complete recovery. There is a one to two per cent mortality, usually due to carditis. There is, however, some tendency for recurrence in chorea.

TREATMENT: The primary aims in therapy are bed rest and quiet. Visiting should be restricted so as to avoid overstimulation. I see no need for hospitalization of the average, mild case if the parents are intelligent and cooperative. If these conditions do not prevail, or if there is overcrowding in the home, hospitalization should be provided. It should also be recommended in very severe cases where protection of the patient from falling out of bed and injuring herself may require better nursing care, and when more drastic procedures such as cortisone therapy may be required.

Sedation, such as phenobarbital gr. ¼ to ½ should be given as needed to provide proper rest and sleep, not more often than three times a day. Anemia should be treated with a nutritious diet and iron.

At present ACTH and cortisone are being tried. They appear to shorten the course, but it is still a question whether cardiac damage is prevented when the chorea is associated with rheumatic fever.

The child should be examined if at home at least once weekly. The handwriting (child's name) should be obtained each time and filed with the record; this is an additional method of judging recovery. The heart should be listened to carefully. As the weeks go by, the child may be allowed a moderate amount of visiting, reading, and television (no horror films, etc.). Subsequently she may go outdoors. If the attack occurs in the spring, no schooling should be permitted until the fall.

Inasmuch as chorea is regarded as a rheumatic manifestation, it is recommended that the children be put on the same prophylactic regime as rheumatic fever patients, using penicillin 300,000 units once a day or sulfadiazine gr. XV. This may help to avoid recurrences of the disease.

Ainger, L. E., Ely, R. S., Done, A. K. and Kelley, V. C.: Sydenham's Chorea: Effects of Hormone Therapy. A.M.A.J. Dis. Child. 89:580, 1955.

Bland, E. F. and Jones, T. D.: Rheumatic Fever and Rheumatic Heart Disease: A Twenty Year Report on 1000 Patients Followed Since Childhood. Circulation 4:836, 1951.

Colony, H. S. and Malamud, N.: Sydenham's Chorea—A Clinicopathologic Study. Neurology 6:672, 1956.

Harris, T. N., Friedman, S. and McLean, D. C.: Determination of some Streptoccal Antibody Titers and Acute Phase Reactants in Patients with Chorea. Pediat. 21:13, 1958.

Jacobsson, E.: Rheumatic Fever with Chorea Minor. Acta Ped. Vol. 33, Suppl. 7, 1946.

Kagan, B. M., Rosner, D. and Rosenblum, P.: Chorea (Sydenham). Am. J. Dis. Child. 78:306, 1949.

Taranta, A. and Stollerman, G. H.: Relationship of Sydenham's Chorea to Infection with Group A Streptococci. Am. J. Med. 20:170, 1956.

Zausner, D. M.: The Treatment of Tics in Childhood. Arch. Dis. Child. 29:537, 1954.

CHAPTER 9

CONVULSIVE DISORDERS

A convulsion is of serious import to a family and is a most frightening experience both for the child and doctor. It should be looked upon as a medical emergency and as such, treated promptly. It is the most frequent condition seen in pediatric neurology.

Various studies, including our own unpublished data on a series of 550 children admitted for seizures to the Long Island College Hospital from 1925-35, are in agreement that febrile convulsion is the most common type in childhood. The greatest number of seizures occur between six months and thirty-six months of age, and those associated with infection account for the largest portion. Other figures suggest that convulsions occur in about six per cent of all children under five years of age.

The age at which a convulsion first takes place is of value in determining its cause. In the newborn and the period of early infancy, birth injury, either due to traumatic intracranial hemorrhage, anoxia, or both, is of primary importance. In addition, congenital cerebral malformations are to be considered. Other lesser factors include kernicterus, infections, such as meningitis, encephalitis, general sepsis, toxoplasmosis and cytomegalic inclusion disease. Chemical considerations include tetany and rarely hypoglycemia. It is to be noted that in the paranatal period the onset of a seizure is liable to indicate a serious cause with probable organic pathology, except for some of the chemical factors. As we get on to the period past three months and up to four years of age, infection with thermal reaction plays the greatest role. These are referred to as febrile convulsions and are most frequently associated with infection extraneous to the nervous system, such as acute pharyngitis, tonsillitis, acute otitis media, pneumonia, or pyuria. Less frequently, seizures occur with infections of the central nervous system such as meningitis and encephalitis. Occasionally in this period one still sees tetany. Seizures due to postnatal trauma, degenerative disease of the nervous system, lead encephalopathy, and following injections such as antipertussis vaccine are also seen. In the period beyond three years of age the factor of febrile convulsion recedes and epilepsy, that is recurrent paroxysmal seizures, becomes the primary problem.

Neonatal Period and Early Infancy. A careful history of the family background should be obtained. It has been shown that there is a familial susceptibility to seizures. When convulsion occurs in a child, there is a greater number of individuals in the family who have abnormal electroencephalographic patterns and seizures than in the normal population. This shall be interpreted more fully in discussing epilepsy. The pregnancy must be evaluated for any factors which might have produced anoxia in the infant, such as severe anemia in the mother, premature separation of the placenta, or maternal infection. Hyperirritability, course tremor, twitching, or generalized seizures associated with a high-pitched, continuous, piercing cry may be present in an infant born of a mother with drug addiction, e.g., heroin, if the last dose was taken within a week of delivery. Birth trauma is important. It may be due to any abnormal obstetrical factor: for example, malposition of the fetus, high forceps application, prolapsed cord, or breech extraction. We have discussed malformations of the brain, cerebral palsy, birth injuries, and mental deficiency in greater detail in other sections. It is necessary here simply to stress that the seizure is a symptom of the more serious organic background disorder. This is also true when there is meningitis, sepsis, or kernicterus.

Tetany of the newborn is suspected in any child who twitches or has more generalized seizures. It should be considered especially when the physical examination is normal and the baby may not appear to be too ill. The seizures appear shortly after birth. However, they may also begin after the baby has left the hospital. In one instance twitching began a month after a normal delivery. The examination is negative for other types of brain damage previously considered. Rarely, there may be a positive Chvostek, carpopedal spasm, and a positive Trousseau sign. The diagnosis is based on the presence of seizures and a blood serum calcium level below 7.5 mg./100 ml. There is usually an elevated serum phosphorus. The higher concentration of phosphorus in cow's milk together with a functional hypoparathyroidism may both play a role in the production of newborn tetany. It has also been suggested that inability of the kidney to excrete phosphorus may be a factor. Tetany has also been noted in prematures born of diabetic mothers. The treatment of tetany in severe cases is the injection intravenously of 5 to 10 cc. of a 10 per cent solution of calcium gluconate at a rate not to exceed 1 cc. per minute. (Do not administer calcium gluconate intramuscularly in infancy.) There can then be added to the daily formula 30 to 60 grains of calcium lactate for three weeks. In mild cases with occasional twitching, calcium chloride, two to three grams in 2 per cent solution added to the formula, may be given for two days, followed by calcium lactate as indicated above. The prognosis is good for complete recovery. Hypoglycemia as a cause for newborn convulsions is rare. Gellis reported that of 800 infants born of diabetic mothers, only two had hypoglycemia with seizures. (Personal communication.) Seizures associated with hypoglycemia have been precipitated in infants by protein administration (amino acids).

In the physical examination fever may be noted. We have emphasized elsewhere, however, that in the neonatal and period of early infancy, sepsis may be present without fever. Examination may show an enlarged head due to congenital hydrocephalus, a bulging fontanel or neck stiffness suggesting meningitis. There may be absent Moro reflex, weakness or paralysis of the extremities; Chvostek sign, carpopedal spasm, or Trousseau's sign as evidence of tetany, and jaundice shortly after birth suggesting erythroblastosis. Ophthalmoscopic study may reveal hemorrhages, which should suggest intracerebral or subdural hemorrhage. Chorioretinitis suggests toxoplasmosis especially if there is an enlarged head (hydrocephalus) or small head (microcephalus) present with the seizures. Lumbar puncture should be done to help rule out intracranial hemorrhage, meningitis, and encephalitis. Blood culture should be taken for sepsis. Blood calcium and phosphorus levels should be determined. If subdural hematoma is suspected, bilateral subdural punctures should be done. An X-ray of the skull may reveal calcification as in toxoplasmosis, abnormal vascular channels, and fracture.

In considering convulsions in the neonatal period we have stressed looking for the organic background, especially in the brain. Sepsis, meningitis, and occasional chemical alterations have been mentioned. However, the other systems should also be thought of. With twitching and cyanosis, an X-ray of the chest may reveal cardiac anomalies, atelectasis, pneumonia, or an enlarged mediastinal shadow (thymus). Adrenal hemorrhage, usually due to breech extraction or high forceps, may produce twitching and elevated fever. Occasionally the masses in the flanks may be palpated. The outlook in this type is very poor. Therapy consists of cortisone, intravenous glucose and saline, transfusions of blood. Jaundice in the newborn period with seizures leads to a consideration of erythroblastosis, sepsis, cytomegalic inclusion disease or toxoplasmosis. Urine examination and blood chemistry will reveal the possibility of an occasional genitourinary anomaly with infection as a cause for seizures. Reference should also be made to the reported instances of pyridoxine (Vitamin B_6) deficiency, due to the fact that these infants were fed a liquid milk deficient in this vitamin. Seizures occurred at an average age of two and one-half months after birth. The workup was essentially negative except for an abnormal electroencephalogram. The addition of Vitamin B_6 corrected the seizures; a normal EEG followed and the infants developed satisfactorily. Recent studies suggest that in some of these infants, both artificially and breast fed, who have developed seizures, there may not only be deficiency of B_6, but in some, a need for a greater than average requirement. The infant's diet should contain 0.2 to 0.3 mg. of Vitamin B_6 daily. If a convulsion is from an inapparent cause, give 5 to 10 mg. of pyridoxine hydrochloride daily as prophylactic procedure.

Finally, attention is called to the problem of hypernatremia as a cause of convulsions. This condition usually occurs in infants under one year. It is due to dehydration, brought on by severe diarrhea associated with vomiting, or lack of fluid intake. Infection may be present. The baby may be comatose and convulsing. Subdural and subarachnoid hemorrhages may occur. The spinal fluid shows no cellular increase, but there is an elevated protein. The diagnosis is made on the basis of a serum sodium above 150 m. Eq./L. Therapy is directed toward restoration of water loss with glucose and dilute solutions of electrolyte. (See references.)

The treatment of seizures at this age would depend on the cause. The specific and detailed therapy is described in the chapters on meningitis, encephalitis, birth injury, kernicterus, etc. If no cause is found or until specific therapy for the known factor becomes effective, general measures such as the injection intramuscularly of sodium phenobarbital, gr. ⅛ to gr. ½ should be employed. In very severe cases ether may be administered by a trained anesthetist. Oxygen is useful at all times.

When we consider the age period of six months to three years we are discussing that time of childhood when most seizures occur.

The majority are febrile convulsions, e.g., they occur in association with a rise of temperature usually at the onset of the acute illness. The cause of the fever is an infection such as acute tonsillitis, bronchitis, pneumonia, adenitis, otitis media, nephritis, etc. In a smaller number meningitis or encephalitis is present. Roseola infantum may be the cause; the convulsion may occur at the onset of the rise in fever or shortly thereafter. Various infectious diseases like pertussis, measles, mumps, and chicken pox must be considered as they may be complicated with a convulsion due to encephalitis. Occasionally seizures occur in infectious mononucleosis. In the child with a febrile convulsion, inquiry should be made concerning familial seizures, the type of delivery, developmental progress of the infant, and the present illness. In the majority of febrile seizures, the past history will be normal and examination will reveal an acute infection extraneous to the central nervous system. The spinal fluid will usually be normal. Therapy is aimed at reducing the fever and stopping the seizures as quickly as possible. For this purpose, sodium phenobarbital, grains one to two, or gr. 1/10 per kg. is injected intramuscularly, immediately. This may be followed within one or two hours by another injection of half the dose previously used. Treatment is continued with ¼ to ½ grain t.i.d. orally for the next few days. The dosage should be maximal, but overdosage with barbiturates should be guarded against. Intravenous injection is hazardous and should only be used as an initial dose, if needed. These measures will usually suffice to control the seizures. The infection is treated with the proper antibiotic drugs, and following termination of the convulsion, the infant should be kept on aspirin to control the rise of fever. If the seizure should continue, other measures, such as paraldehyde 1½ m./kg. injected intramuscularly, oxygen, and chloroform or vinyl ether administered by a trained anesthetist, should be added. In febrile convulsions due to meningitis the major emphasis is on treating the infection directly with specific drugs. In encephalitis there is no drug therapy which is specific, and additional measures consist of the intravenous injection of hypertonic glucose or sucrose (20 per cent), which may have some effect on the cerebral edema. In addition to the general measures for treatment of the febrile seizures, conditions such as lead encephalopathy, tetany, postnatal head injury, tetanus, tumors of the brain, swallowing of poison, nephritis, residual birth trauma, or congenital developmental malformations should be treated specifically. Examples are magnesium sulphate in hypertensive nephritis with convulsions, stomach washings and proper antidotes for poisoning, and calcium disodium versenate in lead intoxication.

In recent years a number of cases of convulsions in children under steroid therapy have been reported, in some instances, even status epilepticus. In none of these was the original condition for which steroids were being given connected with the nervous system. In some of these hypertension was present. Electroencephalographic changes were found in almost every case, especially slowing of activity and changes in alpha rhythm. For a full discussion and references see the article by Good and associates.

When the febrile convulsion is over and the patient is well, what should be the management for the future? Several questions arise in the minds of the parents. Will the seizures recur? Until what age may recurrences be expected? Shall they use any regime to attempt to prevent a seizure with the onset of fever? What are the chances of the child with febrile seizures for developing epilepsy? The majority of seizures of the febrile type are limited to one attack and do not recur. They are associated with a normal intellectual level, both before and after the attack. It is unusual for a febrile seizure to occur for the first time after five years of age or for recurrent febrile seizures to continue after six years. The outlook for children in this group is good, both for cessation of seizures and normal intellectual development. It is important, however, to treat the high fever and seizures actively so as to minimize the risk of vascular accident, anoxia, or the effects of high fever on the brain. After a first convulsive attack it is suggested that phenobarbital be kept in the home. At the earliest sign of a cold or infection, even if no fever is present, the child should be given a teaspoon of the elixir or a ¼ grain tablet of phenobarbital. Others have used dilantin sodium, grains ¾, repeated twice more that day and the following day or two as well if fever does occur. While there are no data of a controlled nature to judge the effect of this routine, it appears to be of value. In any case, at no expense to the child it bolsters the morale of the parents to whom the thought of a recurrence is frightening, and rightfully so. If a second febrile seizure occurs, electroencephalography may be performed and if the EEG is normal, which is the case in over 70 per cent, it reenforces the prospect of a favorable prognosis. This is further enhanced if the seizures are generalized and not focal. When a third seizure occurs, an EEG recording should definitely be made and carefully studied. Abnormalities in the rhythm have been correlated with subsequent epilepsy, and excessively rapid or slow tracings have been found to be associated with a history of birth trauma or the effect of fever on brain tissue. In many of these there may also be a family history of seizures. It may be best to place such children on a short period of daily anticonvulsant therapy, phenobarbital or dilantin sodium, without indicating to the parents that the child has epilepsy. It should be explained that measures are being used in an effort to avoid this development. The actual technique of therapy with phenobarbital and dilantin sodium is described under the treatment for epilepsy.

Most observers are agreed that epilepsy is not likely to follow febrile convulsions. In various reported series the incidence has been 3 to 15 per cent. It is close to 3 per cent or less when seizures are generalized, the I.Q. normal, the EEG normal between seizures and when there is a cause for the excessive fever extraneous to the central nervous system. When the seizure is due to an underlying disease, such as birth injury, lead encephalopathy, postnatal trauma, etc., the prognosis depends on the underlying process.

In seizures originating after three years of age the factor of acute infection decreases until at about ten years of age it is almost non-existent. Occasional cases of meningitis and encephalitis continue to be factors throughout childhood and adolescence. The effects of birth trauma also continue to be noticed to some extent in these age periods. The greatest factor is epilepsy.

Bessey, O. A., Adam, D. J. D., Hansen, A. E.: Intake of Vitamin B6 and Infantile Convulsions: A First Approximation of Requirements of Pyridoxine in Infants. Pediat. 20:33, 1957.

Cochrane, W. A., Payne, W. W., Simpkiss, M. J., and Woolf, L. I.: Familial Hypoglycemia Precipitated by Amino Acids. J. Clin. Invest. 35:411, 1956.

Craig, W. S.: Clinical Signs of Neonatal Tetany: with Especial Reference to Their Occurrence in Newborn Babies of Diabetic Mothers. Pediat. 22:297, 1958.

Finberg, L., and Harrison, H. E.: Hypernatromia in Infants. An Evaluation of the Clinical and Biochemical Findings Accompanying This State. Pediat. 16:1, 1956.

Gittleman, I. F., Pincus, J. B., Schmerzler, E., and Saito, M.: Hypocalcemia Occurring on the First Day of Life in Mature and Premature Infants. Pediat. 18:721, 1956.

Good, R. A., Vernier, R. L. and Smith, R. T.: Serious Untoward Reactions to Therapy with Cortisone and Adrenocorticotropin in Pediatric Practice. (Part 1). Pediat. 19:95, 1957.

Lamm, S. S.: The Danger of Intramuscular Injection of Calcium Gluconate in Infancy. J.A.M.A. 129:347, 1945.

Lennox, M. A.: Febrile Convulsions in Childhood. Am. J. Dis. Child. 78:868, 1949.

Molony, C. J. and Parmelee, A. H.: Convulsions in Young Infants as a Result of Pyridoxine (Vitamin B6) Deficiency. J.A.M.A. 154:405, 1954.

Patrick, H. T. and Levy, D. M.: Early Convulsions in Epileptics and in Others, J.A.M.A. 82:375, 1924.

Peterman, M. G.: Treatment of Convulsions in Childhood. Am. J. Dis. Child. 84:409, 1952.

Steg, N.: Narcotic Withdrawal Reactions in the Newborn. A.M.A.J. Dis. Child. 94:287, 1957.

Toomey, J. A.: Convulsions and Acute Infections, Am. J. Dis. Child. 75:752, 1948.

Weil, W. B., and Wallace, W. M.: Hypertonic Dehydration in Infancy. Pediat. 17:171, 1956.

EPILEPSY

Recurrent paroxysmal seizures are referred to as epilepsy. They occur in four per thousand population. There is usually a loss of consciousness. Instead of or accompanying the seizure there may be alteration of feeling or behavior. There is an area of excitation and excessive neural discharge from which the seizure originates (paroxysmal dysrhythmia). When a child who may have epilepsy is seen by the physician, the following information must be obtained in order to manage the problems properly:

1. Is the etiology of the condition known?
2. What is the type of seizure and may it be correlated with any specific region of the brain?

The first question which arises is the relation of epilepsy to heredity. Lennox reported that of 2,053 epileptic patients a family history of epilepsy or migraine was obtained in 43 per cent. In 122 twin pairs without prior brain damage, 84 per cent of single egg twins showed epilepsy in both contrasted with 10% in double egg twins. In pairs with brain damage the corresponding incidence was 17 per cent and 8 per cent. He concluded that a transmitted predisposition to seizures represented by cerebral dysrhythmia and brain damage was a factor. Lilienthal and Passamanick on the other hand, in reviewing the prenatal and paranatal records of 564 epileptic children, found significantly more complications of pregnancies and deliveries, prematurity, and abnormal neonatal conditions, than in a similar number of matched controls. Furthermore, the abnormalities were just as frequent among epileptic children whose parents did not have epilepsy. They considered that their data raised some doubt as to the genetic basis of convulsive disorders. Frasier states that with a positive family history the risk is 1 to 40 (general incidence in the population is 1 to 250); it is greater if the positive family history demonstrates an idiopathic type of electroencephalogram, early onset of seizures, and no history of brain injury. It is less with a "focal" electroencephalogram, negative family history, late onset, and history of brain injury. Lennox found abnormalities of the electroencephalogram in 50 per cent of near relatives contrasted with 16 per cent of the normal population.

The pregnancy should be studied for evidence of intrauterine anoxia e.g., cardiac decompensation in the mother, maternal infections e.g., german measles, toxoplasmosis, or erythroblastosis.

In the neonatal history one should look for evidence of birth injury (intracranial hemorrhage or asphyxia with resulting anoxia) due to the abnormality of labor e.g., coils of cord about the neck, heavy sedation of the mother, etc.

The developmental history may reveal the association of seizures with cerebral malformation, meningitis or encephalitis, brain abscess, nephritis or tumor of the brain. Chemical studies may reveal tetany, hypoglycemia or phenylketonuria. Data should be obtained concerning postnatal trauma, drugs or metallic poisons. Seizures may follow injections such as pertussis vaccine, or they may be associated with a rise of fever. Grand mal seizure may follow a long period of reading. The development of the child should also be studied to get an idea of the intellectual status.

The final question in the history is the description of the seizure itself. This brings us to the second question, namely the type of seizure and possible correlation with a specific region of the brain. In conjunction with these questions, the age when the first seizure occurred and a complete description of the first attack should be recorded. The story of the seizures should also include how often they have occurred, the interval between attacks, and any specific way in which they began. Did they originate the same way each time, or were there varied onsets? The presence or absence of fever, the parts of the body involved in the attack, and in what order and manner, should be noted. There should also be a statement concerning the presence or absence of consciousness, the loss of urinary or bowel control, and the total length of time of the attack.

Classification of Seizures. Seizures are fundamentally of three types, centrencephalic, focal cerebral, and diffuse unlocalized cerebral (Penfield).

The centrencephalic seizures originate in the reticular substance and central gray matter. There is then usually a spread to the entire cortex resulting in a grand mal seizure. In the petit mal form, however, the onset is initiated in the thalamus, then followed by a spread to the cortex. The centrencephalic seizures are characterized by their symmetry. Aura is evident in the grand mal type particularly. The electroencephalogram shows bilateral synchronous discharges with no focal point of origin. The brain may show no anatomical abnormality.

The second type of seizure is focal. In this case the abnormal discharge originates from a localized area of the cerebral cortex. The cortical site of origin usually shows organic pathology. The electroencephalogram shows evidence of a focal site of origin. The clinical site of onset of the seizure is correlated with the area of cortical disease. The spread to contiguous cortical areas is referred to as Jacksonian.

Finally, there are cerebral seizures with no focal point of origin. Evidence usually suggests diffuse pathology in the brain or the brain may be affected by external factors such as hypernatremia or hypoglycemia.

Grand Mal. Grand mal is the most frequent type of seizure, both alone and in combination with other forms. It is most commonly associated with petit mal. The attack may begin with an aura and is characterized by a sudden loss of consciousness, followed by periods of tonic and clonic spasms of the muscles. The aura may be of a motor or sensory type. It consists of numbness, tingling, dizziness, or pain in the abdomen. During the seizure there may be urinary and fecal incontinence, the eyes may deviate to any direction, the tongue may be bitten, and there may be intense salivation. In the tonic spasm respiration is interfered with so that first pallor, then cyanosis develops. Subsequently the patient falls asleep. On arising there are headache, a feeling of dullness and depression, and confusion. The usual seizure may last several minutes, occasionally much longer. Subsequently the child senses that he has had an attack, except when the seizure has occurred during the night while the child was asleep. In these instances the sheet may be bloodstained or the bed wet. The number of attacks vary; usually one, occasionally two, in a day. There then may follow an interval of weeks, months, or a year or two between seizures. Status epilepticus is the term used when one attack is followed by another in rapid succession without an intervening period of returning consciousness. This results in severe dehydration and unless extreme measures are used may end in a fatality.

Focal epilepsy, as we have previously stated, refers to a seizure coming from a specific pathological area in the gray matter of one cerebral hemisphere. It refers to location rather than anatomic type of pathology. A specific form of focal seizure is the Jacksonian. The seizure begins locally in any part of the body and then spreads in a definite manner corresponding to areas in the precentral gyrus. The seizure is usually contralateral and clonic in type. For example, if the local twitches or clonic movements begin in the fingers, there is a spread to the wrist, forearm, arm, face, and then leg, all on the same side of the body, which is opposite to the focal area of the lesion in the brain. There is usually no loss of consciousness unless there is a spread to the other side in which case there is both a loss of consciousness and the appearance of a grand mal attack. Other forms of focal seizures in addition to the focal motor or Jacksonian type, according to Penfield, are adversive (a coordinated movement of turning the head and body to one side with eyes deviated in the same direction, both usually away from the affected hemisphere), tonic mesencephalic seizures (either similar in appearance to decerebrate rigidity or opisthotonic) and postural seizures. Focal seizures may originate from areas other than the precentral gyrus (motor). They may be sensory with tingling or numbness arising from the postcentral gyrus, visual from the occipital lobe (flashes of light before the eyes), auditory (temporal lobe), or olfactory (uncinate gyrus). Aphasia results from involvement of the dominant hemisphere.

Petit Mal. This refers to a minor seizure in contrast to the major or grand mal type. It occurs essentially during childhood and is a form of centrencephalic seizure, probably originating in the thalamus. There is a brief loss of consciousness accompanied by a vacant stare, all occurring within a few seconds. Along with this there may be blinking of the eyelids or nodding of the head. The involvement is simultaneously bilateral. There is no evident preceding aura or subsequent drowsiness. The child continues his activity, often unaware of the momentary interruption. In addition to the simple form of petit mal with transient lapses, there are the myoclonic and akinetic types, forming a triad with a characteristic electroencephalographic tracing. The myoclonic form is characterized by brief involuntary contractions with sudden jerks of the trunk muscles or those of the extremities. Akenetic seizures are seen as sudden losses of muscle tone. The head and body nod forward or there may be a sudden fall to the ground (salaam or drop seizures). There is no loss of consciousness but slight confusion may be present for a few minutes. The petit mal triad may be present in patients who also have grand mal seizures. While usually classified as being unassociated with anatomic disturbance, petit mal may also be seen in children who have had birth trauma, developmental or degenerative cortical disease, or encephalitis. The akinetic and myoclonic seizures have been located in foci in the basal ganglia (pallidus). Petit mal seizures, in contrast, to grand mal, are repeated many times during the day. They will often appear in school where the child may cease writing or reading momentarily, then continue his task. The term "pyknolepsy" was used to designate a form of petit mal which ceased at puberty, but this is now considered to be ordinary petit mal.

Psychomotor. In these attacks there is a brief period of clouding of consciousness. During this state, which lasts longer than the usual petit mal, there are automatic repetitive stereotyped movements such as mastication, swallowing, chewing, fumbling with objects involuntarily, or laughter for no apparent reason. There is apt to be partial amnesia during and after the attack. During this period the child is unware of his actions, which may take the form of violence or abnormal behavior. These have been referred to as fugue states or psychic equivalents. In a recent study Glaser and Dixon pointed out that these children have auras of anxiety and visceral symptoms associated with varied feelings. Between the seizures there is quite often evidence of a disturbed personality in the form of overactivity and aggression. The electroencephalogram shows either bilateral slow spike waves of diffuse origin or unilateral or bilateral spikes or spike waves arising from the temporal region. Therefore, the temporal, limbic, and centrencephalic systems are involved. Zimmerman has described a group of children who demonstrate periodic and violent outbursts of impulsive behavior paroxysmal in character. In these children there were no seizures but there were abnormal electroencephalogram, organic Rorschach, and marked improvement with dilantin. They did not respond to psychotherapy. He felt these were epileptic equivalents more akin to major seizures of frontal origin rather than psychomotor. Others use the terms interchangeably. The pathology in the psychomotor type is generally considered to be located in one temporal lobe, with evidence of brain damage in 33 to 60 per cent from either birth trauma or infection.

Abdominal. This is referred to as paroxysmal abdominal pain and is of very rare occurrence. The pain is periumbilical and gastric. It comes on suddenly and is associated with vomiting and diarrhea. In many instances the child falls asleep immediately after the attack of pain. In some there may be associated convulsions. The electroencephalogram is abnormal, showing synchronous discharges of high voltage slow waves and spike and wave bursts. The patients have no other reason for their pain. The attacks appear to respond to drugs which are used to treat epilepsy. In some of the reported cases where abdominal epilepsy was first noted, it was followed later by true seizures.

Infantile Spasms (Massive Myoclonic). These seizures occur mainly in the first two or three years of infancy and originate during the first year. The spasms are of short duration, abrupt and generalized, involving groups of muscles, especially of the arms, legs and head, and are not rhythmically repeated as in petit mal. There may be sudden bending or jerking of the head, with simultaneous upward flinging of the arms, and flexion of the thighs upon the abdomen, accompanied by a cry. There may be many spasms per day, each lasting about a second, or a continuous series. In one third of the children there are major seizures as well. The vast majority of these infants are mentally deficient. Encephalitis, prenatal developmental factors and birth injury are the main etiological agents. Some cases have occurred secondary to pertussis immunization. The electroencephalogram is characterized by hypsarhythmia (high voltage waves and spikes which are diffuse and nonrhythmic). The electroencephalographic pattern and seizures usually disappear at about four years. It has recently been reported that if the infantile spasm is associated with a normal electroencephalogram, there is a 55% chance the infant will develop normally. Treatment is unsatisfactory, but some favorable effect on the spasms has followed the use of Gemonil, a ketogenic diet, or ACTH.

Livingston prefers to group massive myoclonic, head nodding and akinetic seizures under the term minor motor epilepsy and reserve the term petit mal for the children with transient lapses and the typical electroencephalogram, namely bilateral synchronous 3-per-second spike and wave forms.

Epileptic Cephalea. These are paroxysmal headaches which may be the sole manifestation of epilepsy. The electroencephalogram reveals epileptic activity particularly under photic stimulation.

PHYSICAL EXAMINATION: There are no physical features characteristic of epilepsy. If the child has symptomatic epilepsy he may have neurological signs characteristic of the underlying disease, for example, brain tumor or encephalitis. Old lesions, such as a traumatic intracranial hemorrhage incurred at birth, may show evidence in the form of a residual hemiplegia. If, however, there is centrencephalic epilepsy, the only neurological findings may be those that are present during and shortly after the attack. There may be abolition of the pupillary light reflexes, Babinski sign, weakness of the extremities, and increased reflexes. Along with the postconvulsive dullness and confusion these all tend to clear.

LABORATORY: As with the physical examination, the laboratory study, including the spinal fluid, is usually normal in centrencephalic, or so-called idiopathic epilepsy. Only in symptomatic or focal seizure will the study reveal abnormalities of the underlying disease, as in lead encephalopathy, brain tumor, or recent head trauma. Roentgenographic study of the skull may detect evidence of fracture or signs of increased intracranial pressure. At the same time one should note any cerebral calcification as in toxoplasmosis, tuberous sclerosis, or angiomatosis. After an electroencephalogram has been recorded, pneumoencephalography or arteriography may be performed when indicated. These are needed only for focal epilepsy when one may wish to localize an area of organic pathology. If tumor is suspected, ventriculography may be of value.

PATHOLOGY: There is no distinctive pathology in epilepsy. There may be anatomical changes related to the underlying disease, such as occur following anoxia or trauma.

ELECTROENCEPHALOGRAPHY: Recording the electrical activity of the brain is a useful procedure in the diagnosis of epilepsy when interpreted in conjunction with the history and clinical findings. It must be remembered that a negative electroencephalogram does not rule out epilepsy since a recording during the seizure-free interval may be normal. However, with repeated examinations and activation methods it will be found abnormal in 90 per cent of cases of epilepsy. Abnormalities in the electroencephalogram may be seen in perfectly normal persons. They may be relatives of epileptics in some instances. Others are potential epileptics. The recording is useful especially in localizing the origin of the pathological process and characterizing to some extent its nature but not necessarily the clinical form of the seizure. In children sedation may be required in order to obtain proper recordings. This is valuable since much more data are obtained with sleep records. In children with epilepsy 80 per cent will show abnormal tracings in their sleep record as contrasted with 35 per cent while awake. In the early period of electroencephalography specific patterns were described. These included grand mal, characterized by "extreme acceleration of the electrical activity of the cortex" with high voltage spikes; petit mal, three per second rounded waves with spike attached and alternate fast and slow activity, and psychomotor or slow high voltage flat topped waves, 4 to 6 per second. The last is generally found in adults with pathology in the temporal lobe. A blunt spike followed by a slow hump occurring at 2 per second is described as a petit mal variant, which Lennox and David interpret as being due to three influences, namely, heredity, extreme youth, and neuropathologic change. In addition to sleep recordings, hyperventilation, flickering light (intermittent photic stimulation), hydration, and metrazol may be used to bring out abnormal tracings. Reference to specific texts will reveal the details of electroencephalography.

The electroencephalogram is used as an aid in the diagnosis of epilepsy; it may indicate where the focus of excitation may be. It may aid in selecting cases of focal cortical seizures which are to be explored surgically and is of help in following drug therapy. A series of wave forms such as petit mal type or petit mal variant is useful in describing the electroencephalographic pattern but the fact that this pattern is found does not necessarily mean that the patient has petit mal. Howell found a variety of clinical pictures with bilaterally synchronous, 3 per second, classic wave and spike discharges, either spontaneous or after ventilation. Similarly, Clark and Knott reported on 178 cases of seizures with a wave and spike form of electroencephalogram. Of these only 16 per cent had seizures classified as belonging to the petit mal triad without any other types of seizures, 22 per cent had grand mal seizures only, and 70 per cent had petit mal and another type as well. When the seizures were of the petit mal variety alone, 78 per cent had a classic electroencephalographic pattern. When seizures were of the grand mal type alone, 50 per cent had 3 per second patterns, 50 per cent showed slow or fast variants. They did find that organic disorder was infrequent with the classic 3 per second pattern. Finally, Glaser and Golub analyzed the interictal and ictal electroencephalographic tracings of 110 children from 1½ to 16 years with psychomotor seizures. They found the wave forms varied. Focal temporal spikes were relatively infrequent and only slightly higher in sleep. The incidence of spike and wave discharges with and without petit mal seizures was high. Their final conclusion was again non-specificity of the spike and wave or any other pattern and that psychomotor seizure is not always associated with temporal lobe pathology.

We may now evaluate our data and arrive at a diagnosis and subsequent management. The history is taken with the object of finding out at what age the first seizure occurred and circumstances under which it took place and this will be correlated with the prenatal, natal, and developmental history. If the seizure occurred in infancy for the first time, birth trauma (anoxia or hemorrhage) and congenital maldevelopment of the brain should be strongly considered. At a later age period one may still consider the effect of damage in the neonatal period, also malformations of the brain, encephalopathy (lead), encephalitis, vascular accidents (thrombosis of cerebral vessels), postnatal trauma, and brain tumor. In many instances no data can be obtained to shed light on a causative factor. A thorough physical is done including neurological and eye ground examination. This may reveal evidence of old damage to the brain or be entirely normal. If possible, one of the seizures should be witnessed by the physican himself. If necessary techniques to bring them out may be used.

1. Hyperventilation (especially useful in petit mal): Sit the child in a chair. Ask him to breathe deeply. By the time he has done this close to 100 times he may develop a petit mal seizure. Continued deep breathing may produce carpopedal spasm and alkalosis tetany but no seizure in nonepileptic patients.

2. Excessive hydration test or pitressin test (McQuarrie): This is especially useful in grand mal. Omit anticonvulsive drugs for a few days before the test. The child should be on a high caloric diet (salt-free). On the morning of the test, give 75 to 100 cc. of water per kilogram body weight over a period of 24 hours. The total amount is divided equally into six periods. Inject .5 cc. of pitressin every two to three hours subcutaneously. Seizure will usually occur within 24 hours (when the patient has gained about 5% of his body weight). The child should be observed by a trained nurse throughout; all data in reference to the seizure should be recorded as well as any untoward side effects such as a fall in blood pressure. This test brings out major seizures primarily. It is of little or no use in petit mal. It should not be used unless absolutely needed to demonstrate the type of seizure or abnormal electroencephalographic tracing.

We have stressed that the onset and type of seizure be carefully studied so that localization in the brain may be aided. The electroencephalographic recording should be used to help along with the clinical studies by showing a focus of electrical abnormality. Activation methods as described above, such as hyperventilation, excessive hydration, or photic stimulation may aid in electroencephalographic localization. Following the history and physical examination, laboratory procedures should be carried out: blood chemistries including sugar and calcium, lumbar puncture and analysis of the spinal fluid, and urine examination. An X-ray of the skull should also be taken. If clinically indicated, as in suspected tumor, ventriculography may be performed to provide positive evidence for surgery. In some instances with a low I.Q. encephalography is done to help evaluate prognosis by revealing areas of cortical or cerebral atrophy with ventricular dilatation.

DIFFERENTIAL DIAGNOSIS: In infants breath holding spells must be considered. These come on during the latter part of the first year and during the second. They may follow fright, anger, disagreement, or frustration. The infant begins to cry, holds his breath, and apnea develops. Pallor and cyanosis result, the spell lasting about ten to twenty seconds. This is followed by inspiration and the symptoms disappear. The electroencephalogram is usually normal in these children, both when awake and asleep. Thus, the history of occurrence only on provocation ending when inspiration occurs, and a normal tracing differentiate these breath holding spells from epilepsy.

Cyclic vomiting (periodic acetonemic) is recurrent vomiting associated with ketosis. It occurs at irregular intervals. There are likely to be fever, marked dehydration, and pallor. A family history of migraine is often present. At times there may be no apparent cause for the onset of vomiting. In others it occurs at the onset of an acute infection. The condition usually disappears around puberty. An exhaustive study must be made to rule out brain tumor, kidney disease, allergic gastrointestinal manifestation, appendicitis, or familial autonomic dysfunction. Recently cyclic vomiting has been considered as a form of autonomic epilepsy because of the family history of migraine or epilepsy, evidence of brain damage in some, abnormal electroencephalogram, and response to therapy of proven value in epilepsy or autonomic dysfunction. In treating this problem each patient will have to be considered separately. Certainly if there are other evidences of brain damage and positive correlation in the electroencephalogram, anti-convulsive therapy should be used. These children are usually alert, have a high I.Q., and are generally physically normal. If there is no evidence of epilepsy, a psychological approach may be of value. The important point in therapy is to use sedation such as Thorazine® or phenobarbital at the onset of the attack along with sugar, lollipops, sips of cola syrup, a teaspoon at a time, or sucking an orange. This may avoid further trouble. The prognosis is good. Most of the attacks disappear by puberty.

Hysterical fits which must be differentiated from psychomotor epilepsy are very rare in children. There is no deep loss of consciousness so that the patient can easily be aroused. These children do not lose urinary or fecal control. There are no postconvulsive phenomena. The electroencephalogram is of value. However, in some instances none of these features is absolute and the experience of the physician must be used to see whether through psychological therapy or anticonvulsant treatment a differential may be made.

Other conditions to be differentiated include abnormal behavior, which is to be distinguished from a "fugue state," ordinary fainting spells (syncope attacks), narcolepsy, and carotid sinus reflex. The latter are all rare in children except for the problem of abnormal behavior. Here a differential must be made from bad behavior due to psychological causes, e.g., poor parental-sibling relationships, or encephalitic personality distortion. The psychomotor or epileptic equivalent type of behavior has electroencephalographic features of epilepsy and the behavior is more paroxysmal or episodic rather than continuous. It responds to Dilantin® or phenobarbital.

TREATMENT: The management of epilepsy includes:

1. Treatment of the cause when known
2. Treatment of the individual seizure (status epilepticus)
3. Drug Therapy
4. Diet
5. Surgery
6. General questions and prognosis

1. TREATMENT OF THE CAUSE WHEN KNOWN: We have stressed the importance of attempting to find any contributing factor which may produce the seizure. Such would be instances of brain tumor, lead encephalopathy, allergy, hypoparathyroidism, hyperinsulinism, nephritis, neonatal birth injury, or postnatal trauma. In these instances therapy would be directed towards the underlying cause

as described in their respective chapters in the text. However, the majority of children either do not fall in this group or have unalterable pathology and will therefore require drug therapy.

2. TREATMENT OF THE INDIVIDUAL SEIZURE: This requires no special procedures except to see that the child does not injure himself during the attack. If he is liable to bite his tongue, a handmade gag may be placed between the teeth, such as tongue depressors wrapped with a piece of cloth or the cloth itself. The child should be placed in a bed or on the floor and the clothes loosened. These attacks are usually over in a couple of minutes, but occasionally they keep on recurring without an intervening free period and we have the condition referred to as status epilepticus. In this situation therapy must be intensive to avoid a fatality or severe brain damage.

The child should be hospitalized. Sodium phenobarbital, 0.2 to 0.5 grams, should be given intravenously according to the weight of the child, to be followed by a similar dose intramuscularly if relaxation does not occur. Ether anesthesia may be used if needed, likewise oxygen. Intravenous glucose should be given to avoid dehydration. In addition to sodium phenobarbital, paraldehyde may also be injected, once, intravenously and intramuscularly, 1.5 cc. to 3 cc. Measures should be used to combat the hyperthermia, such as cold packs, sponging, and salicylates per rectum. The sedation should be carefully controlled to avoid respiratory depression.

3. DRUG THERAPY:

Phenobarbital. This is the drug of choice in grand mal epilepsy. The dosage in the first four years of life is a ¼ grain tablet or a teaspoon of the elixir of phenobarbital (grains ¼), three times a day, once on arising, once during the day, and once at bedtime. In older children, ½ grain three times a day may be used. These beginning doses should be increased up to 0.3 gm. daily in divided doses if seizures are not being controlled provided too much drowsiness does not occur. Drug complications are rare.

Diphenylhydantoin Sodium or Dilantin Sodium (Parke-Davis). This drug is extremely useful in grand mal and psychomotor epilepsy. It may be used in combination with phenobarbital. It does not produce drowsiness or dullness. The dosage in infants and very young children is ½ of a ¾ grain tablet, or 1/3 teaspoon of the liquid suspension (0.1 gm. to tsp.), three times a day after meals. In children three to six years of age one ¾ grain tablet or ½ teaspoon of the liquid suspension may be given three or four times daily. Over six years a maximum of 0.4 gram may be reached, or about two tablets three times a day. The toxic reactions from this drug include nausea, vomiting, restlessness, dizziness, vertigo, nystagmus, ataxia, and hypertrophy of the gums. The last may at times be annoying as the teeth may be overgrown with tissue. As a rule, however, this can be controlled by drug dosage, gum massage, and good care of the teeth. A morbilliform or erythematous rash appears in some of the patients about the tenth day to two weeks following onset of treatment. The white count should be checked periodically to rule out severe leucopenia. Excess growth of hair may occur; if annoying, the drug may be changed. Any of these symptoms can be made to disappear by reducing the drug dosage by about ⅓; the dosage can then be gradually increased again to the desired level. If this is unsuccessful or the seizures cannot be brought under control with the lesser dosage, the Dilantin should be eliminated gradually with the simultaneous introduction of another drug.

Mesantoin, 3-methyl, 5-phenyl, 5-ethylhydantoin, (Sandoz): This drug may be used for grand mal seizure if phenobarbital and Dilantin combined are not efficacious. Mesantoin may be used alone or with other drugs. It is also of aid in petit mal seizure but should not be used with Tridione as the risk of toxicity is increased. Dosage is a 0.1 gram tablet three times a day for one week. It can be increased by one tablet weekly, until a maximum of four tablets, three times a day, is reached. With children under six years the dose is halved. Agranulocytosis and toxic rashes may occur. With this drug, as with all others except phenobarbital, a blood count should be done two weeks after the onset of therapy. It should be repeated monthly, thereafter.

Mebaral - N - methyl - ethyl - phenyl - barbituric acid (Winthrop Stearns): For children up to four years, give one tablet of ½ grain, three times a day. For older children, one grain, three times a day. This is twice the dosage of phenobarbital. The action of both drugs is similar.

Gemonil, 5, 5-diethyl-1-methylbarbituric acid (Abbott); This drug is useful in grand mal, petit mal, and myoclonic epilepsy especially. Dosage: For infants and small children ½ of an 0.1 gram tablet, one to three times daily. Older children; one tablet, one to three times daily. There may be drowsiness, irritability, rash, dizziness, and vomiting.

Mysoline 5-phenyl, 5-ethyl-hexahydropyrimidine-4, 6 dione. (Ayerst). For grand mal and psychomotor seizures, either alone or with Dilantin sodium. Dosage is one tablet, 0.25 grams. The dosage is increased by one tablet weekly until four a day are given. There may be nausea, vomiting, dizziness, and ataxia. In younger children the dose is halved.

Tridione, 3, 5, 5-trimethyl oxazolidine-2, 4-dione. (Abbott). This is the drug of choice of petit mal. It may be used with phenobarbital when major seizures are also present. Dilantin is contraindicated in petit mal since it may aggravate the seizures. Mesantoin is also to be avoided, as toxicity is increased when combined with Tridione. Dosage is 0.3 gram tablet, three times a day for older children. It is increased by 0.3 gram to a maximum of two grams, if necessary. For children under two years, one-half the dose is used. Aplastic anemia, Stevens-Johnson syndrome, agranulocytosis, and photophobia may occur. The drug should be discontinued for any of the above except photophobia. Blood counts should be done monthly and the drug should be stopped at the first sign of toxicity.

Paradione 3, 5-dimethyl-5-ethyl oxazolidine-2, 4-dione. (Abbott). This drug is similar to Tridione but is less toxic. The dosage for infants is 0.3 gram daily; for children two to six years, 0.6 gram daily, and for older children 0.3 gram, three times a day.

Milontin, N-methyl-phenyl-succinimide. (Parke-Davis). This is used in petit mal when Tridione or Paradione are ineffective or toxic. The dosage is 0.5 gram, two or three times a day, to a maximum of two grams. Drowsiness, nausea, and vertigo may occur. These disappear as the dose is decreased. The blood count should be followed.

Miltown-2-methyl-2-n-propyl-1, 3-propanediol dicarbamate. (Wallace). Of especial benefit in akinetic seizures and the massive infantile myoclonic type. Only drowsiness is noted usually. There are few severe toxic reactions. Therefore it may be safer than Tridione. The dose is 200 mg. three times a day. This is increased at the rate of 200 mg. every two weeks, as needed.

Phenurone (Abbott): Especially valuable in psychomotor seizures. Under six years dosage is one 0.3 gm. tablet three times daily. Over six years the initial dose is a 0.5 gm. tablet, twice daily. It may be increased slowly. The patient should be checked for toxic effects, since behavior changes, rash, and hepatitis may occur.

Celontin N-methyl-a, a-methylphenylsuccinimide (Parke-Davis): This drug is used for petit mal and psychomotor seizures. The dose is one 0.3 gm. Kapseal daily for one week. It is increased by one Kapseal each week to a maximum of four Kapseals per day, if needed.

Diamox acetazolamide (Lederle): A carbonic anhydrase inhibitor, which produces an acidosis. It is used mainly in petit mal. The dose is a 0.25 gm. tablet three times a day. Toxic effects may be noted in the blood and kidneys.

Peganone 3-ethyl-5-phenylhydantoin, (Abbott): This drug is useful in grand mal. One 250 mg. tablet is given four times a day after meals. It may be used with other drugs.

Bromides are rarely used today because of their toxicity.

Benzedrine may be used in epilepsy to counteract the lethargy produced by drugs like phenobarbital. The dosage is 5 mg. twice daily, in the A.M. and mid-afternoon.

4. KETOGENIC DIET: This diet, high in fats, low in carbohydrates, is beneficial in reducing seizures. It has been used along with fasting and restricted fluid intake. The ketogenic effect produces an acidosis with loss of tissue fluids. The difficulty in persuading a child to remain on this diet because of the restricted selection of foods (butter, cream, etc., in excess and very little in the way of sweets) and the advent of so many new drugs for the treatment of epilepsy have made this type of therapy obsolescent. However, it may be used in a refractive case, as in myoclonic epilepsy, and according to Livingston it is the best agent for minor epilepsy.

5. SURGERY: When there is evidence of a brain tumor, brain abscess, progressive hydrocephalus, cyst, or hematoma, surgery is indicated. In many of these cases, following surgery drug therapy may need to be continued. In the case of focal epilepsy without an

expanding lesion, if drug therapy is successful, no surgery should be performed. If, however, there is no response to adequate and prolonged medication, then surgery may be required. In psychomotor seizures Penfield and his co-workers have shown that there may be an "incisural sclerosis" of the temporal lobe, especially that part which lies upon the free edge of the tentorium. The tip of this lobe herniates down through the incisura of the tentorium as a result of head compression in birth injury, causing arrest of the flow of blood. This is corrected surgically by partial temporal lobectomy. In other instances hemispherectomy may be done. The procedure is especially valuable in children with infantile hemiplegia accompanied by personality alterations, mental impairment, and severe epilepsy. The procedure is a hemi-decortication of the brain on the side opposite to the hemiplegia. Seizures are usually eliminated or reduced as a result. There may be improvement in mentality and personality subsequently.

SUMMARY OF THERAPY:

Grand Mal. Use phenobarbital and Dilantin sodium singly or combined. Start slowly, using phenobarbital first and work up to maximum dosage. Dilantin is relatively safe, but blood counts should be done monthly at the beginning of therapy. If untoward symptoms of drug toxicity do occur from the Dilantin, reduce the dosage for about a week as previously described. Then as the reactions have abated, gradually increase to maximum dosage. The drugs should be given regularly, daily. If it is desired to substitute one of the other drugs listed, reduce the dosage of phenobarbital or Dilantin slowly and simultaneously begin the use of the new drug. This will avoid bringing on seizures through too rapid withdrawal. Combinations of these drugs are available; these may be used after dosage is standardized. In most instances phenobarbital plus Dilantin sodium will control the grand mal seizures. If not, other drugs like Mesantoin, Mebaral, Mysoline, or Peganone may be tried. Check for drug reactions regularly.

Petit Mal. For the classical petit mal with transient lapses, use Tridione. Miltown should be substituted if there are toxic reactions or no response. Paradione may also be effective. The ketogenic diet is especially useful in minor motor seizures and with Diamox may correct resistant myoclonic seizures. When there are combinations of major epilepsy and the petit mal type, one may use Mesantoin alone or phenobarbital combined with Tridione. All drugs, whether administered singly or in combination, should be used to their maximum dosage.

Psychomotor. Phenurone is especially useful. Dilantin sodium is also a most valuable drug in psychomotor epilepsy and may be used in combination with phenobarbital or any of the other drugs listed for major seizures. Celontin may also be given for psychomotor seizures.

Infantile Myoclonic Spasms. For the infantile myoclonic spasms associated with organic brain disease Gemonil is the drug of choice. A Ketogenic diet is often valuable. Recently ACTH has been reported as helpful.

6. GENERAL QUESTIONS AND PROGNOSIS:

Under what conditions should drug therapy be started?

If the child has had only one seizure, a period of further observation may be tried. In some instances the seizure is not repeated. If there is recurrence, then drug therapy should be begun.

How long should drug therapy be continued?

Therapy once begun should be continued until the child has had no seizures for two years, and then the dosage of the drugs should be reduced gradually. The electroencephalogram may return to normal, but the decision to reduce drug therapy should be made on the clinical absence of seizures; in many cases the electroencephalogram may continue to appear abnormal in spite of clinical cure.

The petit mal type will often disappear by puberty and most are gone by adult life. Many of the children begin with petit mal and later develop major seizures. If so, therapy is continued for the latter.

Reexamine the child periodically. New factors may develop. Continuation of the seizures, especially when the response to drug therapy is not satisfactory in spite of adequate dosage, may be due to some new condition, e.g., brain tumor, or original failure to classify the seizure properly with the resultant use of the wrong drug. Other causes for the lack of good results may be giving a drug insufficient trial or changing the drug too frequently.

What about the mental status?

This depends on the underlying pathology. If the child has had a brain injury at birth, there may be a low I.Q. due to the brain damage of which the seizures and/or paralysis are also manifestations. However, figures generally given indicate that about ten per cent of epilepsy is associated with marked mental retardation. These children are in institutions for their mental deficiency. Of the remaining 90 per cent there is a normal I.Q. in about 65 to 70 per cent with the others just below. When epilepsy is "idiopathic," the mentality is usually normal. With modern therapy one does not see mental deterioration in epilepsy during childhood, and according to adult statistics, when the mental status is normal in childhood it is likely to remain so if the epilepsy is properly treated. The limitations to this favorable outlook depend on the extent of the original brain damage, the frequency and severity of the seizures, and the length of time they have been present. There appears to be no effect on the mental level from the drugs themselves. Bridge, quoting Lennox, gives data on non-institutionalized epileptic individuals to show the inverse relationship between the number of seizures and the duration of the disease and the mental status.

What of the daily routine of the child?

The epileptic child should attend school regularly and participate in all activities. However, until the seizures are well controlled, swimming and bicycle or horseback riding should be done only with other children or adults present. Careers not permissible are those in which the lives of others might be jeopardized, for example, a taxi driver, engineer on a train, or airplane pilot. However, personal driving of a car should be permitted under certain conditions, such as the absence of seizures for at least two years.

What about marriage and children?

This must be evaluated in each instance. In our discussion of heredity, we indicated the importance of epilepsy in near relatives, whether the epilepsy was acquired through injury or cryptogenic, and the significance of the electroencephalogram. Figures usually given indicate that epileptic parents may produce an epileptic child in 1 of 40-60 chances as against 1 out of 250 when there is a normal family history. Epilepsy is not transmissible, but rather the predisposition to seizures is.

What is the prognosis and outcome?

The goal in management is control of the seizures and development of a wholesome child who matures normally—mentally, emotionally, and socially. To this end, when treatment is to begin after the complete workup, the parents should have a full discussion with the physician as to the implications of the disease. The points previously taken up should be explained. While being frank, the doctor should be assuring and hopeful about the prospects.

With adequate therapy the frequency and severity of seizures should be favorably influenced within several months, certainly within a year. In some it may be possible to eliminate drugs completely after freedom from seizure for two years. This does not happen often, and the majority must be on some medication. About 50 per cent can be made free of seizures. In 35 per cent the frequency of seizures can be reduced. Clinical improvement is the guide to therapy. If the electroencephalogram, which should be recorded annually, shows a return to normal, and there is clinical disappearance of the seizures, the outlook for the child is excellent. However, if there is clinical freedom from seizures and the electroencephalographic pattern remains abnormal, the outlook is also considered good, since the clinical absence of seizures is the goal in therapy.

Epileptic children under controlled therapy should live as long as other children. With constant improvement in therapy, and reduction in prenatal and natal brain injury there is good hope for prevention and control of this disease.

Ansell, B. and Clark, E.: Acetazolamide in Treatment of Epilepsy. Brit. Med. J. 1:650, 1956.

Baird, H. W. and Borofsky, L. G.: Infantile Myoclonic Seizures. J. Pediat. 50:332, 1957.

Bridge, E. M.: Epilepsy and Convulsive Disorders in Children. New York McGraw-Hill Book Co., 1949.

Burnett, L. L., Gibbs, E. L. and Gibbs, F. A.: Prognosis in infantile spasms. Pediat. 21:719, 1958.

Clark, E. C. and Knott, J. R.: Paroxysmal Wave and Spike Activity and Diagnostic Subclassification. Electroencephalog. & Clin. Neurophysiol. 7:161, 1955.

DeJong, R. N.: "Psychomotor" or "Temporal Lobe" Epilepsy. A Review of the Development of Our Present Concepts. Neurology 7:1, 1957.

Fraser, F. C. J.: Medical Genetics in Pediatrics. Pediat. 44:85, 1954.

Gibbs, E. L. and Lennox, W. G.: Electroencephalographic Classification of Epileptic Patients and Control Subjects. Arch. Neurol. & Psychiat. 50:111, 1943.

Gibbs, F. A. and Gibbs, E. L.: Atlas of Electroencephalography. Epilepsy ed. 2, Cambridge, Mass. Addison-Wesley Publishing Co., 1952.

Gibbs, E. L., Gillen, H. W., and Gibbs, F. A.: Disappearance and Migration of Epileptic Foci in Childhood. Am. J. Dis. Child. 88:596, 1954.

———, Fleming, MM., and Gibbs, F. A.: Diagnosis and Prognosis of Hypsarhythmia and Infantile Spasms. Pediat. 13:66, 1954.

Glaser, G. H. and Golub, L. M.: Electroencephalogram of Psychomotor Seizures in Childhood. Electroencephalog. & Clin. Neurophysiol. 7:329, 1955.

———, and Dixon, M. S.: Psychomotor Seizures in Childhood. Neurology 6:646, 1956.

Goodall, R. J.: Cerebral Hemispherectomy; Present Status and Clinical Indications. Neurology 7:151, 1957.

Halpern, L. and Bental, E.: Epileptic Cephalea. Neurology 8:615, 1958.

Hoefer, P. F. A., Cohen, S. M., and Greeley, D. McL.: Paroxysmal Abdominal Pain—a Form of Epilepsy in Children. J.A.M.A. 147:1, 1951.

Howell, D. A.: Unusual Centrencephalic Seizure Patterns. Brain 78:199, 1955.

Krynaw, R. A.: Infantile Hemiplegia Treated by Removing One Cerebral Hemisphere. J. Neurol., Neurosurg. and Psychiat. 13:243, 1950.

Lennox, W. G.: Tridione in the Treatment of Epilepsy. J.A.M.A. 134:138, 1947.

————: The Genetics of Epilepsy. Am. J. Psychiat. 103:457, 1947.

———— and Davis, J. P.: Clinical Correlates of the Fast and the Slow Spike-Wave Electroencephalogram. Pediat. 6:626, 1950.

————: The Heredity of Epilepsy as told by Relatives and Twins. J.A.M.A. 146:529, 1951.

Lillienfeld, A. M. and Pasamanick, B.: Association of Maternal and Fetal Factors with the Development of Epilepsy. J.A.M.A. 155:719, 1954.

Livingston, S.: The Use of Peganone (AC 695) in the Treatment of Epilepsy. J. Pediat. 49:728, 1956.

————: Celontin (PM-396) in the Treatment of Epilepsy. Pediat. 19:614, 1957.

———— and Pauli, L.: Meprobamate in the Treatment of Epilepsy of Children. A.M.A. J. Dis. Child. 94:277, 1957.

———— and Pauli, L. L.: Phenacemide in the Treatment of Epilepsy: Results of Treatment of 411 Patients and Review of the Literature. New England J. Med. 256:588, 1957.

————, Eisner, V. and Pauli, L.: Minor Motor Epilepsy. Pediat. 21:916, 1958.

Livingston, S. H.: The Social Management of the Epileptic Child and His Parents. J. Pediat. 51:137, 1957.

Low, N. L., Gibbs, E. L. and Gibbs, F. A.: Electroencephalographic Findings in Breath Holding Spells. Pediat. 16:595, 1955.

McQuarrie, I. and Peeler, D. B.: Effects of Sustained Pituitary Antidiuresis and Forced Water Drinking in Epileptic Children. A Diagnostic and Etiologic Study. J. Clin. Investigation 10:915, 1931.

Merritt, H. H. and Putnam, T. J.: Sodium Diphenyl Hydantoinate in the Treatment of Convulsive Disorders. J.A.M.A. 111:1068, 1938.

————: Textbook of Neurology. Philadelphia, Lea and Febiger, 1955.

Millichap, J. G.: Milontin: A New Drug in the Treatment of Petit Mal. Lancet 2:907, 1952.

————, Lombroso, C. T., and Lennox, W. G.: Cyclic Vomiting As a Form of Epilepsy in Children. Pediat. 16:705, 1955.

Penfield, W. and Jasper, H.: Epilepsy and the Functional Anatomy of the Human Brain. Boston, Little, Brown & Co., 1954.

Perlstein, M. A.: Use of Meprobamate (Miltown) in Convulsive and Related Disorders. J.A.M.A. 161:1040, 1956.

————: Metharbital (Gemonil) in Myoclonic Spasms of Infancy. A.M.A. J. Dis. Child. 93:425, 1957.

Rasmussen, T., Olszewski, J. and Lloyd-Smith, D.: Focal seizures due to chronic localized encephalitis. Neurology 8:435, 1958.

Reed, S. C.: Counseling in Medical Genetics. Philadelphia. W. B. Saunders Co., 1955.

Saltzstein, S. L., Jaudon, J. C., Luse, S. A. and Ackerman, L. V.: Lymph-
adenopathy Induced by Ethotoin (Peganone). J.A.M.A. 167:1618, 1958.
Smith, B. H. and McNaughton, F.: Mysoline, A New Anticonvulsant Drug.
Canad. Med. J. 68:464, 1953.
Snyder, C. H.: Epileptic Equivalents in Children. Pediat. 21:308, 1958.
Stevens, H.: Reading Epilepsy. New England J. Med. 257:165, 1957.
Yahr, M. D. and Merritt, H. H.: Current Status of the Drug Therapy of
Epileptic Seizures. J.A.M.A. 161:333, 1956.
Zimmerman, F. T.: Explosive Behavior Anomalies in Children on an Epilep-
tic Basis. New York State J. Med. 56:2537, 1956.

Migraine

Migraine is characterized by headache, usually limited to one side of the head, which is periodic and recurrent. It is often preceded by visual aura and accompanied by ocular and gastrointestinal symptoms such as nausea and vomiting. Sleep follows the attack. There is a hereditary and familial component, several members of a family being similarly affected. Between the attacks the child appears well. Boys are affected more frequently.

ETIOLOGY: The cause of migraine is unknown. The frequent positive family history (75 per cent) and the influence of tension and emotional upsets in precipitating an attack have been recognized. In some instances allergy has appeared to be a factor, and in others there has been an association with epilepsy. The mechanism of the attack appears to be vascular.

CLINICAL PICTURE: Krupp and Friedman showed that of their fifty children with migraine there was a history of headache in eighty-four per cent of the parents, of whom seventy per cent gave a classical picture of migraine. The onset of the attack is often associated with some type of stress, such as a school exam, a quarrel at home, or attending the movies. The child complains of severe headache, usually unilateral, over the front of the head or over the orbit, and he is bothered by light. Soon he begins to vomit. There may be fever. The nausea and vomiting may go on for varying periods for the next few hours, ending in sleep. In a number of children around three years of age, the picture is primarily one of cyclic vomiting. About twenty-five per cent of various reported series have had their onset at this age. The children are generally of superior intellectual level. However, they may show a number of personality disorders such as undue sensitivity, enuresis, or nail biting. In addition, these children may have psychological conflicts involving both the home and school work. As to the individual symptoms, in children the nausea and vomiting appear to be even more paramount than the headaches. The latter are frontal or orbital in most children, but may be temporal or occipital. There may be visual disturbances which precede or accompany the headache and vomiting. These consist of scintillating scotoma and blurred vision. In children, however, these findings are not common. There may be associated convulsive disorders, aphasia of the expressive type in which the child is confused and cannot speak clearly, paresthesiae, abdominal pain, numbness of fingers, or flushing of the face. The electroencephalogram in about twenty-five per cent of the children shows a dysrhythmic pattern, similar to that seen in epilepsy, usually non-localized. The attacks may recur with some periodicity every two or three weeks or irregularly. It has been noted that they occur much less frequently in the summer.

DIAGNOSIS: The diagnosis is based on the characteristic features of recurrent headache, usually unilateral, vomiting, and familial history. Brain tumor is ruled out by absent neurological signs, normal fundi, and X-ray of the skull, which shows no evidence of increased intracranial pressure. Vascular abnormalities of the cranial vessels are also usually eliminated by the above procedures. If suspected, arteriography may be needed. Common causes for headaches in children include eye strain due to refractive errors and sinusitis. These should be investigated along with abnormalities of the bones in the nose and skull, e.g., platybasia and trauma to the head. Psychological conditions, such as produce hysteria, should be considered, although these are also a great factor in precipitating the migraine attack.

OPHTHALMOPLEGIC MIGRAINE: This is the usual migraine associated with the development of extraocular muscle palsy (third nerve). Aneurysm, hemangioblastoma, and myasthenia gravis should be ruled out.

ABDOMINAL MIGRAINE: This must be distinguished from a surgical abdomen and abdominal epilepsy. In the latter the E.E.G. is characteristic. The family history and a generally normal E.E.G. would suggest abdominal migraine.

MIGRAINE AND EPILEPSY: There is conflict on the relationship between the two. Several authors have reported that twenty-five per cent or more of their children with migraine had electroencephalograms compatible with epilepsy, but Krupp and Friedman, had no abnormal tracings and no clinical evidence of epilepsy in their fifty children with migraine.

PROGNOSIS: This cannot be stated in definite terms. Burke and Peters in their short term follow-up (six years) indicated that the migraine is less severe as the children grow older, but it did not disappear in forty-nine of fifty-eight children.

TREATMENT: At the onset of the attack aspirin should be given orally if vomiting has not begun, otherwise by rectal suppository (twice the oral dose). In addition, one tablet of Cafergot® (which contains 1 mg. of ergotamine tartrate and 100 mg. of caffeine) may be given immediately and every half hour to total four doses. If necessary, this may also be given as a rectal suppository. Dilantin sodium® may be used as a means of prevention or treatment of the attack in those children with a positive electroencephalogram. If seizures are present, the condition should be treated as epilepsy.

Prophylaxis. This is most important. The parents should be told of the significance of emotional upsets, undue tensions, and too hard a daily routine in triggering the attacks of migraine. They must avoid open disharmony. Furthermore, they must not stress their own headaches and anxiety in front of the child. All factors which might have a bearing, such as nasal congestion, sinusitis, ocular difficulties, especially errors of refraction, and food allergies, should be corrected.

Burke, E. C. and Peters, G. A.: Migraine in Childhood. A.M.A. J. Dis. Child. 92:330, 1956.

Friedman, A. P. and Von Storch, T. J. C.: A Review of Headache. New York State J. Med. 56:3883, 1956.

Glaser, J.: Migraine in Pediatric Practice. A.M.A. J. Dis. Child, 88:92, 1954.

Krupp, G. R. and Friedman, A. P: Migraine in Children. A.M.A. J. Dis. Child. 85:146, 1953.

Ostfeld, A. M. and Wolff, H. G.: Arterenol (Norephinephrine) and the Mechanism of Vascular Headache of the Migraine Type. Arch. Neurol. and Psychiat. 74:131, 1955.

Pritchard, J. S.: Abdominal Pain of Cerebral origin in Children. Canad. M.A.J. 78:665, 1958.

Wolff, H. G., Tunis, M. M., and Goodell, H.: Evidence of Tissue Damage and Changes in Pain Sensitivity in Subjects with Vascular Headaches of the Migraine Type. Arch. Int. Med. 92:478, 1953.

CHAPTER 10

INTRACRANIAL TUMORS

In the discussion of intracranial tumors in infancy and childhood, major emphasis will be placed on the characteristics which are peculiar to the age period. The reader will find in the references detailed reports upon which this discussion is based.

LOCATION: The first significant fact about intracranial tumors in children is that the majority are located below the tentorium. In Ingraham and Matson's series of 313 tumors, 185 or 60 per cent were infratentorial. This includes tumors of the medulla, pons, cerebellum, 4th ventricle, and cerebellar-pontine angle. In adults, on the other hand, the opposite is true, that is, the majority are supratentorial.

Secondly, childhood tumors develop especially along the neural axis, often accompanied by obstructive signs (hydrocephalus and increased intracranial pressure).

TYPE: The most common type of neoplasm in the age group up to sixteen years is the malignant glioma. Of 154 cases of intracranial neoplasm, classified pathologically by Bailey, as reported by Cushing, 116 or 75 per cent were gliomas. Bailey and others have since reported similar percentages, stressing further the preponderance of subtentorial location and the infrequency of pituitary adenomas, meningiomas, and acoustic neuromas, which make up a large percentage of adult tumors. Of all the gliomas in childhood the most frequent types are astrocytomas, medulloblastomas, and ependymomas. In the supratentorial region, the most frequent tumor is craniopharyngioma.

AGE: Intracranial tumors occur in infancy. Their number rises to a maximum at five to eight years, with a peak age at six years, and then declines, with a secondary rise at ten to twelve years; then a

265

further decline takes place. Bailey has suggested that this last decline is due to the tapering off of childhood tumors at a time when the adult types have not as yet begun to make themselves apparent.

SYMPTOMS AND SIGNS: The symptoms and signs of intracranial tumor usually develop slowly in infancy and childhood. They are based on evidence of a general increase in intracranial pressure, and secondly, on the focal neurological effects produced by the specific location of the tumor.

The classical signs and symptoms of increased intracranial pressure are vomiting, headache, and papilledema. In infancy, however, the effects of increased intracranial pressure may be delayed, because the open fontanels and suture lines permit enlargement of the head. When the head circumference appears to be expanding too rapidly (over ½ inch a month in infancy) so that hydrocephalus is suspected, tumor should be considered as a cause. This is strongly emphasized because the majority of the tumors of childhood are along the neural axis or midline, producing a block in the flow of cerebrospinal fluid. The onset of symptomatology may follow a fall or injury. Hemorrhage into the tumor and surrounding edema may produce the development of obstructive symptoms. In addition to trauma, infection may also precipitate the onset of symptoms. There may be pleocytosis in the spinal fluid. Tumor must be differentiated from other causes of hydrocephalus, e.g., congenital or due to meningitis. Subdural hematoma must also be ruled out; subdural punctures will reveal the presence or absence of hematoma.

Vomiting. This is extremely common in intracranial tumors of childhood. It is the most frequent sign of subtentorial tumors and is usually no different from that seen in the ordinary gastrointestinal upset so common in infants and children. In pediatric practice such vomiting is most often considered part of a general acute respiratory infection or tonsillitis. When it is recurrent, "cyclic vomiting" is diagnosed, possibly associated with a hypertonic or highly emotional youngster. It must be kept in mind that in gliomas of the brain stem, ependymoma of the 4th ventricle, or medulloblastoma of the cerebellum, vomiting is an early feature, especially in glioma, where it precedes the development of increased intracranial pressure and is due to vagal irritation.

Headache. This is a common complaint in childhood tumor. When recurrent and persistent it is highly significant. Its location is not diagnostic; it may be frontal or occipital. It frequently occurs on arising in the morning. It often accompanies vomiting and may be affected by changes in position. Nausea is not of any moment.

Diplopia. Double vision or diplopia occurs together with internal strabismus. This may be of localizing value prior to any evidence of increased intracranial pressure, when internal strabismus (6th nerve palsy) is associated with impaired conjugate deviation of the eyes, as in glioma of the brain stem (Bailey). Along with this there is often blurred or complete loss of vision. In the latter case, there may be papilledema or secondary optic atrophy.

Papilledema. This is extremely common, occurring at some time in most brain tumors in children. It is followed by secondary optic atrophy and is characterized by failing vision. However, in glioma of the brain stem, papilledema may be lacking or late. Hence its absence does not rule out brain tumor.

There are other general indications of increased intracranial pressure such as extreme drowsiness, alteration in pulse rate, and disturbance in respiration, which appear late. Elevation of blood pressure is also usually a late feature except in brain stem or hypothalamic tumors.

OTHER SYMPTOMS AND SIGNS:

Convulsion. Since most tumors in childhood are infratentorial and thus unassociated with seizures, convulsions do not play a great role in diagnosis. Convulsions occur primarily with supratentorial tumors, especially of the cerebral hemispheres. The seizures are likely to be generalized, but may be focal and Jacksonian. Most instances of seizure in children are due to epilepsy and the cause is other than tumor; however, the latter must always be considered in any case of recurrent seizures. Cerebellar fits may occur, with retraction of the head and rigidity of the extremities. Stiff neck is often seen in children with posterior fossa tumors.

Gait. There may be a staggering gait or Romberg sign, usually due to a subtentorial tumor (cerebellar). The children walk on a broad base and cannot walk a straight line.

Behavior Change. Changes in personality with lack of interest in school work may occur. This is essentially present in adults with frontal and temporal lobe tumors which are not common in children. Hypothalamic tumors are associated with drowsiness and hypersomnia.

LOCALIZING SIGNS: Reference should be made to the subsequent pages, where the individual types of tumors and their locations are described along with the clinical pictures.

LABORATORY: Lumbar puncture should be avoided in the presence of choked discs. In general it should not be done in suspected posterior fossa tumors as there is a marked risk to the child and since the result usually is not a factor in the ultimate diagnosis. If needed for differential, then ventricular puncture may first be done to relieve pressure. In very occasional instances, however, spinal puncture may be done, drawing off slowly only a few cc. of spinal fluid. Pressure is elevated in most cases. Protein is usually increased. When it is, the fluid may be xanthochromic, although generally it is clear. Cell counts over ten per cu. mm., found in a small number of cases, suggest that the tumor has invaded the subarachnoid space or meninges. In this case the clinical picture is one of meningitis and the spinal fluid sugar may be decreased.

Ventricular fluid may be different from that observed by spinal puncture. If there is a block in the posterior fossa with obstructive hydrocephalus, the spinal fluid pressure may be normal, but ventricular pressure will be increased. The protein content may be normal or increased, the latter occurring particularly when the tumor is pressing on the ventricles.

X-RAY OF THE SKULL: Roentgenography may show separation or diastasis of the cranial sutures, enlargement of the head, convolution atrophy with bone resorption, intracranial calcification of the tumor, and erosion of the sella. Tumors within the sella cause ballooning.

ELECTROENCEPHALOGRAPHY: This technique has great value in tumors of the cerebral cortex. It may help to localize a focus of abnormality, especially if repeated electroencephalograms show the same area of pathology. In children, since most tumors are in the posterior fossa and since the electroencephalogram does not reveal any excitation from the deeper areas, the test has limited value.

ANGIOGRAPHY: The injection of radio-opaque dyes into the carotid or vertebral arteries to show first the arterial and, with subsequent films, the venous system is not of much use in infancy, but may be of value in older children where the vessels are larger. In general, angiography may indicate the location, as well as the type of tumor, especially the supratentorial tumors. It is most useful in demonstrating vascular malformations and aneurysms.

RADIOACTIVE SUBSTANCES: These may be injected intravenously in the form of radioactive iodinated human serum albumin (RIHSA). This procedure may detect subdural hematomas or cerebral neoplasms. Its value in children is not too great.

VENTRICULOGRAPHY AND PNEUMOENCEPHALOGRAPHY: When there is obvious indication of increased intracranial pressure, ventriculography is the method of procedure. This technique, however, should only be used when the suspected tumor cannot be localized without it. It is followed by immediate surgery.

Pneumoencephalography or injection of air through the lumbar subarachnoid space is usually reserved for information concerning cortical atrophy and is not used in suspected brain tumor. The reason is that the majority of tumors in children are infratentorial; hence, removal of spinal fluid may permit herniation of the cerebellum and medulla into the foramen magnum, with death resulting. If it is done in unsuspected tumor and the ventricles do not fill with air, ventriculography should be done, as there may be an obstruction.

The value of ventriculography in suspected brain tumor lies in demonstrating dilatation of the lateral and 3rd ventricles due to obstruction of the 4th ventricle or aqueduct. The anterior portion of the 3rd ventricle and the lateral ventricles may show distension, together with a filling defect in the posterior part of the 3rd ventricle, or non-filling of the latter, due to tumor. The lateral ventricle is compressed and shifted to the opposite side in tumor of the cerebral lobe.

Finally some cystic brain tumors may be visualized through needle aspiration followed by injection of dye which will outline the cyst.

GLIOMAS OF THE BRAIN STEM

These tumors comprise about 15-20 per cent of all intracranial neoplasms in childhood. They occur primarily in the pons, but they may involve the medulla and upper cervical cord or extend into the cerebellum or cerebral peduncles.

PATHOLOGY: The tumors are composed of different types of glial tissue and cause a marked increase in the size of the pons. Since the tumor grows within the pons, it rarely blocks the aqueduct. Damage is therefore usually produced through infiltration and destruction of the nerve cells.

CLINICAL PICTURE: In view of the pathology, the significant feature is the development of multiple cranial nerve palsies of the bulbar type. The onset may be slow or insidious, but there is a progressive involvement of the various cranial nerves. There is loss of the corneal reflex and deviation of the jaw to the side of the lesion because of weakness of the temporal and masseter muscles (5th Nerve). Paralysis of lateral gaze is important (6th Nerve). There may be paralysis of movement of both eyes toward the side of the tumor. Facial paralysis of the peripheral type is evident through inability to close the eye, lack of wrinkling of the forehead, and inability to whistle. There may be difficulty in hearing (8th nerve). There may also be involvement of the remaining nerves, including difficulty in speech and swallowing, palatal palsy, and deviation of the tongue toward the side of the lesion (9th, 10th, and 12th nerves). If there is extension of the tumor upward, various ocular palsies may occur. Vomiting is present early, unaccompanied by signs of increased intracranial pressure. Extension to the cerebellar pathways produces difficulty in walking, which is performed on a wide base and with a tendency to fall backwards. The pyramidal tracts may be affected causing paralysis of the extremities, which may be flaccid or spastic, but which is accompanied in either case by hyperactive reflexes, Babinski sign, and ankle clonus. With extension toward the midbrain there is marked somnolence. There may be fever without leukocytosis and also hypertension.

Lumbar Puncture. The spinal fluid is clear, usually under no increased pressure; lymphocytosis to about 50 cells per cu. mm. may be present due to meningeal irritation. There may be a slight elevation of protein. Sugar is normal.

Ventriculogram shows displacement of the aqueduct and 4th ventricle posteriorly and upward.

DIAGNOSIS: The major point in diagnosis is the development of multiple cranial nerve palsies. These are unaccompanied by signs of increased intracranial pressure, even though vomiting may be persistent. There then follow paralysis of the extremities and/or unsteadiness in gait.

DIFFERENTIAL: These cases are often diagnosed as encephalitis because of pleocytosis in the spinal fluid, the development of bulbar palsies, and fever. However, in encephalitis there are other findings indicating more widespread involvement of the brain, positive serology tests such as complement fixation, and sometimes a history of mumps, etc. There may be a history of trauma or previous respiratory infection which confuses the picture. We have mentioned the absence of signs of increased pressure such as headache, papilledema, or enlarged head, although vomiting is present early. In the summertime poliomyelitis is often diagnosed. Diphtheria may be considered. To emphasize again, however, when there is the development of multiple bulbar nerve palsies, tumor, particularly glioma of the pons, must be considered. Differential from other tumors such as of the 4th ventricle, pinealomas, etc., may be suggested by the fact that these present signs of increased intracranial pressure early. Bulbar nerve involvement follows later.

PROGNOSIS: The outlook is poor. Death usually occurs within a year.

TREATMENT: The tumor should be explored and biopsy taken. It cannot be removed because it is not encapsulated. X-ray treatment should be given.

EPENDYMOMA

This tumor originating from the ependymal cells invades the 4th ventricle. It may, however, arise from ependymal cells in other locations, such as the 3rd ventricle. It comprises about seven per cent of childhood tumors.

PATHOLOGY: In the 4th ventricle the tumor has a tendency to occupy the floor and fill up the various spaces. The subtentorial ependymomas also tend to send long projections of tumor tissue toward or into the spinal canal, invading the cord itself. Microscopically, the cells are varied in form and are arranged in solid sheets radially about blood vessels. For classification as to the type of cells see the article by Kernohan.

CLINICAL PICTURE: This is based on obstruction of the flow of cerebrospinal fluid with the development of signs of increased intracranial pressure. There are vomiting, headache, papilledema and cranial suture separation with enlargement of the head. As a result of the projection of the tumor cells toward the spinal canal, there is spasm of the neck muscles. The head is held stiffly, tilted to the side for relief. There are marked pain in the neck and shoulders and limitation of movements. If the cerebellum is displaced or invaded, the "vermis syndrome" picture, similar to cerebellar medullo-blastoma, is seen. This consists of a disturbance of equilibrium in walking (ataxic gait), whereas no incoordination is noted when voluntary movements are made in bed.

LABORATORY: Spinal puncture should be avoided in the presence of papilledema. The X-ray may show midline calcification in the tumor, which is diagnostic, and a widening of the sutures.

DIAGNOSIS: There are no distinctive features separating this tumor from others such as medulloblastoma. Early signs of increased intracranial pressure, dizziness, or the signs of the vermis syndrome should make one suspicious of tumor.

PROGNOSIS: The outcome is poor since the tumor, being invasive, cannot be removed in toto. The site of the tumor, ease of removal, and preoperative duration of symptoms particularly affect the survival period.

TREATMENT: As much of the tumor as possible should be removed without injuring cranial nerve structures; this is followed by deep X-ray therapy, which may prolong life.

CEREBELLUM

MEDULLOBLASTOMA

This gliomatous tumor of the cerebellum is markedly malignant, usually midline, arising in the roof of the 4th ventricle. It is of frequent occurrence in the tumors of childhood.

PATHOLOGY: The tumor is usually located in the midline. It may spread by way of the subarachnoid channels to invade the cerebellar hemispheres and spinal cord. Its growth in the midline produces pressure on the vermis and causes separation of the cerebellar lobes, secondary hydrocephalus, and even pressure on the cervical cord. The medulloblast is of embryonic origin and may develop either as a glial cell or ganglion cell. The tumor it forms is soft and friable.

CLINICAL PICTURE: The onset may occur at any time in childhood, but especially between three and six years. It is essentially a tumor of young life, being rare in adulthood. It is the most frequent or next in order in the various reported series of tumors in children. Its course is rapid, since it is extremely malignant.

The first signs are vomiting and headache, indicative of increased pressure. The vomiting is likely to occur on arising in the morning, and may be projectile. The headaches may be frontal, but are accompanied by suboccipital discomfort. There soon follows a staggering gait. There is lack of equilibrium in walking; while lying down, however, there is no incoordination on movement of the limbs. Papilledema, diplopia, internal strabismus, and enlargement of the head soon follow. Further cranial nerve palsies occur through extension to the cerebrum and spinal cord.

LABORATORY: X-ray shows suture separation, enlargement of the head, and convolutional atrophy. The *ventriculogram* demonstrates symmetrical dilatation of the lateral and 3rd ventricles. The *electroencephalogram* is normal or may show slow waves with bilateral synchrony from the occipital lobes.

PROGNOSIS: The children die usually within two years. There are extension to the meninges and deposits elsewhere in the cerebrospinal axis.

TREATMENT is to reestablish circulation of the spinal fluid by surgery, removing as much of the 4th ventricle mass as possible, using some for a biopsy specimen. Deep X-radiation follows.

ASTROCYTOMA

Astrocytoma of the cerebellum along with the medulloblastoma is the most frequently seen brain tumor of childhood. In contradistinction to medulloblastoma, however, astrocytoma is considered perhaps the most benign type. It comprises about 20 per cent of the childhood group.

PATHOLOGY: The tumor is located usually in the midline (vermis) or nearby. It is either solid or cystic, and slow growing. It may extend into the cerebellar hemispheres, rarely into the brain stem. One of the outstanding characteristics is the cystic nature. The cysts contain a mural nodule, which Cushing felt was the source of the growth of the tumor. This nodule and adjacent cyst wall must be removed to effect complete cure. The cystic fluid is yellow and clots or gels on removal. Microscopically, there are fibrillary or protoplasmic astrocytes in the solid portion of the tumor.

CLINICAL PICTURE: The onset of symptoms, usually insidious, includes the usual evidences of increased intracranial pressure, namely, headache and vomiting. In others the first symptoms include disturbance of gait or impaired vision before the onset of cerebellar signs. In older children there may be lethargy or lack of cooperation with the family. Unilateral cerebellar involvement may be indicated by a slow, coarse nystagmus to the side of the lesion, hypotonicity, dysmetria, and ataxia of the extremity on the side of the lesion. The length of evolution of the clinical picture is greater than in most other tumors, covering a period of three to eight years in the majority of cases. Matson stresses the presence of a wide base to the gait and inability to walk on a line as being more significant for diagnosis than the usual cerebellar signs which may be absent. The tendon reflexes and muscle tone are diminished in intrinsic tumors of the cerebellum. Papilledema is almost always present, diplopia and internal strabismus occasionally.

LABORATORY: X-ray of the skull shows separation of the sutures. The electroencephalogram may show slow wave and slow spike activity with increase of wave amplitude, but this is not diagnostic. The ventriculogram shows dilatation of the ventricles. Ventriculography, if done, must be followed by surgery.

DIAGNOSIS: Since these tumors are slow growing, it may take time to produce block of the cerebrospinal fluid with symptoms of increased pressure. In cases of persistent vomiting or recurrent headache, the optic disc should be looked at for evidence of papilledema. An X-ray of the skull should be taken for suture separation. Other features to be looked for include unsteadiness in gait, apathy, undue irritability, and persistent pain or stiffness of the neck, which may be accompanied by tilting of the head. Strabismus or visual difficulty may be noted.

PROGNOSIS: The outlook is favorable. In Matson's series of 34 cases, the cure rate was 80 to 90 per cent, with normal function in about 80 per cent. About 20 per cent have residual cranial nerve damage.

TREATMENT: This consists of the removal of the tumor in a one stage operation. If the tumor is in the lateral lobes, the results are good with no sequelae. If in the vermis, removal often cannot be accomplished without some cranial nerve damage. There is no response to X-ray or radium.

HEMANGIOBLASTOMAS

These tumors of embryonic origin, often familial, are essentially confined to the cerebellum.

PATHOLOGY: The tumor is of vascular origin with a tendency to become cystic, in which case there is a solid nodule attached to the wall. Some are solid. The tissue consists of capillaries and cellular elements. Rarely the tumor originates in the cerebral cortex as a cavernoma. Hemangioblastma is a benign tumor, but may become malignant.

CLINICAL PICTURE: These tumors occur essentially in adult life. The symptoms and signs are those of all the other types of cerebellar tumors, but often come on late. Early, there may be suboccipital discomfort and headache, later vomiting and papilledema.
DIAGNOSIS: A differential diagnosis cannot be made from other cerebellar tumors when hemangioblastoma exists alone. However, in some instances, when there is a retinal lesion (Von Hippel Disease), examination of the discs will show a tortuous, dilated vein and beading of the accompanying artery which together reach the periphery of the retina to enter a nodule. This finding would suggest that the cerebellar tumor is a hemangioblastoma.

PROGNOSIS: This may be good if the hemangioblastoma is solitary. If, however, there is involvement of the retina (angioma) or angiomatous nodules in either the spinal cord, brain stem, or viscera (Lindau's disease), the outlook is poor.

TREATMENT: The hemangioblastoma should be removed.

GLIOMAS OF THE OPTIC NERVE

These occur mainly in children.

PATHOLOGY: The tumor may cause enlargement of the optic nerve. It grows slowly, and does not metastasize. It usually arises in the intraorbital portion of the nerve and may extend toward the chiasm or advance further into the orbit. It may also be associated with Von Recklinghausen's disease. The glial cell is the spongioblast.

CLINICAL PICTURE: Since most cases are of intraorbital origin, the primary early feature is exophthalmos. This is unilateral. It is often accompanied or preceded by failing vision or diplopia. Ptosis may be present. The tumor may originate intracranially and involve the chiasm. Optic atrophy and progressive loss of vision are noted; occasionally, papilledema precedes the atrophy. The skin should be observed for cafe-au-lait spots as the involvement of the optic nerve may be associated with generalized neurofibromatosis.

DIAGNOSIS: Unilateral proptosis of the eye and progressive decline in vision are major points. Fundiscopic study reveals optic atrophy. X-ray shows enlargement of the optic foramen or thinning of the orbital roof. Visual field study shows irregular defects.

DIFFERENTIAL OF ORBITAL TUMORS: A variety of lesions involving the orbit may need differentiation. These include congenital encephalocele with orbital defect, dermoid, teratoma, metastatic neuroblastoma of the orbit, which may be diagnosed by the association with a palpable mass in the abdomen, and hemangioma. Exophthalmos may occur in orbital abscess, cavernous sinus thrombosis, exophthalmic goiter, Schüller-Christian syndrome, polyostotic fibrous dysplasia, and osteoma of the paranasal sinuses (frontal and ethmoid).

PROGNOSIS: The prospects are dismal.

TREATMENT: Transfrontal craniotomy with an attempt at total excision may be tried. If unsuccessful use radiation.

CEREBRAL HEMISPHERES

GLIOMAS

Gliomas of the cerebral hemispheres comprise about ten per cent of childhood brain tumors. They are composed primarily of astrocytomas and ependyomas. Glioblastoma multiforme, which is the common adult type, is rare. Oligodendroglioma is also infrequent.

CLINICAL PICTURE: In the infratentorial group of tumors the clinical picture is based on signs of increased intracranial pressure and local cerebellar or brain stem pathology. In the cerebral hemisphere tumors there is absence of a cerebellar signs, but localizing signs of pressure in the cortex are present. However, the difficulty in diagnosis lies in the age of the patient. Children are often too young to cooperate, so that more reliance must be placed on objective data than in adults, where a good deal of information is obtained through the study of visual field disturbances, from the presence of aphasia, etc. In addition, the cortical areas in early childhood may not be fully developed and capable of producing reliable focal anatomical diagnosis.

The presenting complaints include persistent headache, vomiting, alteration of personality (psychic disturbances, apathy, disinterest in appearance), and focal, including Jacksonian, seizures. There may be motor weakness, hemiparesis, increased tendon reflexes, and a Babinski sign. Papilledema may be noted. Sensory findings are difficult to elicit.

DIAGNOSIS: When one reviews the clinical picture, it is seen that there is a slowly growing tumor, which is less likely to produce abrupt signs of increased pressure than the infratentorial type. It is likely to be confused with a number of childhood diseases, including birth injury, centrencephalic epilepsy, cerebral palsy, and encephalitis. In any child who has sudden onset of seizures, motor weakness, a change of disposition, or persistent headache, further study should be carried out irrespective of any previous diagnosis, for the tumor may either be primary or complicating a previous condition such as cerebral palsy.

X-ray of the skull may show separation of sutures, calcification in the tumor, or convolutional atrophy. Electroencephalogram may show foci of abnormal electrical discharge. Ventriculography and arteriography may be carried out for localization of the tumor.

PROGNOSIS: This depends on the type of tumor and the time when the diagnosis is made. The slow growing tumors such as the astrocytoma and ependymoma have the best outlook, but in most cases death occurs early.

TREATMENT: This consists of removing as much of the tumor surgically as possible. Drug therapy should be given for the seizures. Radiation should be used for the sensitive types.

CRANIOPHARYNGIOMA

This tumor is the most frequent supratentorial neoplasm in children. It is known also as a Rathke's pouch tumor, adamantinoma, and hypophyseal duct tumor.

EMBRYOLOGY AND PATHOLOGY: The hypophysis is developed from a protrusion downward of a neural portion of the hypothalamus (floor of the 3rd ventricle) and from an epithelial pouch projecting upward from the buccal mucosa (Rathke's). In this process, squamous epithelial cell rests come to lie in the area of the pars tuberalis or infundibulum of the hypophysis. It is from these rests that the tumor is formed, so that actually it is not a craniopharyngioma, but the name is retained because of the long usage. The tumor is usually cystic, containing yellow fluid with cholestrin crystals, often with a solid portion below the cyst. It is usually located in the suprasellar region, occasionally in the sella, and often calcifies. Microscopically, the cells are stratified squamous. Occasionally they are arranged to resemble tooth buds (adamantinoma), or the appearance is that of mucoid cysts lined with secreting cells. Due to its location the tumor compresses or invades the 3rd ventricle. It may lie in the sella and also compress the hypophysis or press into the cerebral hemispheres (frontal or parietal lobes).

CLINICAL PICTURE: The onset of difficulty in children is usually marked by early evidence of increased intracranial pressure due to blocking of the 3rd ventricle by the tumor, so that headache, which is persistent and recurrent, progressive diminution in vision, and vomiting are early complaints. Papilledema is often present. The majority of children develop the clinical picture in the latter half of the first decade and through the second.

The visual defects depend upon the location of the tumor. If it is behind the chiasm there is papilledema; if in front, there may be optic atrophy. The visual field defects may be asymmetrical, but since the tumor is usually suprasellar, there are lower quadrant field defects and a bitemporal hemianopia. Pressure on one tract results in homonymous hemianopia; if on the nerve, there is blindness with atrophy. The 3rd nerve especially and also the 4th and 6th may be involved, producing diplopia and ocular palsies. Inclusion of the 7th results in facial palsy.

With involvement of the pituitary gland there is evidence of retarded skeletal development and growth. In older children there are sexual infantilism, hairlessness, and smooth skin. The syndrome of Simmonds cachexia or Lorain dwarfism with infantilism may be seen. Hypothalamic pressure is noted by the presence of diabetes insipidus, drowsiness, hypothermia, or the adiposogenital syndrome (Fröhlich).

ROENTGENOGRAM: Calcification is evident in most of the cases, usually suprasellar (80 per cent), which is diagnostic. Signs of increased intracranial pressure are present, including suture separation, wide flat sella, and erosion of the posterior clinoid processes.

DIAGNOSIS: The diagnostic features are the age of the child, presence of persistent headache, papilledema, diminution of vision, endocrine changes, and X-ray evidence of suprasellar calcification.

Other considerations include pituitary adenoma. These are extremely rare in children. A differential is made by the presence of suprasellar calcification in craniopharyngioma and visual field defects which are usually not present in the adenomas of childhood. Gliomas of the optic nerve involving the chiasm produce rapid loss of vision, and X-ray shows an enlarged optic foramen. Craniopharyngioma may simulate cerebellar tumor due to pressure backward, causing cerebellar signs of ataxia and difficulty in walking. Tumors of the 3rd ventricle may require differential. It must be remembered that in about 20 per cent of craniopharyngiomas calcification does not occur. In these and in young children whose visual fields cannot be checked, ventriculography may be needed to aid in the diagnosis. Finally reference should be made to the hamartomas and gangliomas of the posterior hypothalamus which produce excessive physical growth and precocious puberty in early childhood. They are demonstrated by pneumoencephalography as an abnormal mass in the interpeduncular space.

PROGNOSIS: The outlook is poor. About 20 per cent may survive five to ten years after surgery.

TREATMENT: Total removal is rarely possible because of the close adherence of the cyst wall to the pituitary and hypothalamus. The cyst is evacuated and removal of the capsule is attempted. When the tumor blocks the flow of spinal fluid by pressing up into the ventricle, a Torkildsen may be performed. Ingraham, Matson, and McLaurin have used cortisone and ACTH to make up for poor adrenal function due to pituitary disturbances, both pre- and postoperative. Deep X-ray therapy may be tried.

PITUITARY TUMORS

ADENOMAS

These are extremely rare in childhood. Of 154 cases of tumors of the brain in preadolescence reported by Cushing there were only two cases. We have discussed the pituitary gland and the effects of hypo and hyperpituitarism in the chapter on endocrinology.

Here it is only necessary to stress that with tumor of the pituitary (adenoma), the effects of pressure of the tumor on the pituitary gland itself and adjacent structures such as the optic chiasm, optic nerve and tracts, 3rd ventricle, hypothalamus, and nearby cranial nerves are added to the endocrine effects of hypo or hyperpituitarism.

The tumors are either chromophobe (most common tumor of the pituitary, but almost always in adults) or chromophile (eosinophilic or basophilic) and arise from the anterior lobe. Chromophobe tumors produce headache, failure of vision, optic atrophy, and bitemporal hemianopia plus signs of hypofunction of the pituitary. The X-ray shows ballooning of the sella plus enlargement and erosion. Treatment is removal of the tumor or X-ray therapy. Eosinophilic tumors produce signs of pressure similar to the chromophobe type plus gigantism due to hypersecretion of growth hormone. Acromegaly occurs in the adult. Basophilic tumors are associated with Cushing's syndrome.

TREATMENT: X-ray therapy should be used if there are slight or no visual disturbances. If there are marked visual changes, decompression is carried out and as much of the tumor as possible is removed.

CHOROID PLEXUS

Papilloma of the choroid plexus is essentially a tumor of childhood, comprising about 3 per cent of all such brain tumors.

PATHOLOGY: These tumors arise most frequently from the choroid plexus of the 4th ventricle, occasionally from the lateral ventricles. They are papillomatous and similar to the normal choroid plexus in structure, cauliflower in appearance, and may be cystic. They may develop malignant tendencies (adenocarcinomas). They may produce hydrocephalus, communicating in type with hypersecretion, if in the lateral ventricle or non-communicating (obstructive) in type in the 4th ventricle by blocking the aqueduct. They do not invade neural tissue. Being highly vascular, they may hemorrhage into the ventricle.

CLINICAL PICTURE: The infant comes to attention mainly because of enlargement of the head (hydrocephalus), bulging fontanel and suture separation, or persistent vomiting. In older children there are headache and unsteady gait. Convulsions may occur. The fundi show papilledema. If hemorrhage into the ventricle should occur, there are signs and symptoms of spontaneous subarachnoid hemorrhage. There are no localizing signs, because the neural tissue is not invaded.

DIAGNOSIS: Since the presenting picture is similar to hydrocephalus, ventriculography must be done. Choroid plexus tumor should be suspected in every case where chronic hydrocephalus, subdural hematoma, or posterior fossa tumor is under consideration. If there is any doubt, ventriculography is preceded by subdural punctures. Ventriculogram may show a mass in the lateral ventricle or obstructive hydrocephalus with the tumor in the 4th ventricle.

Vascular malformation which ruptures to produce spontaneous subarachnoid hemorrhage is usually not associated with signs of increased intracranial pressure. Ventriculography and angiography should help in differential diagnosis.

PROGNOSIS: This is doubtful because of the difficulty of removal of the tumor in toto and the possibility of seeding to other parts of the brain and cord.

TREATMENT: The tumor should be removed. If this is not completely possible, deep X-ray therapy is used. Horrax feels that decompression and X-ray therapy rather than extirpation should be the method of procedure.

PINEAL GLAND

Tumors of the pineal gland comprise about 3 per cent of intracranial tumors in children.

PATHOLOGY: These tumors consist essentially of pinealomas and pineoblastomas but other histological types are described including teratomas, gliomas, and ganglioneuromas. The pineoblastomas, have a tendency to break through into the ventricular system. Gliomas and neuroblastomas may infiltrate the pineal region.

CLINICAL PICTURE: Because of the location of the pineal gland, there is extension into the 3rd ventricle and block of the flow of cerebrospinal fluid with the production of hydrocephalus. This may also occur from pressure down and back involving the aqueduct of Sylvius, cerebellum, and midbrain. Most cases are in males.

The early symptoms are those of increased intracranial pressure, resulting in suture separation and increase in the size of the head in infancy. Headache, vomiting, and papilledema may be noted.

The most significant localizing sign is a paralysis of upward conjugate gaze or movement of the eyes due to pressure on the quadrigeminal plate. The pupils are usually dilated and do not react to light, but accommodate in convergence. Bilateral ptosis may be present. Hearing may be lost due to involvement of the inferior colliculi. Pressure on the cerebellum produces unsteadiness of gait.

In boys, precocious puberty or pubertas praecox may occur. This includes early development of the adult type of penis and testicles with growth of body hair and voice changes. It is seen very rarely and is considered to be due to an involvement of the hypothalamus (not pineal). It is due either to pressure upon or a tumor of the hypothalamus from aberrant pineal rests or invasion through the subarachnoid space. In similar fashion the pinealoma may involve the floor of the 3rd ventricle and hypothalamus and thus produce the symptoms of diabetes insipidus.

X-RAY: Ventriculogram will show a filling defect in the posterior portion of the 3rd ventricle; the anterior part of the 3rd and lateral ventricles are dilated equally.

DIAGNOSIS: The major features of the pineal tumor include signs of increased intracranial pressure with failure of upward conjugate movement of the eyes. When present, signs of precocious puberty suggest hypothalamic involvement. Ventriculography may help.

TREATMENT: Torkildsen procedure is performed to relieve the obstructed flow of cerebrospinal fluid; X-ray therapy for the tumor is employed.

COLLOID CYSTS

Colloid cysts occur in the anterior portion of the 3rd ventricle. They are referred to as paraphysial cysts because the paraphysis of the embryo has been considered to be the site of origin. A mucinous secretion has been found in a number of these cysts.

The clinical picture is based on the block of cerebrospinal fluid flow from the lateral ventricles and foramen of Monro to the 3rd ventricle and pressure on adjacent structures such as the hypothalamic tracts and nuclei. Severe recurrent headaches occur. Since the cyst may shift its position, these headaches may be brought on or relieved by changes in the child's posture or movements of the head. They are intermittent. Hypersomnia (an uncontrollable desire to sleep in which arousal is possible) may be present due to pressure on the floor of the 3rd ventricle. There may also be visual disturbance and epileptiform seizures.

Diagnosis is made by ventriculography which indicates symmetrical dilatation of both lateral ventricles in normal position. If only one ventricle is pictured, there are failure of air to go to the other lateral ventricle or 3rd ventricle, deviation of the septum pellucidum, and a filling defect of the anterior part of the 3rd ventricle. If both are pictured, there is cutting off of the air shadows in the Foramen of Monro and a filling defect of the anterior portion of the 3rd ventricle.

Differential diagnosis from other tumors involving the 3rd ventricle such as craniopharyngiomas, gliomas, and pinealomas must be made.

TREATMENT: The treatment is surgical removal, if possible. If not, the contents are evacuated.

DERMOIDS AND TERATOMAS

Dermoids and teratomas were found by Ingraham and Bailey to include 15 of 231 neoplasms of the central nervous system or 6.5 per cent. Of these, eight were intracranial and seven intraspinal.

PATHOLOGY: These tumors may be composed of any of the three layers of germinal origin. They are firm, but some part of the inner area of the tumor is cystic, containing a pale yellow or cloudy white fluid. The dermoid contains hair and sebaceous material. The teratomas may contain hair, teeth, bone, fat, and gland tissue.

These tumors are located in any part of the central nervous system, usually along the midline, that is, the 4th ventricle, pineal and pituitary regions, occipital area, and spinal cord.

CLINICAL PICTURE: This is similar to that of other tumors, presenting either the effects of increased intracranial pressure or focal signs. X-ray may reveal evidence of pressure or calcification. Ventriculography may show a filling defect. Generally the diagnosis is made at operation.

TREATMENT: The tumor is removed if possible. If it is not malignant, the patient is cured. Some dermoids cannot be removed completely because of their connection with a dermal sinus in the skin over the midline of the posterior fossa. In this case the major dural sinuses are involved and complete removal of the lesion cannot safely be done.

TUMORS OF THE SKULL

These are of various types, including the dermoid and epidermoid, which are congenital, and the osteomas. The latter may involve the inner or outer table of the skull, and also the paranasal sinuses.

In the skull the osteoma has a tendency to reach a great size, growing outward to produce deformities. Rarely, it may grow inward towards the brain to produce pressure on the dura and brain contents. X-ray shows the thickened bone. Treatment is removal of the osteoma and cranioplasty.

Osteoma of the sinuses may involve extension into the orbit or brain. The frontal and ethmoid sinuses are most often involved. When the osteoma extends into the orbit, the development of proptosis and diplopia is seen. If the frontal lobe of the brain is invaded, there are signs of increased pressure and frontal lobe symptoms may develop. Rarely communication with the cerebrospinal fluid system produces rhinorrhea and secondary meningitis.

DIAGNOSIS: X-ray of sinuses and skull reveal the tumor.

TREATMENT: Removal by craniotomy is performed.

Lymphosarcoma or lymphoepithelioma arising from the nasopharynx may invade the skull. They grow rapidly and metastasize early. The tumor may penetrate the orbit or middle or posterior fossa. There may also be a spread by way of the lymphoid tissue (cervical glands) and blood stream. The cranial nerves from the second to the twelfth may be involved. The eustachian tube may be occluded by a pharyngeal wall tumor. The diagnosis is made by the presence of cranial nerve involvement and local findings of nasal obstruction, nasal discharge, and cervical lymphadenopathy. X-ray of the base of the skull may show a tumor shadow. The treatment is irradiation.

Rarely, sarcoma of the bone may arise as a primary neoplasm. It is noted as a rapidly growing, firm tumor of the vault and may erode the bone (X-ray). The disease is fatal due to rapid metastasis, especially to the lungs.

Hemangiomas may produce symptoms by pressure on the brain

after penetrating the bone, or there may be associated intracranial hemangiomas. X-ray shows thinning out of the bone. Angiography outlines the hemangioma.

TREATMENT: X-ray therapy is indicated if the tumor is large or multiple, so that removal is not feasible.

TUMORS OF THE MENINGES

These are not common in childhood. They are classified as meningiomas by Cushing and Eisenhardt, in whose series of 295 cases, six were in the preadolescent age group. Generally, when occurring in children, the meningeal tumors are of a sarcomatous nature and more invasive.

Meningiomas arise from tufts of arachnoidal cells and are likely to be solid, encapsulated, and slow growing. They are most frequently located in the parasagittal area and over the convexity of the cerebral hemispheres. They also arise in the floor of the anterior fossa and sphenoidal ridge. They may undergo calcification (psammoma). The tumor may invade the dura and skull but not the brain.

The clinical picture depends on the location of the tumor. In the convexity near the longitudinal sinus there may be focal paralysis and seizure; in the sphenoidal area, exophthalmos and orbital cranial nerve pathology; in the olfactory groove, anosomia and optic nerve atrophy; and in the anterior fossa, involvement of the tuberculum sellae with compression of the chiasm resulting in bitemporal hemianopia.

Diagnosis is occasionally made by localizing signs and symptoms, but more often by X-ray evidence of erosion into the bones, calcification (psammoma), and ventriculography.

Treatment consists of surgical removal of the tumor and the attached dura.

Sarcoma or melanoma of the meninges may occur. Both of these tumors arise from the leptomeninges. The meningeal sarcoma spreads freely through the subarachnoid space, especially over the base of the brain, including the cerebellum and brain stem. It also spreads over the cerebral cortical areas. The symptoms may be those of increased intracranial pressure, or irritation, simulating meningitis. In the latter case, the spinal fluid shows a cellular increase, elevated protein, and may have a low sugar. Meningeal sarcoma should be considered if cultures and smears of the spinal fluid do not reveal purulent organisms, M. tuberculosis, or yeasts.

In considering the diagnosis of intracranial tumors, an attempt must be made to establish the presence of tumor as differentiated from other conditions. In doing this, the techniques previously outlined will aid not only in differential from other causes, but also in establishing the anatomic location and perhaps the type of tumor.

In infancy, enlargement of the head due to hydrocephalus is a major manifestation of midline tumor. Other causes must be ruled out, such as congenital hydrocephalus due to atresia of the aqueduct or failure of development of the foramina of Magendie and Luschka. Dye tests and ventriculography will usually aid. In macrocephaly there are neither increased intracranial pressure nor enlarged ventricles. Subdural hematoma is ruled out by negative subdural punctures. Thrombosis of the dural sinuses may cause confusion; usually the infant is markedly malnourished and there is a preceding infection. In the neonatal period there may be a relation between angiomatous tumors of the brain and congenital anomalies elsewhere.

DIFFERENTIAL DIAGNOSIS:

a) *Brain abscess.* This is usually secondary to mastoiditis, septic thrombosis of the intracranial venous sinuses, or infection in the lungs or paranasal sinuses. Congenital heart disease may be present. There are spinal fluid changes with mild pleocytosis, or severe, if meningitis is present.

b) *Tuberculosis.* Since the pathology in tuberculosis usually involves the base of the brain, it may produce signs of increased pressure similar to posterior fossa tumors. Tuberculous meningitis is diagnosed by a positive intradermal skin test, positive Ziehl-Neelson stain of the spinal fluid, and culture. The spinal fluid sugar is low.

Tuberculomas. These are now rare. A negative intradermal tuberculin test is evidence against tuberculoma, and conversely, positive signs of tuberculosis as above are significant in conjunction with signs of tumor.

c) *Syphilis.* This is very rare and is ruled out by a negative Wassermann both in the blood and spinal fluid.

d) *Fungi* such as torula, producing chronic meningitis with increased intracranial pressure, need to be differentiated. Occasionally parasites also require consideration.

e) *Viral Encephalitis.* This may produce fever, ocular palsies, and hypersomnia, which may stimulate glioma of the brain stem or 3rd ventricle tumors. However, while glioma produces cranial nerve palsies, encephalitis is not restricted to the brain stem.

f) *Toxic.* (lead poisoning): The major picture is one of generalized convulsion, which is not usual in tumors in children. There is a history of lead exposure, excessive elimination of lead and coproporphyrin in the urine. X-ray of the long bones shows increase in density at the metaphyseal junction. Blood lead is elevated.

g) *Epilepsy.* In every case of recurrent seizure, the work-up must rule out tumor.

h) *Nephritis.* With hypertension and cerebral edema, seizures may occur.

i) *Vascular malformation.* Look for angiomata and nevi on the skin. X-ray of the skull may reval anomalies (injection of contrast media).

j) *Serous Meningitis, arachnoiditis, or pseudotumor cerebri.* There is increased intracranial pressure, with the usual symptoms and signs of vomiting, headache, papilledema, and diplopia but without focal or localizing signs. The ventriculogram is usually normal. In the posterior fossa the picture may simulate cerebellar tumor; arachnoiditis about the chiasm may look like tumor of the sella or pituitary adenoma. If operated upon, relief of the pressure may improve the child.

Metastatic Tumors. These should be differentiated from primary intracranial neoplasms. Metastatic tumors are rare in childhood because carcinoma, the main cause in adults, is uncommon. Metastasis may occur from sarcoma, which may originate primarily in one area of the brain and spread through the meninges, or from the lung, ovary, or thigh. Glioma of the retina, hypernephroma, or a sympathetic system tumor may be primary. There may be spread from the nasopharynx or orbit.

The metastasis may involve the brain, dura, or bone. The spread is by direct extension or hematogenous. The clinical picture may be that of a localized tumor or of a general nature, including fever, vomiting, and drowsiness. It is important to X-ray the other areas of the body, such as the lungs, bones, and abdomen, which may reveal the primary source.

COMMENT

In a general way the importance of the diagnosis of brain tumors in infants or children resides in the fact that there are several neoplastic lesions which are curable by surgery, namely the hemangioblastoma and astrocytoma of the cerebellum. On occasion, meningiomas and more rarely cerebellar-pontine angle tumors are encountered that are relatively curable lesions. A great variety of intrinsic lesions of the brain stem are not curable, although a combination of surgical procedures and radiation therapy may provide palliation.

Of considerable importance is the recognition of lesions which are curable, and which may simulate the unfortunate types of neoplasms. Some types of abnormalities in this category are bilateral subdural hematoma, benign arachnoid cysts of the posterior fossa, and aqueductal insufficiency. Many times the clinical picture presented by these last three lesions may simulate in every way that of a malignant posterior fossa tumor. A child with a bilateral subdural hematoma may have severe cerebellar ataxia, ocular palsies, and marked papilledema and present in every way the features of, for example, a cerebellar medulloblastoma. Although by and large most neoplasms that occur in the infratentorial area are malignant, the only positive method of diagnosis is tissue verification. Clinical, radiologic and other indirect procedures are no substitute for tissue diagnosis. There can be little justification for primary therapy such as radiation without positive identification of the type of neoplasm or other lesion simulating neoplasm. In some midline ventricular tumors it may be preferable at times to perform a short-circuiting procedure such as a Torkildsen and administer X-ray therapy without tissue diagnosis. However, if there is no improvement in the clinical state, the lesion should be verified by open exploration. Certainly, it would indeed be unfortunate to have a child with a potentially benign lesion treated in this fashion. Regardless of what is done to a child with a cerebellar medulloblastoma, the ultimate result is death, so that one's attitude must be to attempt to find a benign lesion rather than to fall back on the diagnosis of a malignant lesion and use therapy which might only have a temporary effect.

From the standpoint of the surgeon, it seems extremely important to emphasize the danger of papilledema in relation to subsequent blindness. On occasion, he has had the unfortunate experience of operating on a benign cerebellar lesion with marked choked disc, only to find out after operation that the child is totally and forever blind. For this reason early treatment of the tumor and verification whether it is a benign or malignant lesion by a surgical approach is urgent. As a general rule ventriculography, pneumoencephalography and arteriography are of no avail and are to be avoided in situations of this character. The diagnosis often can be made on clinical grounds. The reason is obvious in relation to pneumoencephalography; but also in performing ventriculography and then following this with craniotomy and removal of the tumor, the very length of the total operative procedure and anesthesia threatens the life of the child.

Arnstein, C. H., Boldrey, E., and Naffziger, H. C.: A Case Report and Survey of Brain Tumors During the Neonatal Period. J. Neurosurg. 8:315, 1951.

Arseni, C.: Tumors of Basal Ganglia. A.M.A. Arch. Neurol. and Psychiat. 80:18, 1958.

Bailey, O. T. and Ingraham, F. D.: Intracranial Fibrosarcomas of the Dura Mater in Childhood: Pathological Characteristics and Surgical Management. J. Neurosurg. 2:1, 1945.

Bailey, P. and Cushing, H.: Medulloblastoma Cerebelli: A Common Type of Mid-Cerebellar Glioma of Childhood. Arch. Neurol. and Psychiat. 14:192, 1925.

——— and Eisenhardt, L.: Spongioblastoma of the Brain. J. Compt. Neurol. 56:391, 1932.

———, Buchanan, D. N., and Bucy, P. C.: Intracranial Tumors of Infancy and Childhood. Chicago, Ill. Univ. of Chicago Press, 1939.

Bell, R. L., Friedmann, A. B., and Olsen, B. W.: Scintiscanning as a Method for Localization of Cerebral Tumors. J. Neurosurg. 13:344, 1957.

Bray, P. F., Carter, S., and Taveras, J. M.: Brainstem Tumors in Children. Neurology. 8:1, 1958.

Bucy, P. C.: Intradiploic Epidermoid (Cholesteatoma) of the Skull. Arch. Surg. 31:190, 1935.

Casamajor, L., Laidlaw, R. W., and Kozinn, P.: Validity of Pneumoencephalographic Diagnosis, J.A.M.A. 140:1329, 1949.

Cramer, F., and Kimsey, W.: The Cerebellar Hemangioblastomas. Arch. Neurol. and Psychiat. 67:237, 1952.

Cushing, H.: The Intracranial Tumors of Preadolescence. Am. J. Dis. Child. 33:551, 1927.

————: Experiences with Orbito-ethmoidal Osteomata Having Intracranial Complications. Surg. Gynec. and Obst. 44:721, 1927.

———— and Bailey, P.: Tumors Arising from the Blood Vessels of the Brain. Springfield, Ill. Chas. C. Thomas, 1928.

———— and Eisenhardt, C.: Meningiomas. Springfield, Ill. Chas. C. Thomas, 1938.

Davidoff, L. M., aud Dyke, C. G.: Congenital Tumors in the Rostral Portion of the 3rd Ventricle. Bull. Neurol. Inst. 4:221, 1935.

Dunbar, H. S., and Ray, B. S.: Localization of Brain Tumors and Other Intracranial Lesions with Radioactive Iodinated Human Serum Albumin. Surg. Gynec. and Obst. 98:433, 1954.

Globus, J. H., Zucker, J. M., and Rubinstein, J. M.: Tumors of the Brain in Children and in Adolescents. Am. J. Dis. Child. 65:604, 1943.

Grinker, R. R., and Bucy, P. C.: Neurology. Springfield, Ill. Chas. C. Thomas. 1949.

Horrax G.: Treatment of Tumors of the Pineal Body. Arch. Neurol. & Psychiat. 64:227, 1950.

Ingraham, F. D. and Scott, H. W.: Craniopharyngiomas in Children. J. Pediat. 29:95, 1946.

———— and Bailey, O. T.: Cystic Teratomas and Teratoid Tumors of the Central Nervous System in Infancy and Childhood. J. Neurosurg. 3:511, 1946.

————, Matson, D. D., McLaurin, R. L.: Cortisone and ACTH as an Adjunct to the Surgery of Craniopharyngiomas. New England J. Med. 246:568, 1952.

———— and Matson, D. D.: Neurosurgery of Infancy and Childhood. Springfield, Ill. Chas. C. Thomas, 1954.

Kernohan, J. W. and Fletcher-Kernohan, E. M.: Ependymomas. A. Res. Nerv. and Ment. Dis. Proc. 16:182, 1937.

List, C. F., Dowman, C. E., Bagchi, B. K. and Bebin, J.: Posterior hypothalamic hamartomas and gangliogliomas causing precocious puberty. Neurology 8:164, 1958.

Maisel, J. E. and Lamm, S. S.: Ependymoma of the Fourth Ventricle in an Infant Under One Year of Age. Am. J. Dis. Child. 86:604, 1953.

Matson, D. D.: Cerebellar Astrocytoma in Childhood. Pediat. 18:150, 1956.

Marritt, H. H.: Textbook of Neurology. Philadelphia, Lea & Febiger, 1955.

Morley, T. P.: Hypothalamic Tumor and Precocious Puberty. J. Clin. Endocrinol. 14:1, 1954.

Mosberg, W. H. and Blackwood, W.: Mucus-Secreting Cells in Colloid Cysts of the 3rd Ventricle. J. Neuropath. & Exper. Neurol. 13:417, 1954.

Odom, G. L., Davis, C. H., and Woodhall, B.: Brain Tumors in Children. Clinical Analysis of 164 Cases. Pediat. 18:856, 1956.

Palmer, H. D. and Murphy, E. S.: Expanding Intracranial Lesions in Childhood. J.A.M.A. 149:220, 1952.

Poser, C. M., and Tavevas, J. M.: Clinical Aspects of Cerebral Angiography in Children. Pediat. 16:73, 1955.

Rand, C. W. and Reeves, D. L.: Choroid Plexus Tumors in Infancy and Childhood. Bull. Los Angeles Neurol. Soc. 5:31, 1940.

Ringertz, N., Nordenstam, H., and Flyger, G.: Tumors of the Pineal Region. J. Neuropath. and Exper. Neurol. 13:540, 1954.

Schnitker, M. T. and Ayer, D.: Primary Melanomas of the Leptomeninges. J. Nerv. & Ment. Dis. 87:45, 1938.

Tegeris, A. S.: Solitary Tuberculoma of the Medulla Oblongata. Pediat. 21:370, 1958.

Titrud, L. A., and Peyton, W. T.: Nasopharyngeal Tumors and Their Neurological Complications. J. Nerv. & Ment. Dis. 92:727, 1940.

Walker, A. E. and Hopple, T. C.: Brain Tumors in Children. J. Pediat. 35:671, 1949.

PSEUDOTUMOR CEREBRI

This condition is characterized clinically by evidence of increased intracranial pressure, and pathologically by an excessive amount of cerebrospinal fluid. It has been referred to as serous meningitis, benign intracranial hypertension, arachnoiditis, hypertensive meningeal hydrops, and otitic hydrocephalus.

CLINICAL PICTURE: This consists of headache, vomiting, and papilledema. There may also be diplopia with failing vision. Except for occasional sixth nerve palsy and disturbance of gait, there are no abnormal neurological signs or evidence of localized cortical involvement. Following the classification of Foley, Davidoff divided his 61 cases etiologically into three groups: those following otitis media, those associated with infections other than otitis or with injury to the head, and finally a group of cases occurring mostly in adult women with no history of injury or infection.

The group following otitis is probably associated with sinus thrombosis, either lateral or superior longitudinal, with the development of cerebral edema. Other factors such as a toxic effect on the brain from acute infection, allergy, or electrolyte disturbances have been postulated. Two cases were reported which developed two months after an attack of poliomyelitis. Why the increased intracranial pressure occurs is not clear. In some cases where there is elevated protein, it is suggested that the blood-brain barrier is mechanically clogged by the protein molecules, preventing the absorption of cerebrospinal fluid, and hence raising pressure and producing accumulation of fluid. The marked amount of fluid in the subdural space may be a factor (Gardner, et al.).

LABORATORY: There is increased spinal fluid pressure, with usually a normal cell count and protein. However, in some cases there has been marked elevation of protein. The electroencephalogram is normal, or there may be a diffuse, slow, high amplitude pattern following infection or injury. The ventriculogram is usually normal.

DIAGNOSIS: Since the child presents a picture simulating brain tumor, differentiation must be attempted by ventriculography; often exploratory surgery is necessary.

PROGNOSIS: Recovery is expected in most cases, though years may be needed in some instances.

TREATMENT: The danger in this condition is visual impairment or complete loss of vision with optic atrophy. Therefore, in most cases decompression is performed to relieve pressure caused by the increased accumulation of cerebrospinal fluid. In mild cases, repeated lumbar puncture plus dehydration measures may suffice.

Davidoff, L. M.: Pseudotumor Cerebri; Benign Intracranial Hypertension. Neurology 6:605, 1956.

Foley, J.: Benign Forms of Intracranial Hypertension. "Toxic" and "Otitic" Hydrocephalus. Brain 78:1, 1955.

Gardner, W. J., Spitler, D. K., and Whitten, C.: Increased Intracranial Pressure Caused by Increased Protein Content in the Cerebrospinal Fluid. New England J. Med. 250:932, 1954.

Gass, H. H.: Papilledema and Pseudotumor Cerebri Following Poliomyelitis. A.M.A. J. Dis. Child. 93:640, 1957.

Moore, R. B.: Pseudomotor Cerebri, Pediat. 19:266, 1957.

Starkman, S. P., Brown, T. C., and Linell, E. A.: Cerebral Arachnoid Cysts. J. Neuropath. and Exper. Neurol. 17:484, 1958.

ARACHNOIDITIS

In this condition there are localized cystic collections of cerebrospinal fluid in the subarachnoid space, due to adhesions between the pia and arachnoid.

The etiology and pathogenesis are not clear. It has been found in meningitis, acute lymphocytic choriomeningitis, and Boeck's sarcoid. It has also been seen after trauma or hemorrhage. In the spinal cord, arachnoiditis has followed trauma with hemorrhage and has also been present in association with syringomyelia and multiple sclerosis. There may be spinal cord compression.

In the brain and cord the major differential problem is tumor. In all cases where there appear to be symptoms, and signs of increased pressure, tumor must be ruled out. Ventriculography or myelography will aid. If in doubt, exploratory surgery should be performed. If the cyst is unaccompanied by hydrocephalus, the result may be quite favorable.

TUMORS IN THE SPINAL CANAL (SPINAL CORD TUMORS)

Spinal canal tumors are much rarer in children than intracranial neoplasms. Hamby collected 214 cases in children under fifteen years of age in his report in 1944. Ingraham and Matson found 63 spinal tumors in children under twelve years as compared to 313 intracranial tumors in the same period, or a ratio of 1:5.

PATHOLOGY: The types of spinal tumors which are most frequent in children are gliomas, sarcomas, and dermoids. This means a greater prevalence of highly malignant and congenital tumors. In adults, tumors originate more often from the meninges (meningiomas) and nerve roots (neurinoma) and are more benign. The location of the tumor may be intramedullary and is likely to be of the glioma series. The histology is similar to the adult forms described in the section on intracranial tumors, including astrocytoma, ependymoma, and medulloblastoma. Extramedullary tumors are most often sarcomas. Being extensions of the paravertebral area, they may develop an hour-glass constriction by erosion of the bone. They compress several segments of the cord. Congenital tumors include dermoids, teratoma, lipoma, and hemangioblastomas or vascular tumors.

The spinal cord tumors originate primarily in the spinal canal. However, there may be instances in which they are metastatic from intracranial tumors or from a paraganglionic area, as in a neuroblastoma. They may be part of a general disease like the neurofibromatosis of Von Recklinghausen. The vascular hemangioblastoma may be part of a Lindau's disease. The congenital tumors may be associated with defective development of the spine or cord, as in spina bifida. This is especially true in the first year of life when congenital tumors are particularly noted and when there is a great incidence of congenital anomalies such as hydrocephalus, spina bifida, anencephaly, hare lip and cleft palate, and talipes varus.

CLINICAL PICTURE: The presenting complaint depends upon the age of the child and the location of the tumor. Symptoms may occasionally follow trauma or acute infection. When the child is old enough, he will usually complain of sensory disturbances and pain and stiffness in the back because of compression of the nerve roots. As Ingraham and Matson point out, however, the tumors of the meninges and nerve roots are uncommon in children, so that early compression and pain may not be a prominent symptom. If very young, the child may not be able to account for his discomfort or explain his sensory disturbances, which may include anesthesia, numbness, etc. There may be loss of urinary and rectal control.

The motor disturbances are noted quite readily and are often the earliest complaint. There is usually weakness of the muscles, with an inability to walk, stand, or bear weight. When the pyramidal pathways are involved, there is spastic paralysis. Spasticity is accompanied by hyperactive deep tendon reflexes and a Babinski sign. If the anterior cord or cauda equina is affected, there are flaccid paralysis, absent reflexes, and subsequent muscle atrophy.

The first complaint may be the observation of a mass in the lower spinal region. In other instances, the picture may be one of transverse myelitis with progressive paraplegia, pain in the back or extremities, subsequent weakness of the muscles with flaccidity, and dissociated sensory disturbances.

Segmental diagnosis in children is difficult. In general, with tumors in the cervical region there are weakness and atrophy of the arms, whereas the muscles of the lower extremities are spastic with hyperactive reflexes and a Babinski sign. Below the level of the arms, there may be sensory disturbances. Pain and temperature levels may be several segments below touch. In the lumbosacral region the paralysis of the limbs is likely to be flaccid with loss of reflexes. Pain is referred to the back or upper thighs. Involvement of the cauda equina produces severe pain in the back and along the lower extremities, flaccid paralysis, and atrophy of the limbs, loss of anal and cremasteric reflexes, paralysis of the bladder, and sensory loss of the involved segments, buttocks, and thighs.

Spinal Fluid: The most important finding is evidence of block in the flow of spinal fluid. The appearance of the fluid may be xanthochromic, with elevation of protein to several hundred mg/100 ml., and no or few cells (Froin syndrome). Occasionally tumor cells are seen. Pressure is usually decreased. Queckenstedt is positive (compression of jugular vein causes no rise in spinal fluid pressure).

X-ray may show dilatation of the spinal canal and destruction of the vertebral bodies.

Myelography will show the location of the lesion. This should be done only if needed in doubtful cases.

Diagnosis: Since spinal cord tumor is not a frequent cause of pain and motor disability in childhood, it is not likely to be considered at the beginning. In most instances, however, the clinical picture is progressive, advancing slowly but steadily.

There are a number of diseases which need to be ruled out or differentiated from spinal cord tumor. These include poliomyelitis, Guillain-Barré syndrome, spastic paraplegia, birth injury to the spinal cord, congenital anomalies like spina bifida, transverse myelitis, Pott's disease or tuberculosis of the spine, and syringomyelia.

In all instances spinal puncture is performed. If the spinal fluid is xanthochromic, with elevated protein and few or no cells, cord tumor is strongly suggested, since of the above mentioned diseases, only the Guillain-Barré syndrome, transverse myelitis and rarely syringomyelia, give this spinal fluid picture.

In Guillain-Barré there is a history of febrile onset with symmetrical paralysis of a flaccid type; myelography shows no block; recovery is the rule.

Transverse myelitis usually follows vaccination for smallpox or some infectious disease, e.g., mumps.

When the spinal fluid findings are not distinctive of block, other diagnostic points will aid. In poliomyelitis, the season of the year, acute onset, selective motor paralysis, and pleocytosis in the spinal fluid are different from cord tumor. Spastic paraplegia in infancy is a form of cerebral palsy; the birth and developmental history are important. Cord injury due to birth trauma will have a paraplegia present at birth and a history of birth injury. Congenital anomalies such as spina bifida may be associated with neurological disturbances.

In all of these there will be no X-ray findings suggesting destruction or block on myelography. In tuberculosis, X-ray evidence of tuberculosis elsewhere may be present and there is a positive intradermal test. There is often a history of preceding tuberculous meningitis. When this has been present and is followed by localizing neurological signs involving the spinal cord, exploration should be considered. Recently five cases were reported, aged seven to twelve years, of children who had been successfully treated for tuberculous meningitis, three to seven years before, and who had developed spinal cord symptoms. Exploration revealed intraspinal epidermoid tumors in the thoracolumbar region. The authors felt that repeated spinal punctures had implanted epithelial cells in the spinal canal, which subsequently formed these tumors. Metastatic lesions to the cord may be diagnosed by evidences of intracranial tumor or malignancy elsewhere, as in neuroblastoma.

To summarize, the diagnosis is based on keeping in mind the

possibility of spinal cord tumor whenever there are symptoms and signs of pain in the back or extremities, motor weakness with limitation of movements, and bladder or bowel dysfunction. If the clinical picture is progressive, or suggests localization to some segment of the cord, the probability of tumor is increased. If the child has been trained in bowel and urinary control and retrogresses, it is most often probably a problem of disturbed child-parent relationship, but it might be the beginning of a cord tumor, and this should always be kept in mind. I have seen this sequence occasionally in our cerebral palsy clinic, when tumor developed in a cerebral palsied child. The diagnosis should be confirmed or eliminated by spinal fluid studies, X-ray, and myelography.

PROGNOSIS: The outlook generally is poor since so many childhood tumors are malignant. However, in about 25 per cent there may be a good result because some of the congenital and other types are amenable to surgery.

TREATMENT: The tumor should be removed if possible. When not feasible, as in intramedullary gliomas, radiation is used. In spite of the generally poor outlook, individual extradural and subdural tumors may be removed in toto with good results since some of them are benign.

Brion, S., Netsky, M. G., and Zimmerman, H. M.: Vascular Malformations of the Spinal Cord. Arch. Neurol. & Psychiat. 68:339, 1952.

Buchanan, D. N. and Walker, E. A. Vascular Anomalies of the Spinal Cord in Children. Am. J. Dis. Child. 61:928, 1941.

Choremis, C., Economos, D., Papadatos, C., and Gorgoulos, A.: Intraspinal Epidermoid Tumors (Cholesteatomas) in Patients Treated for Tuberculous Meningitis. Lancet, 2:437, 1956.

Cooper, I. S., Craig, W. McK., Kernohan, J. W.: Tumors of the Spinal Cord. Surg. Gynec. and Obst. 92:183, 1951.

Dibble, J. B., and Cascino, J.: Tuberculoma of the Spinal Cord. J.A.M.A. 162:461, 1956.

Grant, F. C. and Austin, G. M.: The Diagnosis, Treatment and Prognosis of Tumors Affecting the Spinal Cord in Children. J. Neurosurg. 13:535, 1956.

Grinker, R. R. and Bucy, P.: Neurology. Springfield, Ill. Chas. C. Thomas, 1949.

Gwinn, J. L., Dockerty, M. D., and Kennedy, R. L. J.: Presacral Teratomas in Infancy and Childhood. Pediat. 16:239, 1955.

Hamby, W. B.: Tumors in the Spinal Canal in Childhood. J. Neuropath. and Exper. Neurol. 3:397, 1944.

Ingraham, F. D. and Matson, D. D.: Neurosurgery of Infancy and Child-hood. Springfield, Ill. Chas. C. Thomas, 1954.
Mosberg, Jr., W. H.: Spinal Tumors Diagnosed During the First Years of Life. J. Neurosurg. 8:220, 1951.
Schwartz, H. G.: Congenital Tumors of the Spinal Cord in Infants. Ann. Surg. 36:183, 1952.

TUMORS OF THE PERIPHERAL NERVES

The major type of tumor of the peripheral nerves in children is Von Recklinghausen's disease or neurofibromatosis. In this condi-tion there are tumors arising mainly, but not exclusively, from the peripheral nervous system. There may be tumors of the central nervous system (spinal and cranial) and meninges as well.

NEUROBLASTOMA

Tumors which arise from cells related to the neural crest are occasionally seen in children. These tumors are referred to as neuro-blastomas or sympathicoblastomas. Various degrees of maturation may be found in different tumors or in the same tumor.

PATHOLOGY: The tumor consists of small cells containing oval nuclei with hardly any cytoplasm. Groups of these cells may be arranged around fibrils to form pseudorosettes. They usually orig-inate in the adrenal medulla but may arise anywhere in the periph-eral or sympathetic chain, e.g., in the retroperitoneal or cervical ganglia.

CLINICAL PICTURE: This usually develops in infancy or within the first two years. A few cases show up in the later years of the first decade. In 25 cases reported by Reiquam, Beatty, and Allen, 18 had primary retroperitoneal tumors, 6 primary retropleural, and in one, the primary site was not ascertained. The initial complaint is often a mass found on routine examination. In other instances or combined with the presence of the mass there are low grade fever, pain in the hip, or refusal to walk. If the child tries to walk, there is a limp. These complaints are due to metastasis. Proptosis of the eye may be noted with metastasis to the orbit. There is often meta-stasis to the skull and liver.

LABORATORY: X-ray shows multiple areas of rarefaction in the skull and long bones. The bone marrow shows pseudorosettes. Urine is usually normal.

DIAGNOSIS: This is based on careful routine examinations in infancy. In the course of such check-ups there may be noted an abdominal mass. Another important point is the presence of a limp or refusal to walk.

DIFFERENTIAL: Neuroblastoma should be separated from Wilms' tumor (embryonal adenosarcoma of the kidney). X-ray differentiates it from Ewing's tumor or osteogenic sarcoma.

PROGNOSIS: If the mass is palpated before symptoms develop, the outlook is much better. If there is X-ray evidence of bone metastasis, the outlook is usually fatal. The survival rate is about 25 to 35 per cent.

TREATMENT: Surgical excision, removing as much as possible, followed by radiation, is the method of therapy.

In adults primarily, but occasionally beginning in adolescence, more mature tumors of the sympathetic system, ganglioneuromas, may occur. They are located in the adrenal medulla, retroperitoneally, in the brain, and peripheral nerves. The tumors are usually benign. Paragangliomas arise in the adrenal medulla and in the paraganglia; they are composed of cells of the chromaffin series. Paraganglioma of the adrenal medulla may be associated with Von Recklinghausen's disease.

Koop, C. E., Kiesewetter, W. B. and Horne, R. C.: Neuroblastoma in Childhood. An Evaluation of Surgical Management. Pediat. 16:652, 1955.
Lindsay, S., and Chaikoff, I. T.: Neuroblastoma and Related Tumors. A.M.A. Arch. Path. 63:451, 1957.
Reiquam, C. W., Beatty, Jr., E. C. and Allen, R. P.: Neuroblastomas in Infancy and Childhood. A.M.A. J. Dis. Child. 91:588, 1956.

CHAPTER 11

NEUROCUTANEOUS SYNDROMES

These include tuberous sclerosis, neurofibromatosis, cerebral angiomatosis and angiomatosis retinae et cerebelli. In a sense these are combined disorders of the skin and brain, both of which are derived from ectoderm.

TUBEROUS SCLEROSIS (EPILOIA)

This disease in its complete form consists of mental deficiency, epileptic seizures, and adenoma sebaceum. The incidence is 1/50,000 in the general population and 0.1% in institutions for the care of the feebleminded and epileptics in the United States.

CLINICAL PICTURE: In infancy there is observed a delay in development. This becomes quite marked since the general level of most of these children (70 per cent) is consistent with idiocy or imbecility. Seizures are present in 80 per cent. These are recurrent and may lead to further deterioration of the brain. Later in childhood the characteristic skin lesions appear on the face in a butterfly distribution covering both cheeks symmetrically and across the nose. They consist of small, slightly raised papules. While referred to as adenoma sebaceum, they are actually fibromata of the sebaceous glands. They have blood vessel elements in them; hence, the color may be pink, red, or dark reddish brown. Other areas such as the forehead, trunk, and back may show fibromata which are either flat or pendulous tags. Other types of skin lesions may also be present, especially cafe-au-lait spots or a shagreen patch, consisting of a rough or leathery thickened area of skin, pinkish or whitish in color. Ophthalmoscopic examination reveals tumors in the retina (phakomas). They are yellow or gray-white, oval in shape and appear to arise from the disc margin or may cover most of the disc.

PATHOLOGY: There is a marked involvement of many organs, including the heart, kidneys, liver, spleen, and brain. In the heart are rhabdomyomata; in the kidney, neurofibromatous and mixed lesions; liver cysts and hemangiomata of the spleen are also seen. These may not give symptoms. The brain contains hard nodules (tubers), within which are few normal nerve cells, but numbers of giant and glial cells. They are mostly over the convexity of the cortex. The walls of the lateral ventricles may be infiltrated with these tumors, which project into the ventricles from the caudate and thalamic nuclei. These tumors may calcify. Many of the gyri are thickened and hypertrophic, others are smaller. In some cases separate tumors (spongioblastomas) are present.

ETIOLOGY: This disease is not common. It is transmitted as an autosomal irregular dominant. Just one of the clinical features may appear in siblings or other relatives, or they may all appear markedly in another generation.

DIAGNOSIS: The diagnosis of tuberous sclerosis may be made with certainty when the triad of mental defect, epilepsy, and adenoma sebaceum are present. But as previously indicated there are variable manifestations in this disease. In some, tuberous sclerosis of the brain alone may be demonstrated post-mortem with no other findings. In others, there may be adenoma sebaceum without mental defect. There may be many similarities with neurofibromatosis (Von Recklinghausen's). The early diagnostic features include retarded mental development and recurrent seizures. These are both of the minor and major types, the latter often beginning focally (Jacksonian). There may be associated anomalies such as spina bifida, cleft palate, and renal tumors. An X-ray film may reveal areas of increased density due to calcification in the brain and skull. These are the multiple and bilateral nodules (tubers) especially noted near the ventricles, which appear as "candle gutterings." This is even more obvious in the pneumoencephalogram. In the differential diagnosis of the X-ray changes in the skull, one must rule out multiple telangiectasis, where calcium deposits occur within the walls of the vessels, Sturge-Weber syndrome, calcified subdural hematoma, toxoplasmosis, and Hippel-Lindau cerebellar tumor. Ophthalmoscopic examination of the retina may show the characteristic tumors near the optic disc. At a later age period in childhood the characteristic skin lesions appear, occasionally earlier. The spinal fluid is normal.

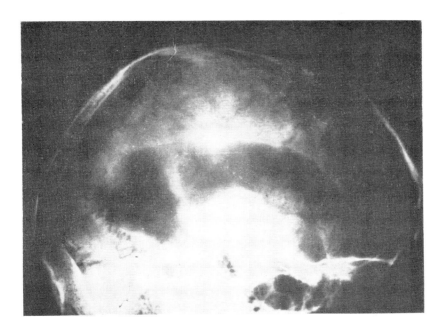

15. Tuberous sclerosis. Ventriculogram showing marked dilation of both lateral ventricles. There are nodular densities in the anterior portions of the bodies of both lateral ventricles. Scattered intracranial calcification is also noted.

PROGNOSIS: The outlook for these patients is poor. They are usually institutionalized because of severe mental defect with seizures. In the very severe forms death occurs in early adult life.

TREATMENT: There is no specific therapy for the underlying condition. The seizures are treated with anticonvulsant drugs. (See under Epilepsy.)

Baird, H. W., Wycis, H. T., and Spiegel, E. A.: Convulsions in Tuberous Sclerosis Controlled by Elimination of Impulses Originating in the Basal Ganglia. J. Pediat. 49:165, 1956.
Berland, H. I.: Roentgenological Findings in Tuberous Sclerosis. Arch. Neurol. & Psychiat. 69:669, 1953.
Critchley, McD. and Earl, C.J.C.: Tuberose Sclerosis and Allied Conditions. Brain 55:311, 1932.
Gibson, R.: Expanding Scope of Oligophrenia: Increasing Range of Syndromes Associated with Mental Defect. Am. J. Dis. Child. 81:803, 1951.
Holt, J. F. and Dickerson, W. W.: The Osseous Lesions of Tuberous Sclerosis. Radiol. 58:1, 1952.
Yakovlev, P. I. and Guthrie, R. H.: Congenital Ectodermoses (Neurocutaneous Syndromes) in Epileptic Patients. Arch. Neurol. & Psychiat. 26:1145, 1931.
Yannet, H.: The Problem of Mental Deficiency in Children. Pediat. 10:223, 1952.

NEUROFIBROMATOSIS (VON RECKLINGHAUSEN'S DISEASE)

Neurofibramatosis has many characteristics similar to tuberous sclerosis, namely pigment anomalies, multiple nervous system tumors, and bone changes. In accord with ectodermal dysplasia, the skin and nervous system are primarily involved. Neurofibromatosis is probably inherited as a simple dominant, occurring in successive generations. This is definitely so in forty per cent. Sporadic types occur due to mutation or failure of gene manifestation in the parents, perhaps due to reduced penetrance.

CLINICAL PICTURE: There are pigment changes similar to those in tuberous sclerosis, including café-au-lait spots, nevi, and moles. Numerous fibromata, either flat or pedunculated, may be seen hanging from the skin. These are diffuse and may be scattered over the entire body.

The neurofibromata grow as nodules just beneath the skin and are of various sizes. They may be as tiny as a pin head or as large as an orange. Their color is pinkish white. They usually feel soft, hence the name, fibroma molluscum. At times the nodules are of firmer consistency, even quite hard. The neurofibromata of nerve trunks form whorls or plexiform arrangements in relation to various nerves; in the neck they occur in conjunction with the vagus; they also appear on the head and face (trigeminal). They are seen in the extremities in relation to the peripheral nerves. There they may produce elephantiasis as a result of the proliferation of the tissues surrounding the plexiform formation of the nerves. The overlying skin is firm and non-tender. Tumors occur in other regions, including the viscera, orbits, and pituitary and pineal regions, producing endocrine changes in the last event. There may be overgrowth of the tongue (Macroglossia). The café-au-lait and other so called mongolian spots over the lumbo-sacral region of the back are noted at birth, but since these may appear in normal individuals, they are not diagnostic. The skin and nerve tumors, however, usually appear at a later age. There are also tumors of the brain, especially acoustic neuromas, meningiomas, and gliomas of various types. Similarly in the spinal cord, tumors may arise. These tumors may produce symptoms in the brain and cord due to pressure, and the presenting picture will depend on the area involved.

A variety of bone changes have been described. They include scoliosis, erosive defects, disorders of growth, bowing and pseudarthrosis of tubular bones, and intraosseus cystic lesions.

Mental deficiency may be associated with the other changes in fifty per cent of cases.

LABORATORY: The spinal fluid is normal, unless there is tumor formation in the brain or spinal cord.

DIAGNOSIS: During infancy reliance must be placed on the multiple skin lesions previously described. They are of two types, either the pigmented lesions or the subcutaneous nodules. There are usually no symptoms with these, but occasionally the nodules may be very painful. The presence of any localized area of elephantiasis in an extremity is also helpful. In most instances the various forms of peripheral nerve and central (brain and cord) tumor formation occur in later childhood and adult life. These central tumors may not be differentiated except by surgical exploration. X-ray of the skeleton is very useful to reveal the bone changes. Mental deficiency, when present, should be differentiated from other forms. A family history should be obtained for any genetic background.

PROGNOSIS: The prognosis is good and the clinical picture is benign, except when cord or brain tumors produce pressure symptoms, in which case surgery may be necessary. In these, there is a poor outlook.

TREATMENT: There is no specific therapy except when tumor growth produces pressure symptoms or pain and requires removal.

Benda, C. E.: Developmental Disorders of Mentation and Cerebral Palsies, New York, Grune & Stratton, 1952.
Crowe, F. W., Schull, W. J., Neel, J. V.: A Clinical Pathological and Genetic Study of Multiple Neurofibromatosis. Bannerstone Div. of Amer. Lect. in Derm. Springfield, Ill. Chas. C. Thomas, 1956.
Holt, J. F., and Wright, E. M.: Radiologic Features of Neurofibromatosis. Radiology 51:647, 1948.
Penfield, W., and Young, A. W.: The Nature of Von Recklinghausen's Disease and the Tumors Associated With It. A.M.A. Arch. Neurol. & Psychiat. 23:320, 1930.
Schönenberg, H.: Zum Erscheinungsbild der Recklinghausenchen Krankheit im Kindesalter. Monatschr. Kinderh. 100:499, 1950.
Schull, W. J. and Crowe, F. W.: Neurocutaneous Syndromes in the M Kindred. A Case of Simultaneous Occurrence of Tuberous Sclerosis and Neurofibromatosis. Neurology 3:904, 1953.

CEREBRAL ANGIOMATOSIS (STURGE-WEBER SYNDROME)

This represents another of the ectodermal dysplasias since the major features include cutaneous lesions (birth marks) associated with angiomatosis of the brain on the same side. As a result of the pathology in the cortex there are usually focal convulsions, contralateral to the side of the brain involved. The condition is probably hereditary, possibly due to a single dominant gene.

CLINICAL PICTURE: The skin lesion consists of a flat, port wine type of stain extending over one side of the face, neck, and forehead. The cutaneous angiomata are either telangiectatic nevi or cavernous in type. Their distribution follows the 1st and 2nd parts of the 5th cranial nerve. The cortex also contains angiomatous formations. These are present on the same side as the skin lesions. Along with these is cortical atrophy. X-ray of the skull shows intracerebral calcification. This is most often in the occipital area. The gyri and sulci are outlined by the calcifications in the form of a doubly contoured mass, a sort of sinusoidal arrangement. The calcification is presumed to be due to a lowered metabolic state in this area, brought on by stasis in the pial veins overlying the sclerotic cortex. In the very young there may be no evidence of calcified plaques but only calcium collections in the vessels. Glaucoma due to angioma of the choroid may occur. Convulsions are usually on the side opposite to the involved cortex. They may begin as focal seizures, then become generalized. Hemiplegia may also occur, spastic in type and on the side opposite to the cortical area involved (contralateral hemiplegia). Mental deficiency is present in about sixty per cent.

In some instances the facial skin lesion may be bilateral while the brain lesion is unilateral.

DIAGNOSIS: The diagnosis of this condition is based on the skin lesion, intracranial calcification (X-ray), contralateral convulsion, and frequently associated mental deficiency. Air study early in the disease may be normal, but arteriogram shows collections of calcium in the vessels.

TREATMENT: Since the malformation of the cortex is diffuse, the vascular anomaly cannot be removed surgically. Therapy in the form of phenobarbital and Dilantin sodium® should be used to control the seizures. It is suggested, however, that with continuing seizures which are uncontrollable with drugs, hemiplegia, and the possibility of subsequent mental deterioration, hemispherectomy should be considered. This procedure usually eliminates the seizures. If there is uncontrolled seizure alone and no hemiplegia, the latter will follow the hemispherectomy. But the procedure may be worthwhile in spite of the resultant hemiplegia since it eliminates the seizures and permits the child to enjoy normal mental development, if this has not been previously affected. This type of problem and the choice of procedure must be considered carefully in each case.

Cohen, H. J. and Kay, M. N.: Associated Facial Hemangioma and Intracranial Lesion. (Weber-Dimitri Disease.) Am. J. Dis. Child. 62:606, 1941.
Falkinburg, L. W., Silver, M. L., Kay, M. N. and Stoll, J.: Sturge-Weber-Dimitri Disease. Pediat. 22:319, 1958.
Ingraham, F. D., and Matson, D. D.: Neurosurgery of Infancy and Childhood. Springfield, Ill. Chas. C. Thomas, 1954.
Krabbe, K. H.: Facial and Meningeal Angiomatosis Associated with Calcification of the Brain Cortex. A Clinical and Anatomopathologic Contribution. Arch. Neurol. & Psychiat. 32:737, 1934.

Lichenstein, B. W.: Sturge-Weber-Dimitri Syndrome; Cephalic Form of Neurocutaneous Hemangiomatosis. A.M.A. Arch. Neurol. & Psychiat. 71:291, 1954.

Peterman, A. F., Hayles, A. B., Dockerty, M. B., and Love, J. G.: Encephalotrigeminal Angiomatosis (Sturge-Weber Disease). J.A.M.A. 167:-2169, 1958.

ANGIOMATOSIS RETINAE ET CEREBELLI (VON HIPPEL-LINDAU)

The Von Hippel-Lindau syndrome consists of angiomatosis of the retina (Hippel) and cerebellum (Lindau). The condition is considered to be heredofamilial.

The retinal lesion consists of a pair of dilated tortuous vessels, with beading of the artery accompanying the enlarged vein. Together the vessels enter a nodule or tumor mass in the periphery of the retina. The cerebellar lesion is a hemangioblastoma. Accompanying the retinal and cerebellar angiomata there may also occur cysts of the kidney, adenomas of the pancreas, angiomas of the liver, spleen or adrenals or hemangioblastomas of the spinal cord.

The clinical manifestations are most often seen at a later age than the Sturge-Weber syndrome. Seizures and skin manifestations are extremely rare.

For the ocular lesion with loss of vision radiation has been used. The cerebellar hemangioblastomas present signs of increased pressure and should be removed. However, because of the multiple lesions, the outlook is not favorable.

Kirby, T. J.: Ocular Phakomatoses Am. J. M. Sc. 222:227, 1951.

Levin, P. M.: Multiple Hereditary Hemangioblastomas of the Nervous System. Arch. Neurol. & Psychiat. 36:384, 1936.

Lindau, A.: Studien über Kleinhirncysten; Bau, Pathogenese und Beziehungen Zur Angiomatosis Retinae. Acta Path. et. microbiol. scandinav., supp. 1, 1926, p. 1.

Von Hippel, E.: Ueber eine sehr seltene Erkrankung der Netzhaut. Arch. f. Ophth. 59:83, 1904.

CHAPTER 12

HEREDOFAMILIAL
AND DEGENERATIVE

There are a number of conditions which may be included under the hereditary ataxias. These are characterized by involvement of the pathways leading to and from the cerebellum or in the cerebellum itself. The various entities are degenerative and passed on in successive generations in affected families. While they are described separately, there are a number of authors who feel that the differences are more apparent than real. This applies to Friedreich's and the Brown, Marie group, for example. Predominantly spinal, spinocerebellar and cerebellar forms of spino-cerebellar degenerations have been described (Greenfield).

HEREDITARY SPINAL ATAXIA (FRIEDREICH'S)

Friedreich's ataxia is a slowly progressive, heredofamilial disease in which there is degeneration of the posterior columns of the spinal cord and of the spinocerebellar and corticospinal pathways. The cerebellum may also show involvement.

CLINICAL PICTURE: The onset is usually noted in childhood with the observation that the youngster is not walking well. This may appear as a new feature in a previously normal child, or on close questioning it may be found that he has always been clumsy or slow in walking. The child walks on a broad base with his feet apart or may stagger. With progression of the disease the ataxia becomes obvious in the upper extremities. There are jerky and uncoordinated movements of the arms, finally extending to the trunk and all voluntary musculature. Speech becomes slow, slurred, dysarthic and incomprehensible. There is a general loss of muscle tone and in the later stages there may be flexion contractures of the lower limbs. The child may develop scoliosis. There is also a characteristic deformity of the foot, pes cavus, and dorsiflexion of the metatarsal-phalangeal joints (hammer toe). There may be associated equinovarus. There is loss of position and vibratory senses, more marked at first in the lower extremities. Romberg sign may be positive. Two point discriminatory sense is lost. Stereognosis, that is, recognition of the size and shape of objects, is also lost.

Nystagmus is usually present at some time late in the disease. The nystagmus occurs just as the eyes are coming to rest (fixation type) or is of the horizontal type upon lateral gaze. Rarely, optic atrophy occurs. The deep tendon reflexes are lost early in the lower and later in the upper extremities; plantar extension may be present. Intelligence is usually preserved; occasionally however, deterioration or psychic symptoms occur. In a number of patients there may be symptoms of cardiac involvement with palpitation and pain, but in others, even without symptoms, electrocardiographic changes have been noted. The spinal fluid is normal.

PATHOLOGY: The spinal cord is small. There is evidence of degeneration and glial proliferation in the posterior columns and roots, especially in the lumbosacral area, the spinocerebellar pathways, both ventral and dorsal, the lateral corticospinal tract, cerebellum, and Clark's column.

ETIOLOGY: The disease is transmitted along familial lines. Schut considers it to be a hereditary ataxia, in which the trait is transmitted directly to one-half the children (dominant inheritance). Other authors have postulated both dominant and recessive genes. There is no distinct sex predilection, but males are slightly more affected. In various families studied a number of cases occurred in the offspring of the affiliated members at about the same time, although not necessarily with the same manifestations.

DIAGNOSIS: The heredofamilial character of the disease, its early onset in childhood, and steady slow progression with physical signs of ataxia, both spinal and cerebellar, and foot deformity make the diagnosis. In addition there are absent deep tendon reflexes, extensor toe sign (Babinski) and posterior cord pathology with loss of proprioceptive sense.

DIFFERENTIAL: Multiple sclerosis, cerebellar tumor, and congenital and other forms of cerebellar ataxia must be considered and differentiated.

PROGNOSIS: The course is usually steadily progressive until the patient is completely incapacitated and dies. There are, however, abortive cases which seem to develop some degree of stabilization without too much disability. A reference to Schut's study indicates that in the family constellation there are variations with regard to the extent of involvement and rapidity of progress.

TREATMENT: There is no specific therapy. Orthopedic operations should be performed for deformities if the disease is not too rapidly progressive.

HEREDITARY CEREBELLAR ATAXIA WITH SPASTICITY (BROWN-MARIE)

This comprises a group in which there are differences from the classical Friedreichs ataxia with further variations within the group itself.

The families described by Brown and Marie are examples of this group of cerebellar ataxia. The condition is inherited mainly as a dominant form. The age of onset is in adult life, and there is no sex predilection. Incoordination develops in the muscles, beginning with ataxia in walking and followed by lack of coordination in use of the upper extremities. This is associated with ocular palsies, ptosis of the eyelids, and optic nerve atrophy. Spasticity of the legs develops, accompanied by hyperactive deep tendon reflexes, an extensor plantar response, and ankle clonus. There is disturbed speech, and in the later years mental deterioration may set in.

OTHER FORMS OF HEREDITARY ATAXIA: Various authors have described other forms of hereditary cerebellar ataxia depending upon the anatomical pathways involved. They occur more often in later adult life, but may begin in childhood occasionally. In some of these increased amounts of aspartic acid were found in the spinal fluid.

Spinocerebellar: This type is based upon spinocerebellar tract degeneration, and is differentiated from Friedreich's because the degeneration in the latter is mainly in the posterior columns.

Roussy-Levy syndrome: (a variant and abortive form of Friedreich's ataxia with marked wasting of the muscles.)

HEREDITARY SPASTIC PARAPLEGIA

This form is included by Schut and Haymaker among the hereditary ataxias on the basis of a common genetic background and a belief that the same morbid process underlines both, with a difference of emphasis on the location of the lesions. There are present spastic paraplegia and ataxia.

CLINICAL PICTURE: The disease is dominantly transmitted. The child between three and six years shows evidence of spasticity of the lower extremities. He walks stiffly on his toes, is awkward, and cannot run well. With time there are weakness and lack of development of the lower extremities; later this is noted in the muscles of the upper extremities and trunk. The tendon reflexes are active. Along with the features of paraplegia, ataxia develops. This is accompanied by nystagmus and scanning speech. Mentality may be affected. There are no sensory defects.

PATHOLOGY: The pyramidal tracts show degeneration in the spinal cord (corticospinal). The Purkinje cells are destroyed, and the spinocerebellar tracts show degeneration.

DIAGNOSIS: The diagnosis is based on the presence of spastic paraplegia in some members of the family of a child who has developed spastic paraplegia along with ataxia.

In some children there may be evidence only of spastic paraplegia. Landow and Gitt found twenty-one clinically affected members of a family group numbering two hundred and eighty-three.

PROGNOSIS: The course is slowly progressive and variable.

TREATMENT: There is no specific therapy.

Bell, J.: Hereditary Ataxia and Spastic Paraplegia. The Treasury of Human Inheritance, Cambridge University Press 4:141, 1939.
Brown, S.: On Hereditary Ataxy with a Series of Twenty-one Cases. Brain 15:250, 1892.
Greenfield, J. G.: The Spino-Cerebellar Degenerations. Springfield, Chas. C. Thomas, 1954.
Hassin, G. B. and Harris, T. H.: Olivopontocerebellar Atrophy. Arch. Neurol. & Psychiat. 35:43, 1936.
———, Friedreich's Ataxia: Histopathologic Study (differentiation from Marie's Ataxia). Arch. Neurol. & Psychiat. 39:116, 1938.
Landow, W. M., and Gitt, J. J.: Hereditary Spastic Paraplegia and Hereditary Ataxia. A.M.A. Arch. Neurol. & Psychiat. 66:346, 1951.
Logothetis, J.: Cerebrospinal Fluid Free Amino Acids in Neurologic Diseases. Neurology 8:374, 1958.

Malamud, N. and Cohen, P.: Unusual Form of Cerebellar Ataxia with Sex-linked Inheritance. Neurology 8:261, 1958.

Marie, P.: Sur L'Heredo-ataxie Cerebelleuse. Semaine Med. 13:444, 1893.

Marie, P. and Foix, C.: Lesions Medullaires dans Quatre Cas d'Heredo-ataxie Cerebelleuse. Rev. Neurol. 27:797, 1914.

Rhem, J. H. W.: Family Spastic Paralysis. J. Nerv. and Ment. Dis. 44:115, 1916.

Schillero, A. J., Antzis, E. and Dunn, J.: Friedreich's Ataxia and Its Cardiac Manifestations. Am. Heart J. 44:804, 1952.

Schut, J. W.: Hereditary Ataxia. Arch. Neurol. & Psychiat. 63:535. 1950.

————, and Haymaker, W.: Hereditary Ataxia, J. Neuropath. & Clin. Neurol. 1:183, 1951.

Wilson, S. A. K.: Neurology. Baltimore, Williams and Wilkins, 1940.

ATAXIA-TELANGIECTASIA

This entity, recently described, is a familial syndrome, consisting of cerebellar ataxia, telangiectasia and sinopulmonary infection. The various features are slowly progressive leading to gradual deterioration during childhood.

CLINICAL FEATURES: The onset usually takes place in late infancy after an apparently normal neonatal period. When the child begins to walk, there is noted an ataxic gait. The movements are unsteady and clumsy. There is tilting and swaying of the head and trunk. Choreoathetoid movements may be seen early. Subsequently there develop intention tremor, hypotonia and diminished or absent tendon reflexes. The telangiectasia usually appear after ataxia has occurred. They are especially noted on the bulbar conjunctivae and in a butterfly distribution over the face. They also involve the ear lobes (See articles by Boder and Centerwall.) The children are susceptible to frequent sinopulmonary infections resulting in bronchiectasis. Other features which may be present include rapid blinking, nystagmus, drooling and slurred speech. The posture is poor, shoulders drooped and the face may assume a sad impassive expression until the child smiles. Growth is retarded in some cases. The intelligence level is normal, but in later childhood levels off so that the child does not perform satisfactorily.

LABORATORY: Blood count, urine and spinal fluid are normal. Lead and copper levels in the blood and urine are also normal. The electroencephalogram shows no abnormality. Pneumoencephalography may show cerebellar atrophy.

PATHOLOGY: The meninges and brain are grossly normal. Microscopically there is a chronic progressive degeneration of the Purkinje cells in the cerebellum. The venules of the cerebellum are enlarged and thin-walled. The mechanism may be anoxia or a primary disorder. The spinal cord is normal. The lungs may show bronchiectasis.

ETIOLOGY: The cause of this condition is not established but from the cases thus far reported it would appear that the disorder is heredofamilial, probably transmitted through a simple autosomal recessive gene.

Because of the onset with ataxia the disease has been described in the section on hereditary ataxias. However, the combination of ataxia and telangiectasia also permits classification under the phakomatoses or neuroectodermal dysplasias such as Sturge-Weber syndrome, von Hippel-Landau disease and neurofibromatosis.

DIAGNOSIS: The essential features of this entity include ataxia with scleral-cutaneous telangiectasia which are slowly progressive and chronic pulmonary infection. In the early stages, the presence of ataxia and occasionally of choreoathetoid movements requires that cerebral palsy be considered. However, the progressive nature of the disease eliminates this diagnosis. With the onset of telangiectasia, Friedreichs ataxia, Pelizaeous-Merzbacher disease, encephalitis, cerebellar tumor and extra pyramidal disorders, such as, Hallervordenspatz disease, are ruled out, but other entities must now be thought of. Von Hippel-Lindau consists of progressive retinal and cerebellar angiomata producing loss of vision and ataxia. However, there is apt to be tumor (hemangioblastoma) demonstrable by arteriogram whereas in ataxia-telangiectasia there is cerebellar atrophy. In Hartnup disease there is a pellagra-like photosensitive skin lesion and ataxia, but there is also aminoaciduria.

PROGNOSIS: The course is slowly progressive. Of about twenty cases thus far reported there have been six deaths, usually due to the bronchiectasis.

TREATMENT: There is no specific therapy to influence the progression of the neurological features or the telangiecstasia. Antibiotics should be used to prevent the recurrent pulmonary infections.

Roder, E. and Sedgwick, R. P.: Ataxia—Telangiectasia. Pediat. 21:526, 1958.
Centerwall, W. R. and Miller, M. M.: Ataxia, Telangiectasia, and Sinopulmonary Infections. A.M.A.J. Dis. Child. 95:385, 1958.
Hallervorden, J. und Spatz, H.: Eigenartige Erkrankung im Extrapyramidalen System mit besonderer Beteiligung des Globus Pallidus und der Substantia nigra. Zeitschr. f. d. ges. Neurol. u. Psychiat. 79:254, 1922.
Kirby, T. J.: Ocular Phakomatoses. Am. J. Med. Sc. 222:227, 1951.
Wells, C. E. and Shy, G. M.: Progressive Familial Choreoathetosis with Cutaneous Telangiectasia. J. Neurol. Neurosurg. Psychiat. 20:98, 1957.

AMYOTROPHIC LATERAL SCLEROSIS

This is a rare disease in childhood. A few cases of a familial type have been reported in children, with previous generations possibly affected.

CLINICAL PICTURE: This condition is characterized by atrophy and spasticity of the extremities, usually symmetrical, resulting in muscular weakness. The process often begins first in the hands, including wasting of the thenar eminences. The upper extremities may show atrophy and wasting, particularly the deltoid, and the muscles of the neck and back. When the motor nuclei of the brain stem are involved, there is weakness and atrophy of the tongue, pharynx, and palate leading to difficulty in swallowing and speaking. Fasciculations of the muscles usually are noted. Evidence of lateral tract disease of the spinal cord develops in the form of spasticity of the lower extremities. This may precede the atrophy and be the first symptom. The tendon reflexes are hyperactive and the Babinski sign and ankle clonus are present. As the process continues, causing complete wasting of the muscles, the reflexes may disappear.

PATHOLOGY: There are degeneration and sclerosis in the anterior horns of the spinal cord, brain stem, motor cortex (Betz cells), and in the fibres of the corticospinal tract.

ETIOLOGY: The cause of this disease is unknown.

DIAGNOSIS: There may be a familial history. The diagnosis is based on the presence of muscular atrophy and weakness of the extremities, together with spasticity and hyperactive reflexes or bulbar signs.

If there is no familial evidence, amyotrophic lateral sclerosis must be differentiated from poliomyelitis, the infantile muscular atrophies, cord tumor, family spastic paralysis, myelitis, post-vaccination encephalitis, syringomyelia, and myasthenia gravis.

PROGNOSIS: The course is slowly progressive, resulting in a fatal outcome.

TREATMENT: There is no specific therapy.

Gordon, R. G. and Delicati, J. L.: The Occurrence of Amyotrophic Lateral Sclerosis in Children. J. Neurol. and Psychopath. 9:30, 1928.
Robertson, E. E.: Progressive Bulbar Paralysis Showing Heredofamilial Incidence and Intellectual Impairment. Arch. Neurol. & Psychiat. 69:197, 1953.

HEREDITARY ATROPHY OF THE OPTIC NERVE (LEBER)

This is a progressive, primary optic atrophy which is heredofamilial, being transmitted as a sex linked recessive, occasionally dominant. It may appear in several generations of a family. Males are preponderantly affected.

CLINICAL PICTURE: The onset is usually around puberty. There is loss of vision, which gradually worsens, occasionally ending in complete blindness. At times the onset and course are more acute. There are bilateral central scotomas for white and colors, or for color alone, due presumably to early degeneration of the maculopapillary bundle. There is little or no peripheral constriction of the visual field. The optic discs may appear normal or show evidence of neuritis; later atrophy may be seen. Accompanying the optic atrophy there may be spasticity and ataxia of the extremities (Marie type), nystagmus, convulsive seizure, and mental defect.

PATHOLOGY: There is primary degeneration of the neurons of the retina and optic nerve.

DIAGNOSIS: This is made on the familial-hereditary history of optic atrophy.

PROGNOSIS: After the early onset and advance of visual impairment the condition usually remains stationary.

TREATMENT: There is no specific therapy.

Ferguson, F. R. and Critchley, M.: Leber's Optic Atrophy and Its Relationship with the Heredofamilial Ataxias. J. Neurol. and Psychopath. 9:120, 1928.

Kwittken, J. and Barest, H. D.: The Neuropathology of Hereditary Optic Atrophy (Leber's Disease); The First Complete Anatomic Study. Am. J. Path. 34:185, 1958.

Leber, T.: Üeber Hereditäre und congenital angelegte Sehnervenleiden. Arch. f. Ophth. 17:249, 1871.

Lodberg, C. V. and Lund, A.: Hereditary Optic Atrophy with Dominant Transmission. Acta Ophth. 28:437, 1950.

Merritt, H. H.: Hereditary Optic Atrophy (Leber's Disease). Arch. Neurol. & Psychiat. 24:775, 1930.

SYRINGOMYELIA

Syringomyelia is a progressive disease of the spinal cord, in which gliosis occurs with the formation of cavities. The process takes place in the region of the central canal. When the brain stem is involved, the term syringobulbia is used.

CLINICAL PICTURE: The onset usually occurs in early and middle adult life. Cases are very rarely seen in childhood. The early clinical features are related to the cervical segment of the cord. There is loss of pain and temperature sense in the hand so that the patient may be burned and not be aware of it. There is no loss of light touch. Atrophy of the muscles of the fingers and hands is noted, due to destruction of the motor horn cells. Later, the shoulder girdle muscles are affected. The muscles are wasted and claw-like hands develop. There are paralysis, loss of reflexes, and a reaction of degeneration. Vasomotor and trophic changes consisting of cold, blue extremities and thickening and ulcerations of the skin are associated with the atrophic muscles. When the pyramidal tracts are involved, the reflexes may be hyperactive with the development of spasticity and the Babinski sign. Extension of the process to the posterior column will cause ataxia. With spread to the medulla there are atrophy of the tongue and paralysis of the palate, pharynx, or vocal cords, with difficulty in swallowing, chewing, and speech. Nystagmus may be present. Anesthesia of the face due to involvement of the descending sensory fifth nerve in the upper cord may occur. Kyphosis and scoliosis are almost always present due to the muscular imbalance. A variety of anomalies have been found associated with syringomyelia, such as cervical rib, hydrocephalus, platybasia, Arnold-Chiari syndrome, Klippel-Feil syndrome, and spina bifida.

While the clinical picture as noted is primarily of the cervical segment of the cord, similar features develop elsewhere, depending on the location of the cord pathology.

LABORATORY: The spinal fluid shows increased pressure with a normal cell count. The protein is variable.

PATHOLOGY: There is a proliferation of glial elements with cystic cavitation. The most common areas are in the cervical region of the spinal cord, with extension toward the medulla or lumbar segments. The gray matter is primarily attacked. In the medulla various cranial nuclei may become involved. In the cord, fibre tracts, especially those of the anterior commissure carrying pain and temperature sense, and cells in the anterior horns are affected. There may be further extension to the posterior and lateral columns of the cord.

ETIOLOGY: The cause of syringomyelia is unknown. Perhaps there is prenatal pathology, either genetic or acquired, in view of the frequent association with other anomalies.

DIAGNOSIS: This is based on the loss of pain and temperature sense with preservation of touch together with atrophy of muscles supplied by the same cord segment. There are a number of conditions which must be differentiated.

(a) *Spinal cord tumor:* This may give the same picture, but progression is more rapid in tumor. When it is suspected, spinal puncture may show the yellow fluid of the Froin syndrome, and myelography will show complete block in the case of an intramedullary tumor (usually glioma). In syringomyelia, the cord is swollen and may block the flow of fluid, but this is not usually so complete. In case of doubt, an operation should be performed.

(b) *Cervical rib* usually originates from the seventh cervical vertebra, and produces its neurological picture by pressure on the brachial plexus. This is rarely manifest until late puberty or thereafter. Because the subclavian artery runs between it and the scalenus anterior muscle, vascular symptoms are also noted. The neurological symptoms consist of sensory changes with atrophy of the muscles of the hand in the ulnar distribution. There are vascular and vasomotor changes, including loss of radial pulse and cold, cyanotic extremities. X-ray will show the cervical rib. Occasionally cervical rib and syringomyelia are combined. If there is a widespread clinical picture, including the medulla and other fibre pathways of the spinal cord, syringomyelia is more likely.

(c) *Progressive spinal muscular atrophy.* There are no changes of sensibility.

(d) *Amyotrophic lateral sclerosis.* There are atrophy and spasticity which are symmetrical, and no sensory changes.

(e) *Hematomyelia.* There is a history of injury and subsequent improvement.

(f) *Tabes.* A history of syphilis is present along with positive tests of the spinal fluid and blood.

PROGNOSIS: The course is usually one of gradual progression in terms of muscular atrophy and sensory disturbances. In syringobulbia, death may occur rapidly due to involvement of the vital medullary centers.

TREATMENT: X-ray therapy is given to the spinal cord to prevent glial proliferation. In some cases the cavities have been drained to relieve pressure on the cord. Neither procedure appears to have much effect.

MORVAN'S SYNDROME

Morvan described seven cases with loss of pain and temperature sensation of the extremities, muscular wasting, palsies, trophic disturbances of the skin and joints, and mutilation of the fingers and toes. This syndrome is now considered to be a form of syringomyelia. In a number of cases a familial pattern has been shown.

These patients must be differentiated from Raynaud's disease, in which there may be gangrene of the extremities, but in the latter there are no sensory changes or muscle atrophy.

In leprosy there are thickened nerve trunks due to peripheral neuritis and no sensory dissociation. The organism can be demonstrated.

PROGNOSIS: This is poor since the course is slowly progressive.

TREATMENT: X-ray therapy to the spine is of no value. The skin and joints should be looked after.

Bassoe, P.: The Coincidence of Cervical Ribs and Syringomyelia. Arch. Neurol. & Psychiat. 4:542, 1920.

Bermann, E. J.: Die Syringomyelie im Kindesalter. Monatschr. f. Kinderh. 37:1, 1927.

Hassin, G. B.: Histopathology and Histogenesis of Syringomyelia. Arch. Neurol. and Psychiat. 3:130, 1920.

Holley, E. B.: Syringomyelia, Morvan's Syndrome. J. Pediat. 30:96, 1947.

Lichtenstein, B. W.: Cervical Syringomyelia and Syringomyelia-like States Associated with Arnold-Chiari Deformity and Platybasia. Arch. Neurol. & Psychiat. 49:881, 1943.

MacKay, R. P. and Favill, J.: Syringomyelia and Intramedullary Tumor of the Spinal Cord. Arch. Neurol. and Psychiat. 33:1255, 1935.

PERONEAL MUSCULAR ATROPHY

Also known as neuritic muscular atrophy or Charcot-Marie-Tooth muscular atrophy, this disease may occur in a hereditary form through generations or there may be a history of several members of the same family being affected. It is usually transmitted as a dominant, occasionally as an autosomal or sex-linked recessive.

CLINICAL PICTURE: The onset occurs between ten and twenty years, sometimes earlier. There is atrophy of the peroneal muscles and extensor digitorum longus. As a result, foot drop occurs and the feet may turn inward, with varus or finally even club feet developing. Steppage gait follows. As atrophy of the legs continues, their thinness compared to the normal upper thighs makes them appear as "stork legs."

In the upper extremities, the small muscles of the hands are first involved. The onset is usually later than in the legs. This is followed by atrophy of the forearms. The upper arms, shoulders and trunk are usually not affected or else very late. Fasciculations are noted. Subsequently the upper arms and lower thighs may atrophy.

The deep tendon reflexes are absent. Sensory changes may occur in the distal portions of the extremities in the form of hypesthesia, but pain is not prominent. Electrical reactions may be absent or show a reaction of degeneration.

There have been a number of reports of the association of peroneal muscular atrophy with other conditions, such as Friedreich's ataxia, Roussy-Levy hereditary areflexia (an abortive form of Friedreich's), and optic atrophy.

PATHOLOGY: There is degeneration of the peripheral nerves, which is probably primary, with secondary involvement of the anterior and posterior roots, ventral horns, and posterior columns of the cord. The atrophy of the muscles follows the peripheral nerve lesion.

DIAGNOSIS: When the peroneal muscular atrophy occurs with a positive familial history, typical atrophy of the feet, legs, and hands, and deformity of the foot, the differential is not difficult. When it occurs sporadically, a differential diagnosis must be made from interstitial hypertrophic neuritis (Dejerine-Sottas) which has thickened nerve trunks, poliomyelitis, the infantile myopathies, and various forms of polyneuritis.

PROGNOSIS: The disease is slowly progressive.

TREATMENT: There is no specific therapy, except orthopedic correction.

Bell, J.: On the Peroneal Type of Progressive Muscular Atrophy. Treas. Hum. Inher. 4:69, 1935.
Brugsch, H. G. and Hauptman, A.: Familial Occurrence of Friedreich's Ataxia with Charcot-Marie-Tooth Neural Muscular Atrophy. Bull. New England Med. Center 6:42, 1944.
Charcot, J. M. and Marie, P.: Sur une forme particuliére dátrophie musculaire progressive, souvent familiale débutant por les pieds et les jambes, et atteignant plus tard les mains. Rev. de. Méd. Par. 6:97, 1886.
Ross, A. T.: Combination of Friedreich's Ataxia and Charcot-Marie-Tooth Atrophy in Each of Two Brothers. J. Nerv. & Ment. Dis. 95:680, 1942.
Spillane, J. D.: Familial pes cavus and absent tendon jerks: Its Relationship with Friedreich's Disease and Peroneal Muscular Atrophy. Brain 63:275, 1940.
Tooth, H. H.: The Peroneal Type of Progressive Muscular Atrophy. London, H. K. Lewis, 1886.

HYPERTROPHIC INTERSTITIAL NEURITIS

(FAMILIAL HYPERTROPHIC POLYNEURITIS)

This condition was described as a clinical entity by Dejerine and Sottas in 1893. It is a chronically progressing polyneuritis with both motor and sensory symptoms and is heredofamilial, transmitted as a simple dominant.

CLINICAL PICTURE: The onset occurs in childhood and the disease progresses slowly. It usually begins in the lower extremities with progressive weakness, deformity, and difficulty in walking. Later, after many years, the upper extremities are likewise involved. The peripheral nerves are palpable and thickened. There are atrophy of the muscles of the distal portions of the extremities (foot-drop), absent tendon reflexes, and diminished electrical excitation. There may be sensory disturbance, either pain or sensory loss. Ataxia, scanning speech, and nystagmus are noted in some. Kyphoscoliosis may be seen. The spinal fluid usually shows an elevation of protein.

PATHOLOGY: The peripheral nerves and posterior roots are markedly hypertrophied and thickened. There is an interstitial hypertrophic neuritis (proliferation of perineural and endoneural connective tissue and proliferation of cells of the sheath of Schwann, producing concentric laminated structures called "onion bulbs"). Secondary atrophy and sclerosis of the posterior columns of the cord and to some degree of the anterior horns are also present.

ETIOLOGY: The cause of this condition is unknown.

DIAGNOSIS: This is based on the heredofamilial history, clinical picture of polyneuritis, and the thickened and palpable peripheral nerve trunks. Histological sections of a nerve may be needed. The relationship to Charcot-Marie-Tooth peroneal atrophy has been raised. For a full discussion refer to the article of Croft and Wadia. Refsum's disease, "heredopathia atactica polyneuritiformis" or polyneuritiform ataxia also presents a picture of chronic polyneuritis, but there are also retinitis pigmentosa with night blindness, high protein in the spinal fluid, and absence of palpable enlarged peripheral nerves.

PROGNOSIS: The course is slowly progressive and chronic, but patients may live to advanced ages.

TREATMENT: Orthopedic correction of deformities should be carried out.

Croft, P. B. and Wadia, N. H.: Familial Hypertrophic Polyneuritis. Review of a Previously Reported Family. Neurology 7:356, 1957.
DeBruyn, R. S. and Stern, R. O.: A Case of the Progressive Hypertrophic Polyneuritis of Dejerine and Sottas with Pathological Examination. Brain 52:84, 1929.

Fleming, R.: Refsum's Syndrome. An Unusual Hereditary Neuropathy. Neurology 7:476, 1957.

Wolf, A., Rubinowitz, A. H. and Burchell, S. C.: Interstitial Hypertrophic Neuritis of Dejerine and Sottas, Bull. Neurol. Instit. 2:373, 1932.

DYSTONIA MUSCULORUM DEFORMANS

This disease, also referred to as torsion spasm or torsion dystonia, is a rare progressive syndrome consisting of involuntary movements of the skeletal musculature, especially the trunk and proximal muscles of the extremities.

CLINICAL PICTURE: The onset is gradual, at about five to fifteen years in most cases, without any antecedent history. Herz collected 105 cases up to 1944. He divided them into three groups, with a few beginning soon after birth, a juvenile form originating between five and fifteen years, and those with an onset after fifteen years. In some there is first observed an inversion of the foot with adduction of the thigh due to spasm, thus producing an abnormal gait. Soon there occur rotation and torsion of the body with slow, twisting movements of the trunk muscles so that the child assumes bizarre postures and attitudes. There may be such hypertonicity during the spasm that the child may develop lordosis or opisthotonos. Between spasms there is some diminution of tone. The movements differ from those of chorea or athetosis in which more of the distal muscles are involved. The movements disappear during sleep. There are no paralyses. Mentality is usually normal at the onset but may subsequently deteriorate.

PATHOLOGY: Degenerative changes have been described in the striatum, globus pallidus, substantia nigra, cortex, and cerebellum.

ETIOLOGY: The cause of torsion spasm is unknown. It has occurred mostly in Russian Jews. There is a familial factor.

DIAGNOSIS: There has been doubt in the minds of some whether this condition should be described as a distinct entity. These children have dystonia and no history of trouble before the onset of the clinical picture. Torsion spasm must be separated from other known causes of dystonia such as epidemic encephalitis, hepatolenticular degeneration (Wilson's Disease), Huntington's Chorea, brain tumor, vascular disturbances, and birth injury.

PROGNOSIS: The course is steadily downhill so that the child is eventually bedridden, and death ensues after several years. Occasionally the clinical picture remains fairly stationary.

TREATMENT: There is no specific therapy. Surgery has been used to eliminate the flow of stimuli (see under Cerebral Palsy).

Herz, E.: Dystonia, II Clinical Classification. A.M.A. Arch. Neurol. & Psychiat. 51:319, 1944.

LAURENCE-MOON-BIEDL SYNDROME

This condition was described in 1866 by Laurence and Moon, who observed its presence in four patients of one family. There were obesity, hypogenitalism, mental deficiency, and retinitis pigmentosa. Biedl in 1922 added polydactyly. Ross, Crome, and Mac-Kenzie collected 300 cases up to 1955.

CLINICAL FEATURES: In a number of instances there is a familial history, but this is variable. The obesity is noted in childhood, at times associated with retardation in growth so that the child remains a dwarf. There is failure of sexual development with genital hypoplasia. Retinitis pigmentosa, with degeneration of the retina and loss of vision leading to blindness, is another feature. In some cases cataracts are present. The children are mentally retarded. Polydactylism is present in almost half the cases. Other characteristics noted less often are deformities of the skull or vertebral column and atresia ani. Some authors have reported an association with congenital heart disease and spinocerebellar degeneration.

PATHOLOGY: There are no characteristic changes. Ross and his associates reported that only ten autopsies previous to theirs had been done. In their case, there was no evidence of pituitary or hypothalamic disease. There were a reduction in the number of cortical cells and a lipofuscin-like pigment in all of the nerve cells. The ocular pathology was similar to any form of retinitis pigmentosa, showing primary pigment degeneration. The kidneys showed pyelonephritis.

ETIOLOGY: The disease is believed to be inherited as a recessive condition. Heterozygous carriers may have polydactyly or deaf-mutism.

PROGNOSIS: Of the primary features, the loss of vision is progressive. These patients often develop uremia, which causes their death. The uremia appears to be due to glomerulonephritis and other types of kidney pathology.

TREATMENT: There is no therapy.

Burn, R. A.: Deafness and the Laurence-Moon-Biedl Syndrome. British J. Ophth. 34:65, 1950.
Ross, C. F., Crome, L. and Mackenzie, D. Y.: The Laurence-Moon-Biedl Syndrome. J. Pathol. & Bacter. 72:161, 1956.

MYOCLONUS EPILEPSY

(UNVERRICHT'S FAMILIAL MYOCLONIC EPILEPSY)

This is a heredofamilial disease in which myoclonic contractions occur in conjunction with seizures. The onset is in the early years of childhood. Convulsive seizures may precede by years or follow the onset of myoclonus. They are usually major, but may be petit mal in character. The myoclonic or muscular contractions are sudden, irregular, short, lightning-like jerks, affecting the muscles of the extremities most often. The trunk, diaphragm, and less frequently the muscles of the face and neck are also affected. The myoclonic contractions are most marked on voluntary movement. They do not occur in sleep. As the course of the disease continues, there is mental deterioration. There are also signs of basal ganglia and cerebellar involvement, with rigidity, tremor, and ataxia.

PATHOLOGY: There is neuronal degeneration in various parts of the brain. Amyloid inclusion bodies, spherical in shape, are present within the cell bodies of the neurons. They are most numerous in the dentate nucleus, substantia nigra, pallidum, and rolandic cortex.

LABORATORY: Electroencephalography may show a 3 per sec. or a 4-6 per sec. wave and spike or a rapid series of spikes with a focus in the cortex (frontal) associated with myoclonic jerks.

ETIOLOGY: The disease is inherited and usually transmitted as a recessive, occasionally dominant.

DIAGNOSIS: This is based on the presence of a heredofamilial disease associated with recurring seizures, myoclonic jerks, and dementia. Myoclonic jerks may be associated with grand mal epilepsy or may be a part of a petit mal triad. In these cases, however, there is lack of a heredofamilial history, the contractions occur sporadically rather than almost constantly, and mental deterioration is not observed. Paramyoclonus multiplex (Friedreich) occurs primarily in adults without any of the other manifestations of myoclonic epilepsy. Encephalitis, as in Schilders disease or the inclusion body form, may require differential. Degeneration of the cerebral gray matter should also be considered.

COURSE: This is slowly progressive with gradual deterioration.

TREATMENT: Anticonvulsive drugs should be used such as phenobarbital and Dilantin sodium®.

Ajuriaguerra, J. de., Sigwald, J. and Piot C.: Unverricht's Familial Myoclonus Epilepsy: Clinical, Electroencephalographic and Anatomic Study. Presse Méd. 62:1813, 1954.
Grinker, R. R., Serota, H., Stein, S. I.: Myoclonic Epilepsy. Arch. Neurol. & Psychiat. 40:968, 1938.
Unverricht, H.: Ueber Familiäre Myoclonie. Deutsche Ztschr. Nervenh., 7:32, 1895.
Watson, C. W. and Denny-Brown, D.: Myoclonus Epilepsy as a Symptom of Diffuse Neuronal Disease. A.M.A. Arch. Neurol. and Psychiat. 70:151, 1958.

FAMILIAL DYSAUTONOMIA

This condition is congenital and characterized by diffuse involvement of the central nervous system with particular dysfunction of the autonomic system. It is a familial disease occurring primarily in Jewish children. It is also known as the Riley-Day syndrome.

CLINICAL PICTURE: One of the outstanding symptoms is defective lacrimation so that the children do not produce tears when crying. Other features usually present include transient blotching of the skin, which is of an erythematous type appearing over the face and chest with excitement or eating, excessive perspiration, constant drooling, and emotional instability. The neurological finding which are most constant include motor incoordination, hyporeflexia, and relative indifference to pain.

While the above group of clinical features is almost always present, there are an additional number which though less frequent are significant. They include hypertension, cyclic or periodic vomiting, frequent pulmonary infections, bouts of unexplained fever, breath holding spells in infancy, corneal ulceration, mental retardation, and convulsions associated with an abnormal electroencephalogram. The blood pressure is poorly regulated, labile, and may exhibit postural hypotension; after the child has been in bed, he is asked to rise; following several minutes on his feet, the blood pressure (diastolic especially) may fall (10-60 mm.). Speech is poor due to lack of control of the tongue and lips. In infancy there are evidences of feeding difficulties, poor sucking and swallowing, regurgitation of milk, and respiratory infections simulating aspiration pneumonia.

PATHOLOGY: The brain appears normal. The major lesion thus far noted is a destruction of the reticular formation of the pons and medulla. In one instance parts of the thalamus were also destroyed. In another, the Purkinje cells of the cerebellum showed agenesis and destruction. The nature of the lesion is degenerative. There is, however, no consistent abnormality (Riley).

PATHOGENESIS: Some of the clinical features such as excessive perspiration, drooling and skin blotching seem to be due to parasympathetic stimulation or sympathetic inhibition. Others, such as defective lacrimation, hyperthermia, and hypertension appear to be due to a reverse mechanism, namely sympathetic stimulation or parasympathetic inhibition. Mecholyl, a parasympathetic stimulating drug, when injected subcutaneously produced tears in three patients, showing that defective lacrimation is not due to a defective gland but rather to defective nerve pathways.

ETIOLOGY: The cause of dysautonomia is unknown. It is a familial disease, transmitted as a Mendelian recessive condition, and occurring almost exclusively in Jewish families. Consanguinity of the parents is often present. However, there have been a number of cases recently reported in which the disease has been noted in non-Jews. It may be that the condition accidentally occurs in these or is a developmental error not genetically transmitted, because the four non-Jewish patients have seven siblings, all of whom are normal.

DIAGNOSIS: The major points in early diagnosis are feeding difficulties, defective lacrimation, skin blotching, excessive perspiration, and absent or hypoactive deep tendon reflexes. There is a history of Jewish extraction, at times an affected sibling. Differential must be made from birth trauma and cerebral palsy because of the slow motor development. Later in infancy, familial dysautonomia must be differentiated from acrodynia; if the patient is non-Jewish, the former is less likely. A history of mercury ingestion should be looked for in acrodynia. Pheochromocytoma in older children produces hypertension and should be ruled out by specific tests. In congenital analgia, where there is indifference to pain, reflexes are normal.

PROGNOSIS: About one-third of the reported cases have died. There are retardation in physical growth and development and no change in the individual symptoms. Mentally these children develop satisfactorily, but appear slow due to motor incoordination. They show difficulty in dealing with concrete situations and inadequate adjustment to daily life. At the same time they learn to manipulate their parents, who have developed fears and guilt feelings. Group therapy has helped the parents understand their problems better. These children must be separated from brain-injured children, whom they resemble, and possibly from childhood schizophrenia.

TREATMENT: There is no therapy for the primary condition. Chlorpromazine intramuscularly may be used to control vomiting.

Cohen, P. and Solomon, N. H.: Familial Dysautonomia. Case Report with Autopsy. J. Pediat. 46:663, 1955.

Fanconi, G. and Ferrazzini, F.: Congenital Analgia (Congenital Generalized Indifference to Pain). Helvet. paediat. acta. 12:79, 1957.

Freedman, A. M., Helme, W., Havel, J., Eustis, M. J., Riley, C. and Langford, W. S.: Psychiatric Aspects of Familial Dysautonomia. Am. J. Orthopsychiat. 27:96 1957.

Kroop, I. G.: The Production of Tears in Familial Dysautonomia. J. Pediat. 48:328, 1956.

Linde, L. M.: Diagnosis and Management of Dysautonomia, Pediat. 18:692, 1956.

Moloshok, R. E. and Reuben, R. N.: Familial Autonomic Dysfunction. J. Mt. Sinai Hosp. 21:137, 1954.

Riley, C. M., Day, R. L., Greeley, D. McL, and Langford, W. S.: Central Autonomic Dysfunction with Defective Lacrimation. Report of Five Cases. Pediat. 3:468, 1949.

————, C. M.: Familial Dysautonomia. Advances in Pediatrics, IX, Chicago, Year Book Publishers, 1957.

CHAPTER 13

CEREBRAL SCLEROSES
(DEMYELINATING DISEASES)

These include a group of diseases which have in common a diffuse, nonspecific demyelinization of the cerebral white matter. The lipid content has been found to differ in the various forms of diffuse sclerosis, but the significance of this in relation to the cause or form of sclerosis is yet to be determined. Greenfield feels that the glial cells are the factor in the deficient anabolic myelinization process.

Poser and Van Bogaert have classified the cerebral scleroses into three main groups. The first is the primary demyelinating, such as multiple sclerosis, Schilder's cerebral sclerosis, Balo concentric sclerosis and Devic's disease. The Schilder type has many features similar to multiple sclerosis. There may be recurring clinical and pathological episodes, selective destruction of myelin, inflammatory reaction, and slight axonal involvement. The second embraces the leucodystrophies, including Pelizaeus-Merzbacher disease, the group with "glial insufficiency," the globoid cell type (Krabbe), and the form associated with spongy degeneration of the neuraxis. These forms are heredodegenerative, begin in infancy, usually following a normal birth and early satisfactory development. In this respect they are similar to the lipidoses. There is a diffuse demyelinization of the cerebral white matter which is symmetrical. In the group with glial insufficiency, the abnormal products replacing myelin may stain a dull red, instead of brilliant red (Sudanophilic). The group with spongy degeneration of the neuraxis is characterized by the presence of soft, cystic areas in the cortex due to the intense edema and infiltration of the tissues by a protein rich fluid. The third group includes the subacute encephalitides such as Van Bogaert's and Dawson's (Chap. 8).

In the present state of our knowledge no completely acceptable classification can be made or followed, since there is difficulty in differentiating the various forms of sclerosis clinically or through the use of the ordinary laboratory procedures. A hopeful step is the use of chemical data based on the lipid abnormalities in demyelinating diseases. For this purpose, biopsy of less than one gram of brain tissue is necessary (Cummings). Analysis of the lipid abnormalities of the brain with this technique reveals that in multiple sclerosis there is a loss of phospholipid and the presence of cholesterol esters. In Krabbe's and Pelizaeus-Merzbacher's disease, there are no cholesterol esters. However the cerebroside content is increased in Krabbe's disease, whereas it is reduced in Pelizaeus-Merzbacher's disease. In amaurotic idiocy there is a marked increase in neuraminic acid and no cholesterol esters. In addition to chemical analysis, the biopsied cortical tissue may also be subjected to histological examination for the presence of diffuse sclerosis or cerebral lipidosis.

Descriptions of the individual forms of cerebral sclerosis follow. There is however, the problem, not only of differentiating the various entities, but also of separating the group from other cerebral degenerations such as the lipidoses, the inborn errors of metabolism, and infections of the newborn such as toxoplasmosis. For this purpose the physician may require a careful genetic history, the use of specific laboratory tests, and chemical and histologic study of biopsied brain tissue.

Benda, C. E. and Melchior, J. C.: Progressive Deteriorating Diseases of Infancy. J. Neuropath. and Exper. Neurol. 17:205, 1958.
Cummings, J. N.: Lipid Chemistry in Demyelinating Diseases. Brain 78:554, 1955.
Masland, R. L.: The Prevention of Mental Retardation. A Survey of Research. Am. J. Ment. Def. 62:991, 1958.
Poser, C. M. and Van Bogaert.: Natural History and Evolution of the Concept of Schilder's Diffuse Sclerosis. Acta Psychiat. et. Neurol. Scandinav. 31:285, 1956.
Stevens, H. and Dekaban, A.: Progressive cerebral degenerations of childhood. Neurology 8:677, 1958.
Van Bogaert, L.: Cerebral Lipidoses. A symposium. Springfield, Illinois. Chas. C. Thomas, 1957.

ACUTE INFANTILE FORM OF CEREBRAL SCLEROSIS (KRABBE)

In 1916, Krabbe reported five cases of diffuse brain sclerosis. The infants were born normally, developed satisfactorily up to four to six months, and then began to show clinical evidence of disease. Death occurred at nine months in one, three died at eleven to thirteen months, and one at two years.

CLINICAL PICTURE: The clinical picture is one of normal development in the first few months after birth. There is then an onset of general restlessness, constant crying, lack of appetite, and gradually developing stupor. Associated with this picture is universal rigidity of the body and limbs associated with epileptic seizures, both tonic and clonic in character. These are precipitated by various stimuli such as light or noise. Soon the child cannot swallow and must be fed by tube. Blindness, due either to cortical involvement or optic atrophy, and deafness may occur.

PATHOLOGY: The gross feel of the brain is hard. Microscopically, there is diffuse symmetrical demyelination of the white matter of the brain and cord. Large globoid cells are present. The axis cylinders are also affected. There are replacement of the destroyed tissue by neuroglia and relative intactness of the nerve cells.

DIAGNOSIS: This condition should be differentiated from amaurotic idiocy. The latter occurs in Hebrews and is diagnosed by the cherry-red spot in the macula.

PROGNOSIS: The prognosis is poor, death occurring rapidly within a few months.

TREATMENT: There is no specific therapy.

Blackwood, W. and Cumings, J. N.: A Histological and Chemical Study of Three Cases of Diffuse Cerebral Sclerosis. J. Neurol. Neurosurg. Psychiat. 17:33, 1954.
Jervis, G. A.: Early Infantile "Diffuse Sclerosis" of the Brain (Krabbe's Type). Am. J. Dis. Child. 64:1055, 1942.
Krabbe, K.: A New Familial Infantile Form of Diffuse Brain Sclerosis. Brain. 39:74, 1916.

CHRONIC INFANTILE FORM OF CEREBRAL SCLEROSIS
(PELIZAEUS-MERZBACHER)

The description of this condition may best be given by referring to the titles of the papers of the two authors after whom it is named. Pelizaeus reported a peculiar form of spastic paralysis with cerebral symptoms on a hereditary basis, and Merzbacher referred to a peculiar hereditary disease form. The onset is in early infancy, around the third month of life. There are noted nystagmus, tremor of the head, and inability to hold it up. As the years go by, the infant develops spasticity, first of the lower and then of the upper extremities associated with hyperactive tendon reflexes, a Babinski sign, and absent abdominal reflexes. Other features include ataxia, intention tremors, and scanning speech, suggestive of cerebellar pathology. There may also be extrapyramidal features such as mask-like facies, cog-wheel rhythm of the muscles, and athetoid movements, as well as postural disturbances. Deformities of the bones and disturbances in their nutrition are evident. The progress of these clinical features is usually rapid for the first six years. It is also evident that the child is deteriorating mentally. However, later there are periods during which there is no further progression or where even remission of symptoms occurs, so that the individual may live on to a ripe age. There are many variations of the original clinical picture. While males are mostly affected, females have also been reported with the disease. It is transmitted by a healthy mother. Sporadic cases and onsets in late childhood and adult life have also been reported.

PATHOLOGY: There is a diffuse demyelination in the white matter of the cortex, cerebellum, and brain stem especially, and also in the cord. Within this widespread process, however, there is one distinctive feature, namely, that there are areas or islets of preserved myelinated fibres, mostly around blood vessels. In other types of demyelinating disease, the process is most obvious in the perivascular areas, so that the difference in this disease is outstanding. The process of demyelination is symmetrical, with marked overgrowth of glial cells (sclerosis) in the affected areas.

DIFFERENTIAL DIAGNOSIS: Since this disease occurs in early life, it must be differentiated from the other diffuse scleroses. In Krabbe's, the onset is at a similar age, but death follows quickly. In the sclerosis of Scholz, the onset is later and death occurs rapidly in one or two years. The cardinal features of Pelizaeus-Merzbacher disease must be kept in mind, namely, onset in early infancy, slow progress, heredofamilial incidence, brain stem signs early, and multiplicity of systems involved, namely cortical, cerebellar, and extrapyramidal. Schilder's disease can be ruled out by its more rapid course. Furthermore, in Pelizaeus-Merzbacher there is no visual disturbance. In spite of the apparent clinical differences, an autopsy may be required to make the differential among these various forms of sclerosis.

TREATMENT: There is no specific therapy.

Merzbacher, L.: Eine eigenartige familiär hereditäre Erkrankungsform (Aplasia Axialis Extra-Corticalis Congenita). Zeitschr. Neurol. u. Psychiat. 3:1, 1910.

Pelizaeus, F.: Über eine eigentümliche Form spastischer Lähmung mit Cerebralerscheinungen auf hereditörer Grundlage (Multiple Sklerose). Arch. f. Psychiat. 16:698, 1885.

Tyler, H. R.: Pelizaeus-Merzbacher Disease. A.M.A. Arch. Neurol. & Psychiat. 80:162, 1958.

SUBACUTE JUVENILE FORM OF CEREBRAL SCLEROSIS
(SCHOLZ)

These children are well until eight to ten years of age, when deafneses develops. Soon aphasia and blindness follow. These manifestations are due to cortical pathology; occasionally, however, the loss of vision may be due to optic atrophy. The pupillary reflexes are intact. About a year later spastic quadriplegia develops, beginning first in the legs, then the arms. In others, choreoathetosis may occur. Uncontrollable emotional fits of laughing and crying take place, and finally complete dementia. Death occurs in a few years. The pathology involves the white matter of the brain and is similar to Krabbe's.

Scholz, W.: Klinische, Pathologisch-Anatomische und Erbbiologische Untersuchungen bei Familärer, diffuser Hirnsklerose im Kindesalter. Zeitschr. f. d. ges. Neurol. u. Psychiat. 99:651, 1925.

SCHILDER'S ENCEPHALITIS PERIAXIALIS DIFFUSA
(DIFFUSE CEREBRAL SCLEROSIS)

This disease may be described after Schilder as a diffuse subcortical involvement of the white matter resulting in demyelinization of the cerebral hemispheres, with a variety of clinical features.

CLINICAL PICTURE: The onset of the illness may be acute or more gradual. It occurs in a child who has previously been healthy. There is no sex predilection. While two or more in a generation of one family may be affected, suggesting a genetic basis, probably recessive, sporadic cases also occur.

Depending on the areas involved, a variety of symptoms and signs are present. There is marked apathy. Sooner or later, other psychical manifestations appear in the form of hallucinations, disorientation, and dementia. Neurological examination reveals mono-

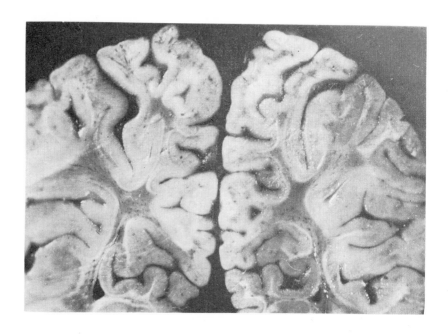

16. Diffuse cerebral sclerosis (Schilder).
Irregular patterns of white matter are seen.

plegias, hemiplegias, and especially quadriplegias of the spastic type. Hyperactive tendon reflexes and a Babinski sign are present. Seizures are an accompanying feature. In some instances rigidity may be noted. Loss of vision is an important development; the blindness is central, that is cortical, due to occipital lobe involvement. The pupils and optic discs usually are normal. Occasionally deafness of a cortical type is present, in some cases combined with blindness. The course is steadily downhill. Aphasia, apraxia, and dysarthria may be present. Cerebellar ataxia may occur. In some instances there may be headache, vomiting, and papilledema; in these the spinal fluid instead of being normal, which is usually the case, shows evidence of increased pressure with excess protein and some cells. The picture thus simulates tumor and these patients have been subsequently explored. Finally, mutism, emotional fits of crying and laughing, and disturbances in swallowing follow. There may be fever and complete dementia ending in death. Occasionally remissions occur for long periods.

PATHOLOGY: The white matter of the brain shows the greatest amount of pathology. There are bilateral, symmetrical softenings. These appear as patches, which stop a short distance from the cortex, where the white matter is preserved (arcuate fibres). The process is diffuse, involving primarily the cerebral hemispheres, and may extend to the brain stem or spinal cord. Microscopic examination reveals destruction of the myelin sheath and to a lesser degree the axis cylinder. There is proliferation of the glial cells, but they may also undergo destruction with cavities resulting. There is some perivascular proliferation.

DIFFERENTIAL DIAGNOSIS: In a clinical picture so varied in character it is difficult to make a clear-cut diagnosis or differential. However, the major features should be kept in mind: the child is well, with nothing to suggest trouble at birth or for a period thereafter; then follow disorders of motility (spastic paralysis), fits, psychic symptoms, cortical blindness, rapid downhill course with disturbed intellect, and occasionally signs of increased pressure like headaches, vomiting, and papilledema. Brain tumor must be differentiated when papilledema with increased pressure appears. Surgical exploration following air studies may be needed. The various forms of diffuse sclerosis, such as Pelizaeus-Merzbacher, Scholz's, and Krabbe's must be considered. Sclerosis similar to Schilder's has been described by Balo. Multiple sclerosis usually begins at a later age.

PROGNOSIS: The course of the disease is progressively downhill, patients succumbing in a few days or surviving as long as thirteen years.

TREATMENT: There is no therapy which will influence the outlook.

Balo, J.: Encephalitis Periaxialis Concentrica. Arch. Neurol. & Psychiat. 19:242, 1928.
Bouman, L.: Encephalitis Periaxialis Diffusa. Brain 47:453, 1924.
————: Diffuse Sclerosis (Encephalitis Periaxialis Diffusa). Bristol, John Wright & Sons, 1934.
Gasul, B. M.: Schilder's Disease (Encephalitis Pariaxialis Diffusa) Am. J. Dis. Child. 39:595, 1930.
Környey, S.: Early Stage of Schilders Disease and Relation to other Forms of Leucoencephalomyelitis. Arch. Neurol. & Psychiat. 68:683, 1952.
Poser, C. M. and Van Bogaert, L.: Natural History and Evolution of the Concept of Schilder's Diffuse Sclerosis. Acta psychiat. et neurol. Scandinav. 31:285, 1956.
Schilder, P.: Zur Kenntnis der Sogenanten Diffusen Sklerose. Ztschr. f.d. ges. Neurol. u. Psychiat. 10:1, 1912.

METACHROMATIC FORM OF DIFFUSE CEREBRAL SCLEROSIS

This form of diffuse sclerosis is similar to the others previously discussed in that there is extensive demyelination of the cerebral white matter along with destructive changes involving the axones, cells, and glial fibres. However, in addition there are granular clumps of abnormal material (lipid-carbohydrate) in the degenerated areas which stain various shades of red with basic blue aniline dyes. The assumption of a color different from that of the dye is referred to as metachromasia.

The clinical picture is one of normal birth, followed by gradually developing paralysis with increased deep tendon reflexes and a Babinski sign, stupor leading to dementia, loss of vision, either cortical or due to optic atrophy, and convulsions. There may be incoordination and nystagmus. Rigidity is usually marked. The course has been as short as six weeks and as long as twenty-two years. There is a strong familial trait, siblings being similarly affected. The spinal fluid shows elevated protein.

The diagnosis may now be made during life by staining the centrifuged urine sediment with one or two drops of a two per cent aqueous solution of toluidin blue. Six distinctive granular forms may be seen with a golden-brown metachromatic color. An additional diagnostic aid is the demonstration of red metachromatic lipid-containing substances in the urine.

Austin, J. H.: Metachromatic Form of Diffuse Sclerosis.
1. Diagnosis During Life by Urine Sediment Examination. Neurology 7:415, 1957.
———: Metachromatic Form of Diffuse Cerebral Sclerosis.
2. Diagnosis During Life by Isolation of Metachromatic Lipids from Urine. Neurology 7:716, 1957.
Brain, W. R. and Greenfield, J. G.: Late Infantile Metachromatic Leuco-Encephalopathy with Primary Degeneration of the Interfasicular Oligodendroglia. Brain 73:291, 1950.
Feigin, I.: Diffuse Cerebral Sclerosis (Metachromatic Leuko-Encephalopathy). Am. J. Path. 30:715, 1954.

MULTIPLE SCLEROSIS

Multiple or disseminated sclerosis is a chronic, progressive disease, with periods of remission and exacerbation and a variety of clinical symptoms and signs.

It is uncommon in childhood, but verified cases have been reported. Low and Carter recently reported seven and reviewed the literature.

CLINICAL PICTURE: The onset may be quite sudden, in some instances appearing to follow an acute infection or injury, in others, with no preceding complaints. The more frequent presenting clinical features include sudden loss of vision, weakness with paraplegia or hemiplegia, vertigo, and ataxia. These may clear completely only to be followed by recurrences and further progression of symptoms. As a rule, a variety of manifestations occur together.

The spastic paraplegia is due to pyramidal tract involvement. Along with it there is muscular weakness. Tendon reflexes are increased, abdominal reflexes absent. Together with the paraplegia, there is likely to be ataxia due to posterior column involvement.

Retrobulbar neuritis produces blurring of vision with central scotomas. The optic discs are usually normal. With subsequent attacks, pallor of the nerve head, especially on the temporal side, occurs. In addition to retrobulbar neuritis, there may be ocular palsies and diplopia.

Cerebellar signs such as ataxic gait, incoordination of muscles, slow scanning speech, and intention tremor are noted. Bladder disturbances usually occur, including retention and incontinence.

Sensory changes may be present, but are not noteworthy in children.

LABORATORY: The spinal fluid pressure is normal. Cells are slightly increased to about 20 per cu. mm. Protein in the spinal fluid is slightly elevated with a relative increase in gamma globulin. There is a paretic (1st zone) or meningeal (2nd zone) gold curve. The electroencephalogram shows slow waves.

PATHOLOGY: Grossly the brain and cord may appear normal. On section, however, there are patches of gray, referred to as plaques of sclerosis, especially evident in the white matter. They are not related to blood vessel distribution. With staining these are seen to consist of disintegrated myelin sheaths with relative preservation of the axis cylinders. In older lesions glial proliferation is noted. The processs is diffuse, involving the spinal cord, especially the pyramidal tracts, medulla, pons, cerebellum, and optic nerve. The phospholipid content of the brain is diminished.

ETIOLOGY: The cause of multiple sclerosis is unknown. It is especially prevalent in areas where there is a moderately cold winter climate; it is rare in the tropics.

DIAGNOSIS: Multiple sclerosis is to be suspected in childhood whenever there are multiple manifestations of central nervous system involvement. These will usually include spastic paraplegia or hemiplegia, cerebellar ataxia, and retrobulbar neuritis with central scotoma. It is to be considered even more strongly when there are periodic remissions and exacerbations. Finally, it is liable to be an exclusion diagnosis, awaiting the test of time, since the patient usually survives into adult life.

The cerebral palsies are ruled out by their presence at birth or shortly thereafter. They tend to improve without exacerbations and remissions. Pelizaeus-Merzbacher is a familial disease, which occurs early in infancy and progresses rapidly at first, later slowly. There are tremors, nystagmus, and later scanning speech.

Schilder's has a rapid course, papilledema, seizures, and cortical blindness. Some have considered it an infantile form of multiple sclerosis.

The presence of retrobulbar neuritis means a consideration of other causes of the condition, including Leber's disease which is familial and usually confined to the eyes. Other causes of retrobulbar neuritis to be differentiated include metallic poisons, sinusitis, and tumors of the sella, chiasm, and optic nerve.

Neuromyelitis optica (Devic's disease). In this condition there is optic neuritis with edema, similar to a picture of increased intracranial pressure. This is rare in multiple sclerosis. Associated with the ocular pathology is a transverse myelitis with flaccid paralysis and absent reflexes below the level of the lesion. It is considered to be a form of multiple sclerosis or disseminated encephalomyelitis, and there is a question whether it is a separate entity. In neuromyelitis optica there are plaques with demyelinating lesions of the brain and cord as well as of the optic nerve.

In post-vaccination and infectious encephalitis there is a history of previous vaccination or of some infectious disease such as measles.

Tumor is to be ruled out when papilledema is present. This may at times require an exploratory operation.

PROGNOSIS: The patients live for long periods, but there is slow progression. Remissions may occur. Eventually disability results. The life span is around twenty years.

TREATMENT: There is no specific therapy. Physiotherapy and psychotherapy may be used to encourage the patient. Recently large amounts of galactose have been given to overcome the myelin disintegration, which is explained on the basis of galactose deficiency. This procedure is still experimental.

Carter, S., Sciarra, D. and Merritt, H. H.: The Course of Multiple Sclerosis as Determined by Autopsy Proven Cases. A. Res. Publ. Ass. Nerv. Ment. Dis. Proc. 28:471, 1950.

Cummings, J. N.: Lipid Chemistry of the Brain in Demyelinating Disease. Brain 78:554, 1955.

Freedman, D. A. and Merritt, H. H.: The Cerebro-Spinal Fluid in Multiple Sclerosis. A. Res. Publ. Ass. Nerv. Ment. Dis. Proc. 28:428, 1950.

Gall, Jr., J. C., Hayles, A. B., Siekert, R. G. and Keith, H. M.: Multiple Sclerosis in Children. Pediat. 21:703, 1958.

Hartstein, J., and Ulett, G. A.: Galactose Treatment of Multiple Sclerosis. (A Preliminary Report). Dis. Nerv. Sys. 18:255, 1957.

Jasper, H., Bickford, R. and Magnus, O.: The Electro-Encephalogram in Multiple Sclerosis. A. Res. Publ. Ass. Nerv. Ment. Dis. Proc. 28:421, 1950.

Leinfelder, P. J.: Retrobulbar Neuritis in Multiple Sclerosis. A. Res. Publ. Ass. Nerv. Ment. Dis. Proc. 28:383, 1950.

Lhermitte, F.: Leuco-encephalites, Paris, Ernest Flammarion, 1950.

Low, N. L. and Carter, S.: Multiple Sclerosis in Children, Pediat. 18:24, 1956.

Zimmerman, H. M. and Netsky, M. G.: The Pathology of Multiple Sclerosis. A. Res. Publ. Ass. Nerv. Ment. Dis. Proc. 28:271, 1950.

DEGENERATION OF THE CEREBRAL GRAY MATTER (ALPERS)

In 1931, Alpers reported a case of an infant who developed seizures, hyperkinesias, and rigidity beginning at three months of age and who died two months later. Examination of the brain showed defective development of the cortex and widespread degeneration of the gray matter in most of the cortical hemispheres, especially the third and fourth layers. There were lesions also in the striatum, pallidum, pons, and thalamus. There were extensive destruction of neurons and proliferation of astrocytes.

CLINICAL PICTURE: In most of the cases the onset occurs during the first year. The birth and family history are usually normal. In some there may be evidence of retarded development before the acute features appear. These consist of myoclonic contractions or twitchings of the muscles, convulsions, rigidity, and hyperkinesias. The seizures consist of head-dropping spells or generalized loss of consciousness. There is another group of cases which originate in later childhood, between three and six years. These have similar clinical features to the infantile group. In addition there may be hemiplegia as a result of the seizures, choreoathetosis, and cerebellar ataxia. The optic discs are normal. Subsequently rigidity, deafness, blindness, and complete dementia occur.

The spinal fluid is normal, or there may be some increase of protein. The electroencephalogram is abnormal. The pneumoencephalogram shows dilatation of the lateral ventricles due to cortical atrophy.

PATHOLOGY: The pathological changes are essentially as described in the original case of Alpers. There may be cortical atrophy and lack of organization of the architecture of the cortex, indicative of defective development. The gyri are reduced in size and show loss of nerve cells. In addition there is diffuse degeneration of the cerebral gray matter. This includes the cortex especially, but also the striatum, thalamus, pallidum, pons, and cerebellum. However, in some cases only the cortex is involved. There is an accompanying astrocytosis. The degeneration in the cortex is the most constant pathological feature. There is some degeneration of the white matter.

ETIOLOGY: The cause is unknown. Some cases are familial.

DIAGNOSIS: The onset may occur in infancy or childhood. The major features are myoclonias, convulsions, spasticity, ataxia, and hyperkinesias. Later deafness and blindness occur progressing to complete dementia.
Myoclonus epilepsy and a family described by Van Bogaert require differential. Ford feels that the cases of Van Bogaert are closely related to the group described here.

PROGNOSIS: The course is steadily progressive. Ford and his associates reported that the infantile cases die before two and one-half years; the juvenile cases end in death between six and nineteen years of age.

TREATMENT: There is no specific therapy.

Alpers, B.: Diffuse Progressive Degeneration of the Cerebral Gray Matter. Arch. Neurol. and Psychiat. 25:469, 1931.
Christensen, E. and Krabbe, K. H.: Poliodystrophia Cerebri Progressiva Infantilis. Arch. Neurol. and Psychiat. 61:28, 1949.
Ford, F. R., Livingston, S. and Pryles, C. V.: Familial Degeneration of the Cerebral Gray Matter in Childhood. J. Pediat. 39:33, 1951.
Wolf, A. and Cowen, D.: The Cerebral Atrophies and Encephalomalacias of Infancy and Childhood. A. Res. Publ. Ass. Nerv. Ment. Dis. Proc. 34:199, 1954.

CHAPTER 14

POLYNEURITIS (PERIPHERAL OR MULTIPLE NEURITIS OR NEUROPATHY)

Polyneuritis is a multiple involvement of the peripheral nerves resulting in pain, motor weakness, and sensory disturbance. Some specific types are described in this section. Others, for purposes of classification, are described elsewhere in the book.

LANDRY-GUILLAIN-BARRÉ SYNDROME; INFECTIOUS NEURONITIS; POLYRADICULONEURITIS

Originally described as a disease of the peripheral nerves with albuminocytologic dissociation in the spinal fluid, the concept has been enlarged as indicated by the terminology of the title, and the spinal fluid picture is considered incidental.

CLINICAL PICTURE: The onset may occur at any age in both sexes. It is probably the most frequent form of polyneuritis. Under a variety of names, a varied type of symptomatology may develop. In some cases there may first be an acute infection involving the respiratory or gastrointestinal tract. This is followed about a week later by the sudden onset of symmetrical weakness of the lower extremities together with paresthesiae and sensory loss. The muscles are tender. Other segments soon are involved in ascending fashion, including the muscles of the trunk, upper extremities, diaphragm, and cranial nerves, especially the facial. The tendon reflexes are diminished, then lost. There is no Babinski sign or loss of sphincter control.

In others, there may be no prodomata, but the disease develops in an insidious manner progressing for days to weeks. It may begin in any of the peripheral nerves. Both motor and sensory neurons may be involved, or one type may predominate. In some the paralysis ascends the cord; in others it may begin in the cranial nerves and descend. Boshes and Sherman reported four cases, the first of which began as a simple spinal form and gradually developed facial paralysis; the second began with midthoracic cord and root symptoms, then the lower extremities became involved, next the uppers, and finally there was a slight facial; the third was a brain stem type which required a respirator and tracheal suction; the fourth case involved the cranial nuclei.

There is rarely significant fever. Of the cranial nerves, the facial is quite frequently involved. There may also be dysphagia, dysarthria, and aphonia. Malignant hypertension may occur in the severe and fatal types.

There may be flaccid paralysis alone with no sensory findings, in which case the anterior roots are affected. On the other hand, when there is hypesthesia, the posterior roots are correspondingly involved. In some instances papilledema may occur.

The duration of the illness is variable. The very acute cases may die within two weeks with involvement of the respiratory muscles and/or bulbar pathology. The majority show signs of increasing paralysis for the first two weeks; then slow recovery sets in, requiring weeks to several months for completion. In some, relapses occur.

LABORATORY: The major finding is in the spinal fluid, consisting of an elevated protein unaccompanied by an increase in cells. This is referred to as an albuminocytologic dissociation. The protein may be normal, although it is more often elevated.

PATHOLOGY: Changes depend on the individual course in each patient; if the disease progresses rapidly there may be few findings. There is degeneration of the peripheral nerves, which is maximal where the anterior and posterior roots fuse. In the spinal cord there may be chromatolysis of the motor neurons. The cranial nerves are also affected. Inflammatory infiltrations are seen in the liver, kidneys, and adrenals. The increased protein in the spinal fluid is presumed to be due to increased permeability of dilated radicular and spinal meningeal vessels. The clinical picture is probably the result of edema of the nerve roots and trunks with resulting compression.

ETIOLOGY: The clinical picture occurs with a variety of conditions, and there is no known specific etiology. It is thought to be viral by some; this has no confirmation. Infectious neuronitis may complicate measles, chicken pox, or mumps. Others hold that it is due to a toxic effect of the original infection. Finally, some cases have been considered allergic phenomena following smallpox or rabies vaccine injection or serum sickness.

DIFFERENTIAL DIAGNOSIS: The Landry-Guillain-Barré syndrome is essentially a clinical picture of polyneuritis in which any peripheral nerve, spinal root, or cranial nerve may be involved. Of the last, bilateral facial paralysis is most common. The albuminocytologic dissociation in the spinal fluid is incidental since it may also occur in other diseases, and is therefore not diagnostic of Guillain-Barré. In some instances it is not present.

Infectious mononucleosis can be ruled out by the heterophile reaction.

In poliomyelitis there are fever, stiff neck and back suggesting meningeal irritation, increased cell count early in the disease, and asymmetrical paralysis. In the second week there is a high protein, but the history and asymmetrical paralysis should permit a differential.

Diphtheritic polyneuritis may present a problem when the presenting complaint is the polyneuritis. The latter is liable to appear many weeks after the initial attack of diphtheria. A previous diagnosis of diphtheria in the acute stage will make the diagnosis. If this was not noted, involvement of the muscles of accommodation, or a preceding history of regurgitation of fluid through the nose or a nasal twang to the voice (pharyngeal or palatal palsy) will help in the differential.

Acute intermittent porphyria, associated with excessive amounts of type III uroporphyrin and coproporphyrin in the urine, is of rare occurrence in childhood. The characteristic onset of acute abdominal pain, followed by a picture of polyneuritis and psychotic manifestations, suggests the diagnosis. The urine shows pink fluorescence in the Wood's lamp, and the Watson-Schwartz porphobilinogen test is positive.

In the peripheral neuropathy due to lead, there is a history of ingestion and excess lead is present in the blood and urine.

Encephalomyelitis due to other causes, e.g., viral or post-vaccinal (smallpox), can be differentiated by serological tests or a history of vaccination.

PROGNOSIS: Mortality figures around fifteen to twenty per cent have been reported, but until the etiology of each case is known, it will be difficult to place an exact estimate on the outlook in so diffuse a syndrome. Aylett collected ninety-nine cases in the literature with seven deaths.

Death usually is due to paralysis of the muscles of respiration, and in many cases bronchopneumonia has been found at autopsy. After two to three weeks of survival, there is usually slow recovery over many months, with recurrent attacks in some cases. There may remain residual weakness or paralysis of the face or of the muscles of the extremities.

TREATMENT: Cortisone and ACTH have been tried on the assumption that the disease is allergic. The results vary. There appears to be shortening of the length of the illness in some. The occurrence of the syndrome while patients were on cortisone for arthritis does not appear to support an allergic basis. BAL has been used in some cases.

Nonspecific therapy consists essentially of the use of the respirator and tracheal suction or tracheotomy in instances of bulbar involvement or respiratory muscle paralysis. Antibiotic therapy should be used for intercurrent infections.

Polyneuritic residuals are treated with physical and occupational therapy, high vitamin diet, and orthopedic devices in an effort to prevent deformities.

Aylett, P.: Five Cases of Acute Infective Polyneuritis (Guillain-Barré Syndrome) in Children. Arch. Dis. Child. 29:531, 1954.

Boshes, B. and Sherman, J. C.: Variability of the Course of the Guillain-Barré Syndrome. Neurology 3:789, 1953.

Byers, R. K. and Taft, L. T.: Chronic Multiple Peripheral Neuropathy in Childhood. Pediat. 20:517, 1957.

Grant, H. and Leopold, H. N.: Guillain-Barré Syndrome Occurring During Cortisone Therapy. J.A.M.A. 155:1252, 1954.

Haymaker, W. and Kernohan, J. W.: The Landry-Guillain-Barré Syndrome. Medicine 28:59, 1949.

Jackson, R. H., Miller, H. and Schapera, K.: Polyradiculitis Landry-Guillain-Barré Syndrome), Treatment with Cortisone and Corticotropin. Brit. Med. J. 1:480, 1957.

Joynt, R. J.: Mechanism of Production of Papilledema in the Guillain-Barré Syndrome. Neurology 8:8, 1958.

Lysaught, J. N. and McCleery, J. M.: Acute Intermittent Porphyria. J. Pediat. 46:552, 1955.

Reye, R. D. K.: Neuropathology of Landry-Guillain-Barré Syndrome. Med. J. Australia 2:386, 1954.

ARSENIC

Arsenical polyneuritis is rare in children since arsphenamine for syphilis has been abandoned in favor of penicillin and since Fowler's solution is no longer used in chorea. When the drug is swallowed accidentally as in the case of the child who takes a rat poison off the shelf, there are signs of acute poisoning. If the child survives, polyneuritis may follow several weeks later. In the chronic form, where small amounts of arsenic are ingested over a period of time, as may happen with food sprayed with insecticide, the onset is more gradual, with headache, gastrointestinal upset, vomiting, diarrhea, loss of appetite and weight, and anemia. The skin shows pigmentation, keratosis, ridging of the nails, and loss of hair. Edema may be present. Together with these features is evidence of polyneuritis. Sensory symptoms are pronounced, including paresthesias, pain, and hyperesthesia. This is followed by weakness and paralysis of the distal portions of the extremities with resultant foot and wrist drop. There may be complete loss of sensation, wasting of muscles, and loss of deep tendon reflexes. Ataxia occurs in some cases.

PATHOLOGY: The changes are those of polyneuritis in general with degeneration affecting the myelin and axis cylinders.

LABORATORY: Arsenic may be found in the urine, but this is not diagnostic as it may be present in normal persons. It is also present in the hair, nails, and feces.

PROGNOSIS: This is good if the source is removed. Gradual recovery takes place in about a year.

DIAGNOSIS: This is based on a history of ingestion of arsenic, the presence of peripheral polyneuritis, changes in the gastrointestinal tract and skin, and possibly recovery of arsenic chemically from the excreta, nails, or hair.

TREATMENT: Remove the source and inject BAL, 2.5 to 3 mg/kg, intramuscularly, four times a day for the first two days. Then the dose is reduced to twice daily for one or two days and then once a day for a week more. The effect of BAL is noted by an increased arsenic output in the urine. Supportive treatment should be given in the form of good nutrition, vitamins, bed rest, and physical and occupational therapy, the last as function returns.

Longcope, W. T. and Luetscher, J. A.: The Use of BAL (British Anti-Lewisite) in the Treatment of the Injurious Effects of Arsenic, Mercury, and other Metallic Poisons. Ann. Int. Med. 31:545, 1949.

THALLIUM

Thallium may produce toxic symptoms by its presence in rat poisons, which are ingested accidentally by children, or in salves for ringworm. The acute form in which large amounts are absorbed at once may result in death. Of eleven such cases reported by Ginsberg, six died. The major symptoms are in the central nervous system, with lethargy, convulsions, ataxia, and tremors. In the chronic form, polyneuritis and optic neuritis may develop alone or together. There is loss of central vision first, later optic atrophy. The clinical features are those of polyneuritis in general, with paresthesias, pain in the distal portions of the extremities, loss of reflexes, and muscle weakness. There may be convulsions. Associated features include alopecia.

DIAGNOSIS: The diagnosis is made on the history of thallium ingestion or exposure, and the demonstration of thallium in the urine.

PROGNOSIS: In the chronic form recovery is the rule. However, there is usually some remaining loss of vision.

TREATMENT: Remove the source of thallium. Sodium thiosulfate, BAL, cortisone, and versenate are not effective. Chamberlain and his associates report the beneficial use of oral dithizone with glucose, 10 mg/kg twice daily. Of ten cases with nervous system involvement, two died; one of those who recovered was decerebrate.

Chamberlain, P. H., Stravinoha, W. B., Davis, H., Knicker, T. and Panos, T. C. Thallotoxicosis: Neurologic Manifestations and Methods of Treatment. A.M.A. J. Dis. Child. 94:489, 1957.
Committee on Pesticides—Council on Drugs of A.M.A. Thallotoxicosis—A Recurring Problem. J.A.M.A. 165:1266, 1957.
Ginsberg, H. M. and Nixon, C. E.: Thallium Poisoning. A Preliminary Report of 11 Cases. J.A.M.A. 98:1076, 1932.

DIPHTHERIA

Polyneuritis occurs in diphtheria from the effect of the toxin elaborated by the Corynebacterium diphtheriae (Klebs-Loeffler bacillus), which has a strong affinity for the peripheral nerves.

CLINICAL PICTURE: The incidence of neuritis as a complication in diphtheria is listed at about fifteen per cent. Generally, the frequency of involvement and the degree depend upon the severity of the diphtheritic attack and the length of time which has elapsed prior to the administration of antitoxin. Occasionally the illness is so mild that the family considered the child to have had a simple cold. A few weeks later, however, paralysis is observed. It is this latter type in which differential diagnosis may be difficult.

Usually the first manifestation is involvement of the soft palate. This occurs toward the end of the first week. There are regurgitation of fluids through the nose and a nasal tone to the voice. Either accompanying the palatal palsy or shortly thereafter, paralysis of accommodation occurs due to involvement of the ciliary muscle. There is difficulty in reading when the book is held close because vision is blurred. Spread to other cranial nerves occurs, resulting in pharyngeal palsy, dilatation of the pupils, strabismus, and facial palsy. After the third or fourth week following the cranial nerve palsies, signs of polyneuritis appear. These are evident in the extremities. The changes include loss of vibratory, joint, and stereognostic senses. To a lesser degree there are also loss of touch, pain, and temperature. The motor phenomena include muscle weakness, hypoactive to absent deep tendon and abdominal reflexes, and in some, muscular incoordination. Foot and wrist drop may occur. In other instances there is weakness of the muscles of the neck with head drop. The most severe type includes paralysis of the phrenic nerve, with dyspnoea and thoracic breathing.

After paralysis occurs, the peak is reached in one or two weeks and then slow improvement sets in which may take months. In most of the children there is full recovery, but in some there may remain atrophy of some of the muscles.

LABORATORY: The spinal fluid is negative except for the marked increase in protein, which together with absence of cells is similar to some cases of the Landry-Guillain-Barré type.

PATHOLOGY: There is degeneration of the myelin sheath and axones of the peripheral nerves. The motor cells of the cord and brain stem may show chromatolysis.

DIAGNOSIS: The recognition of diphtheritic polyneuritis is dependent upon evidence of diphtheria in the acute stage of the disease. When this has been mild and missed, so that the presenting picture is that of a child with peripheral neuritis, the examiner may elicit a previous history of palatal or ciliary muscle palsy. We have discussed under Landry-Guillaine-Barré the differential from diphtheritic polyneuritis. In the latter there are a positive smear and culture for the diphtheria bacillus and an orderly spread to the palate, ciliary muscles, and finally peripheral nerves. Hence, there is a longer interval of several weeks before the onset of peripheral neuritis in diphtheria as compared to Guillain-Barré.

PROGNOSIS: The outlook is good except for the bulbar type.

TREATMENT: Recovery from the peripheral neuritis will be aided by rest. Later physical and occupational therapy should be offered.

Gammon, G. D.: The Effects of Bacterial Toxins on the Nervous System. A. Res. Publ. Ass. Nerv. Ment. Dis. Proc. 32:506, 1953.
Hertz, M. and Thygesen, P.: Nervous Complications in Diphtheria. Acta Medica Scandinav. (Suppl. 206), 541, 1948.
Perkins, R. F. and Laufer, M. W.: A Clinical Study of Postdiphtheritic Polyneuritis. J. Nerv. & Ment. Dis. 104:59, 1946.

DIABETES

CLINICAL PICTURE: The onset of diabetic neuropathy usually does not occur before the tenth year in juvenile diabetes. Generally it takes from five to fifteen years after the onset of diabetes for neuropathy to develop. White has reported that in 702 cases of juvenile diabetes where there was survival of at least twenty years, there were 96 cases of diabetic neuropathy or fourteen per cent.

The clinical features of the neuropathy include sensory and motor manifestations. There are cramps, aching, and tenderness of the muscles. Numbness, tingling, and paresthesiae are also present. The motor features include muscle weakness, especially of the lower extremities, with diminished or lost tendon reflexes. Other lesions include loss of the light reflex with retention of accommodation (Argyll-Robertson pupil) and a paralytic bladder with urinary retention.

Sullivan describes two distinct forms of diabetic neuropathy. One form is a symmetric, distal neuropathy, predominantly sensory, occurring in diabetes which is either uncontrolled or of long duration. The second is an asymmetric, predominantly motor neuropathy which tends toward spontaneous recovery.

LABORATORY: The blood and urine are consistent with diabetes. The spinal fluid shows an increased protein content.

DIAGNOSIS: This depends on demonstrating neuropathy together with the clinical and laboratory signs of diabetes. Other causes of polyneuritis must be differentiated, also tabes dorsalis in which there is a positive spinal fluid Wassermann.

PROGNOSIS: The onset of polyneuritis often follows bouts of uncontrolled diabetes. However, White has pointed out that resumption of control and large amounts of Vitamin B complex have not resulted in rapid recovery. There does, however, appear to be some gradual improvement.

TREATMENT: The diabetes should be controlled. BAL and ACTH have been tried for the neuropathy; also B12, pregnant mammalian liver extract, and adenosine triphosphate with thiamine. The results have not been successful.

Joslin, E. P., Root, H. F., White, P., Marble, A.: Treatment of Diabetes. Chapter on Diabetic Children and Their Later Lives. Philadelphia, Lea and Febiger, 9th ed., 1952.

Rundles, R. W.: Diabetic Neuropathy, General Review with Report of 125 Cases. Medicine 24:111, 1945.

Shuman, C. R. and Gilpin, S. F.: Diabetic Neuropathy. Am. J. M. Sc. 227:612, 1954.

Sullivan, J. F.: The neuropathies of diabetes. Neurology 8:243, 1958.

REACTION OF THE NERVOUS SYSTEM TO INOCULATION OF SERA, VACCINES, DRUGS, AND ANTIBIOTICS

A clinical picture of neuritis, polyneuritis, or cerebral or meningeal irritation may develop following injection procedures in children. This has occurred following injection of sera, such as tetanus or diphtheritic antitoxin, scarlet streptococcic antiserum, and human antipoliomyelitis serum. It has also occurred after immunization against pertussis, rabies, and the typhoid-paratyphoid group and following injection of antibiotics, such as penicillin.

SERA (TETANUS OR DIPHTHERIA ANTITOXIN)

When serum is administered, especially horse serum, the patient may develop signs of serum sickness, usually about seven to ten days following the injection. A wheal is noted at the site, which is followed by a general urticarial eruption, intense itching, fever, angioneurotic edema with swelling of the face and extremities, enlarged, tender lymph nodes, and joint pains and swelling. At the height of the reaction or following the manifestations of serum sickness, neurological complications may develop. Miller and Stanton have divided their cases into four clinical types:

		No. of Cases
a)	Radiculitis (including brachial plexitis)	59
b)	Polyneuritis and Polyradiculoneuritis (Guillain-Barré)	10
c)	Myelitis and Landry's ascending paralysis	6
d)	Meningeal and cerebral forms	10

Irrespective of where the injection is given, the brachial plexus is most frequently involved. The onset is marked by severe stabbing pain across the shoulders, radiating down the arms and along the course of the affected nerve trunks, which are tender. In two or three days weakness and flaccid paralysis appear, followed rapidly by loss of the tendon reflexes, diminished response to electrical stimulation, wasting, and perhaps a reaction of degeneration. The muscles supplied by the 5th and 6th cervical segments of the spinal cord are particularly involved (Erb-Duchenne palsy), including the biceps, pectoralis major, infraspinatus, deltoid, and rhomboid. With polyneuritis there are pain, weakness, diminished deep tendon reflexes, paresthesias, and loss of sensation. The spinal fluid may show albuminocytologic dissociation (Guillain-Barré).

Other reactions include evidence of myelitis, with paralysis developing in an ascending manner (Landry's). Finally, there are severe instances in which marked focal cerebral and meningeal manifestations are present, including seizures, hemiplegia, and signs of increased intracranial pressure. The spinal fluid contains some increase of cells, but the chemistry is essentially normal.

PATHOLOGY: There appears to be some congestion in the brain, spinal cord, and meninges. Edema and small areas of hemorrhage have been reported, and occasionally some necrosis.

PROGNOSIS: Recovery occurs in most instances. In some, damage to the nervous system may remain evident for years. The worst outlook is in the cerebral and myelitic types.

TREATMENT: The ideal situation would have all individuals immunized with diphtheria and tetanus toxoid. This would eliminate the need for antitoxin, which contains horse serum. Exposure would mean booster doses of the toxoid, which is almost entirely free from severe reaction. However, if antitoxin must be used, tests should be done to see whether sensitivity exists. Inject intradermally 0.1 cc of 1:100 horse serum (diluted with physiological saline solution) or use the ophthalmic reaction, one drop of a 1:10 solution. In any event, adrenalin 1:1000 sol. should be available at the time the skin test is performed and used for treatment if a reaction occurs. If there is a positive test or a history of allergy and the antitoxin must be administered, it should be given by a series of small doses. If polyneuritis does occur, cortisone should be given along with the usual treatment, including rest. Later, massage, physical and occupational therapy, and orthopedic devices to avoid deformity until healing occurs, should be utilized.

VACCINES

Typhoid-Paratyphoid Vaccine. The neurological sequelae occur most often after the second injection, rather than the first, according to Miller and Stanton. In their 50 cases they noted plexitis and mononeuritis in twelve, polyneuritis in eight (three of the Landry-Guillain-Barré type), nine cases of ascending Landry's paralysis, one of myelitis, and fifteen with cerebral, and five with meningeal manifestations. In these cases there are not likely to be allergic features such as "serum sickness" preceding the neurological sequelae. Cortisone may be tried in this group.

Tetanus or Diphtheria Toxoid. Meningeal reactions following injections of tetanus or diphtheria toxoid are extremely rare.

Pertussis. Reaction of the nervous system following pertussis immunization manifests itself as a cerebral form, rather than spinal or peripheral. The onset may follow the 1st, 2nd, or 3rd injection, within a few minutes to days following the procedure. The usual picture is one of convulsions, but there may be somnolence followed by paralysis. The spinal fluid may show increased numbers of cells and an elevated protein, or may be normal.

When death occurs, the brain is soft and edematous with some areas of perivascular demyelinization.

The reaction has often occurred in those who seem to have a constitutional predisposition and in whose families a high incidence of abnormalities has been noted. There is a preponderance of males.

PROGNOSIS: Residual damage in the central nervous system is present in most of the children who recover. The pneumoencephalogram may show ventricular dilatation with cortical atrophy. The children are paralyzed, blind in some instances, function at a lowered mental level, and have recurrent seizures. Their behavior is similar to that of the brain injured child.

TREATMENT: The aim in therapy should be prevention of the "cerebral reaction." The possibility of the latter can be lessened by immunizing around the third month of infancy. It should be part of the procedure to question mothers after the first injection as to any undue rise of temperature or other constitutional symptoms. Aspirin gr. ½ should be given orally following an injection to minimize the reaction. If a seizure or somnolence occurs after the first injection, discontinue further injections for several months; then diphtheria-tetanus toxoid alone may be given in smaller doses (4-6 injections). Pertussis injections may subsequently be tried separately, also in smaller doses, or omitted entirely.

Rabies Vaccine. Antirabies vaccine injection is followed by neurological sequelae ten to fifteen days after therapy is begun. These are primarily polyneuritic and myelitic and to a lesser extent cerebral. The prognosis is good except in the ascending Landry form. (See the chapter on rabies.)

In all the forms previously discussed there is a suggestion of constitutional idiosyncrasy or anaphylactic hypersensitivity.

We have omitted reference to the occurrences of paralytic poliomyelitis following injection with DPT in the summertime and of encephalomyelitis following vaccination against smallpox as these problems have been discussed in the sections on poliomyelitis and post-vaccinal encephalomyelitis.

Brody, M.: Neurologic Complications Following the Administration of Pertussis Vaccine. Bklyn. Hosp. J. 5:107, 1947.

Byers, R. K. and Moll, F. C.: Encephalopathies Following Prophylactic Pertussis Vaccine. Pediat. 1:437, 1948.

Miller, H. G. and Stanton, J. B. Neurological Sequelae of Prophylactic Inoculation. Quart. J. Med. 23:1, 1954.

Park, A. M. and Richardson, J. C.: Cerebral Complications of Serum Sickness. Neurology 3:277, 1953.

Smith, H. and Smith, Jr., H.: Dramatic Response to Cortisone Therapy in a Case of Serum Neuritis. J.A.M.A. 157:906, 1955.
To The Editor: Queries and Minor Notes. Serum Neuritis Following Tetanus Immunization. J.A.M.A. 161:297, 1956.

DRUGS

Isoniazid, used in the treatment of tuberculosis, may produce a polyneuritis. The symptoms are predominantly sensory and usually symmetrical. Paresthesiae, hyperalgesia in the soles of the feet, impairment of postural sensibility, and loss of vibratory sense may occur. The lower limbs, especially the distal parts, are usually affected with weakness and paresis. Optic neuritis resulting in atrophy has been reported. The onset may be noted about two months after the start of drug therapy.

The toxic neuritis appears to be related to an alteration in the metabolism of pyridoxine. There is marked loss of pyridoxine in the urine when patients are put on isoniazid therapy. Particularly in adults and in those children with long continued isoniazid therapy, pyridoxine, 1-2 mg. daily, should be given to minimize the possibility of neurotoxic effects. When symptoms have already occurred, the isoniazid should be stopped and pyridoxine together with the entire B-complex group should be administered.

In adults, phenobarbital has been taken in large doses for suicide, with coma and occasional death resulting. The use of the drug in childhood for epilepsy and as a sedative for hypertonic infants is usually free of toxic effects on the central nervous system. The danger from other anticonvulsive drugs such as the hydantoins is discussed under Epilepsy. The effects of alcohol, carbon monoxide, and carbon tetrachloride poisoning are essentially problems of adult neurology.

ANTIBIOTICS

Peripheral neuritis has been observed following the injection of penicillin and streptomycin. In some children injected repeatedly in the gluteal musculature there followed lack of movement of the extremity on the same side, atrophy of the leg muscles, and loss of reflex action and sensation; in other words, peripheral neuritis of the sciatic nerve. Faradic stimulation to the nerve produced no response. In other instances, the axillary and suprascapular nerves may be affected following use of the deltoid muscles for injection. The problem of neuritis following injection is especially prevalent in the premature.

PATHOLOGY: There are two theories as to the cause. One is traumatic, the other toxic. In the former there is direct injury by the needle; in the latter, undue concentration of the chemical agent at the site.

TREATMENT: Injections should be avoided when possible, especially in young and malnourished infants and in prematures who have poorly developed gluteal musculature. If neuritis is present, use physical therapy. If there is no improvement, surgical neurolysis may be needed. Scheinberg and Allensworth suggest conservative therapy for a year; Matson allows a much shorter period before undertaking neurolysis.

PROGNOSIS: The outlook for recovery is variable.

Höök, O.: Polyneuritis Caused by Hydrazide of Isonicotinic Acid. Acta Med. Scandinav. 147:167, 1953.

Jones, W. A. and Jones, G. P.: Peripheral Neuropathy Due to Isoniazid. Lancet 1:1073, 1953.

Kass, I., Mandel, W., Cohen, H. and Dressler, S. H.: Isoniazid as a Cause of Optic Neuritis and Atrophy. J.A.M.A. 164:1740, 1957.

Matson, D. D.: Early Neurolysis in the Treatment of Injury of the Peripheral Nerves Due to Faulty Injection of Antibiotics. New England J. Med. 242:973, 1950.

Scheinberg, L. and Allensworth, M.: Sciatic Neuropathy in Infants Related to Antibiotic Injections. Pediat. 19:261, 1957.

NEUROPATHY OF THE FACIAL NERVE (BELL'S PALSY)

Paralysis or neuropathy of the facial nerve is often referred to as Bell's Palsy after Sir Charles Bell, the Scottish physiologist who described the course and motor function of the facial nerve and presented cases with facial paralysis.

CLINICAL PICTURE: Facial paralysis may be observed without any previous symptomatology, coming on either suddenly or gradually. In other instances there is preceding pain in the area of the ear and cheek. Only one side of the face is usually involved. The corner of the mouth droops on the affected side. The skin of the forehead and cheek is smooth, with loss of the nasolabial groove. The ability to perform voluntary movements is impaired so that the child cannot whistle, smile, or speak properly. There is constant drooling of saliva. The eye cannot be closed, and hence tears overflow. The upper lid droops; the lower lid is everted. There is no corneal reflex. The child cannot wrinkle his forehead or retract the corner of his mouth. Other features depend on the location of the pathology. If the lesion is between the geniculate ganglion and the nerve to the stapedius, there are loss of taste on the anterior two-thirds of the tongue and hyperacusis. If the lesion is between the pons and the internal auditory meatus or in the canal above the geniculate ganglion, there is no lacrimation or taste, and hyperacusis is present. If the lesion is supranuclear, the muscles of the lower face are particularly affected, and there are also pyramidal tract signs. Voluntary movements of the upper face and emotional movements such as laughing or crying are normal. If the nucleus of the facial nerve is the site of pathology, voluntary and emotional movements of the entire face are lost, taste is retained, and hyperacusis is absent. The sixth nerve may be involved. A reaction of degeneration may occur about two weeks after the onset, indicating a lesion of the lower motor neuron.

ETIOLOGY: The cause of Bell's Palsy in children is not clear. In the majority it is idiopathic. It has followed local chilling, such as sitting near an open window. In these, vasospasm and ischemia of the nerve sheath may occur, followed by vasodilatation with edema and pressure on the nerve. Otitis has been incriminated because of the close relationship of the nerve to the middle ear, but actually the association is rare. Furthermore, the ear in most cases of Bell's Palsy is normal. Other rarer causes are trauma, osteomyelitis of the skull, infections such as diphtheria, mumps, and perhaps herpes zoster, and tumors. It may also be associated with edema of the lip or face (Melkersson's syndrome). For a complete discussion of the etiology of facial paralysis in children refer to the article by Paine. He concludes that it is usually due to a neuritis, either toxic, ischemic, or edematous.

DIAGNOSIS: Observation of the child reveals the picture of complete paralysis of the facial nerve. In the differential, supranuclear lesions must be ruled out. In true Bell's palsy the attack is mild and the cause usually obscure. One should check the ear and mastoid and eliminate tumor of the pons, local lymphadenitis, poliomyelitis, polyneuritis, and tuberculosis.

PROGNOSIS: In general, the outlook is favorable in children, with reports of 90 per cent recovery. If after eighteen days there is no electrical reaction of degeneration, recovery will be complete in about four weeks. If there is a reaction of degeneration and complete paralysis, recovery will be slow and may be incomplete. There may be manifestations of misdirected regrowth in which nerve fibres go to muscles other than those which they originally supplied. This results in tics or "crocodile tears," that is, food in the mouth is followed by lacrimation rather than salivation.

TREATMENT: In the acute stage, heat in any form to produce vasodilatation and thus avoid nerve compression and analgesics for pain are very useful. The eye should be rinsed twice daily with isotonic sodium chloride, and at night a drop of mineral oil should be placed in it to avoid dryness. A patch should be placed over the eye if the child goes outdoors. Adhesive may be placed from the corner of the mouth to the front of the ear to support the sagging muscles.

Cortisone appears to speed recovery; 75 to 150 mg. daily should be given for a week or two. Electrical stimulation by galvanic current and exercise before a mirror should be used as adjuncts. If there is no recovery within two months, surgical decompression of the diseased nerve should be considered. Nerve grafts and plastic surgery may be used later for cosmetic effects.

Jongkees, L. B. W.: Treatment of Bell's Palsy. Neurology 7:697, 1957.
Keeler, K. C.: Conservative Therapy in Peripheral Nerve Dysfunction. J.A.M.A. 162:1596, 1956.
Paine, R. S.: Facial Paralysis in Children. Review of the Differential Diagnosis and Report of Ten Cases Treated with Cortisone. Pediat. 19:303, 1957.

CHAPTER 15

POST-NATAL TRAUMA

CRANIAL

Trauma to the head is quite common in infancy and childhood. In infancy it usually is the result of a fall from a table or crib. In childhood, the usual types of adult etiology are found, such as falls, automobile accidents, and blows on the head. There are some variations in the response of the infant and child to trauma as compared to the adult because the bones are softer and there are suture lines which may give. Since the infant brain must expand and grow, there is great danger in unevacuated collections of blood from the standpoint of future mental development. Children generally react to injury quite well. However, when there is a preceding pathological state like hydrocephalus in equilibrium or nonsymptomatic tumor, injury precipitates new and greater symptomatology.

CLINICAL PICTURE: In the case of infants the injury usually occurs in the home from a fall. The infant is likely to be stunned momentarily and then recover consciousness. The baby will cry for an interval, appear pale, may vomit, and then becomes quiet. When the injury is mild, this period will soon be followed by normal lively behavior; at other times, the baby will desire sleep.

In all instances the baby should be examined not only for evidence of brain injury, but also for trauma to other organs. The spine and extremities should also be checked for evidence of fracture with accompanying spinal cord or peripheral nerve damage.

If all seems in order, the infant may be left at home and the mother instructed to check the child's color and breathing while asleep. He should be awakened once or twice to be sure he is not unconscious. In other instances, although the infant has recovered from his momentary period of stupor immediately after the fall and has appeared lucid and active, if he should return to a drowsy state and become pale again, there is very likely epidural or other hemorrhage with much blood loss, and the baby should be hospitalized. Other serious signs to be looked for are recurrent vomiting, seizures, pupillary inequalities, and weakness of the extremities. Any such changes should call for entrance to the hospital.

In the older child the injury is likely to be due to an automobile, a fall from a horse or fence, or a baseball or bat. These children are usually brought to the hospital directly, often with a compound skull fracture. The child should first be looked over generally to determine the degree of consciousness. If there is a cold, clammy skin and low blood pressure, the child may be in shock.

Frequent observations should be made with respect to changes in blood pressure, pulse, temperature, respiration, and general orientation. The reflexes are often hyperactive, and a Babinski sign may be present. The extremities are weak, show paresis, and may be spastic. The pupils may show irregularity. When there is dilatation of the pupil on one side, it suggests brain hemorrhage on the same side or possible temporal lobe herniation with midbrain and oculomotor nerve compression.

Many children make a dramatic recovery after appearing desperately ill immediately following the injury. Others following their injury have a period of temporary loss of consciousness, then a lucid or clear state, which in turn is followed by drowsiness, hyperreflexia, a Babinski sign, and pupillary inequality, which together suggest intracranial pathology. Often, however, after a period of about an hour, the child may suddenly recover consciousness and be well even though the neurological signs remain for a time. If drowsiness does not disappear, however, surgery should be performed for intracranial hemorrhage.

Fractures of the skull may be associated with cranial nerve palsies and blood or spinal fluid leakage. Hemorrhage into the orbit may occur with fracture of the sphenoid or base of the frontal bone; blindness may follow. Bleeding may occur into the nose or through the middle ear. Leakage of cerebrospinal fluid may occur similarly through the nose or ear with the development of pneumocephaly. This can be recognized by roentgenography showing air within the cranium. In these, there is usually fracture of the base. These fractures should all be treated with antibiotics and chemotherapy.

LABORATORY: X-ray will outline any fracture. Lumbar puncture may show bloody spinal fluid and increased pressure.

TREATMENT:

Cerebral Concussion. The child is unconscious following the injury, but there is no permanent damage to the brain. Prompt recovery is the rule. Only supportive treatment is required.

Fractures of the Skull. Linear fractures are demonstrated by X-ray as simple line cracks. They need no therapy and heal spontaneously. Depressed fractures of the vault are of significance if they lacerate brain tissue or blood vessels producing a hematoma. Under these circumstances elevation of the bone should be performed.

Compound Fracture. These should be completely debrided. When the fragments of bone have been removed and the dura closed, antibiotics should be given to prevent brain abscess and meningitis.

We have discussed the clinical pictures in craniocerebral injury as it may occur in closed head injury and where fracture is present. One of the major complications of either type is intracranial hemorrhage. This may be extradural, subdural, subarachnoid, or intracerebral.

Extradural Hemorrhage. This may result from a tear of the middle meningeal artery or in infancy from rupture of one of the dural sinuses or neighboring veins. The clinical picture has been described at the beginning of the chapter; it includes evidence of the original injury to the skull, deepening loss of consciousness, occasionally as in adults after a lucid interval, and neurological findings of contralateral hemiplegia, pupillary dilatation on the same side as the hematoma or irregular pupils, hyperactive reflexes, a Babinski sign, and occasionally seizures. When there is bleeding loss, signs of shock may supervene. X-ray may show a fracture line in the path of the middle meningeal artery. Ingraham and Matson point out that in their series extradural hemorrhage also occurred with diastasis of the lambdoid or squamosal suture, with or without fracture. The treatment is immediate surgery to remove clots and stop bleeding.

Subdural Hemorrhage. This occurs primarily in infancy, occasionally in later childhood. In contradistinction to extradural hematoma, the subdural is likely to develop more slowly due to oozing from the veins entering the superior longitudinal sinus. There is also the factor of associated intracerebral damage. Therefore, a longer period of time usually elapses before headache, vomiting, and drowsiness develop and surgery is required.

In some instances, instead of a hematoma there may be a subdural hygroma, that is, a collection of cerebrospinal fluid due to a rent in the arachnoid which permits the fluid to penetrate into the subdural space. This fluid is evacuated by puncture. Rarely surgery may be necessary if the fluid recurs. In other instances the rent includes the dura, allowing spinal fluid to lie under the scalp. In this event the X-ray shows an even density. The fluid is usually absorbed.

Subarachnoid Hemorrhage. Hemorrhage into the subarachnoid space may produce symptoms of an irritative meningitis, and the child may appear quite ill. The bleeding occurs because of lacerations of the brain surface. The symptoms include headache, vomiting, stiff neck, high fever, Kernig's sign, and lethargy. Lumbar puncture reveals bloody spinal fluid, which completes the diagnosis. The treatment is lumbar puncture, repeated as needed, to remove the bloody spinal fluid.

Intracerebral Hemorrhage. Hemorrhage into the brain tissue may occur with any type of trauma; it may accompany subdural and extradural hemorrhage. There may be focal symptoms and signs, including cranial nerve palsies and contralateral hemiplegia. Because of subsequent cortical scarring, seizures may occur. As with any of the pathological types of trauma, mental and behavioral changes may follow. This problem is discussed under epilepsy.

PROGNOSIS: In general the outcome is good. Children with concussion or simple fracture usually recover completely. The subdural hematoma of infancy responds satisfactorily provided it is recognized and treated early. Today this is usually the case. In the complicated fractures and the various forms of hemorrhage, extradural, subdural, subarachnoid, and intracerebral, the outlook depends upon the amount of damage and the treatment. In some cases, cranial nerve palsies, hemiplegia, or seizures persist, or there is alteration of behavior. (See the section on the brain injured child.)

TREATMENT: This has been discussed under each type. In general it involves early recognition of the extent and type of craniocerebral pathology and repeated and careful observation for changes in the child's condition, which are liable to be frequent and rapid. The management of the child includes:

a. General examination for the extent of the craniocerebral injury and involvement of other areas.

b. Maintenance of the airway with suction of secretions and tracheotomy, if needed; also oxygen.

c. Correction of shock, using blood plasma and i.v. saline or glucose.

d. For increased intracranial pressure:
   1. Lumbar puncture—drain off spinal fluid slowly.
   2. Intravenous hypertonic glucose or sucrose 50%—25-50 cc. periodically as indicated, or 30% urea solution. (See White.)

e. For subarachnoid hemorrhage: lumbar puncture may be used to drain off bloody fluid if there is persistent headache, unexplained fever, or severe neck rigidity.

f. For extreme restlessness phenobarbital or paraldehyde may be used.

g. For convulsions use phenobarbital and Dilantin sodium®.

h. Antibiotics should be given to prevent infections.

i. Artificial hibernation has been used when the foci of the injuries were not accessible.

Brock, S. (Editor). Injuries of the Brain and Spinal Cord and Their Coverings. Baltimore, Williams and Wilkins, 1949.

Browder, E. J. and Cook, A. W.: Indications for Surgical Intervention in Head Injuries. Surg. Clin. N. A. Philadelphia, W. B. Saunders, 1955, p. 577.

Foreign Letters: Hibernation for Cranial Injuries.: J.A.M.A. 167:1658, 1958.

Harris, P.: Head Injuries in Childhood. Arch. Dis. Child. 32:488, 1957.

Ingraham, F. D., Campbell, J. B. and Cohen, J.: Extradural Hematoma in Infancy and Childhood. J.A.M.A. 140:1010, 1949.

——— and Matson, D. D.: Neurosurgery of Infancy and Childhood. Springfield, Ill., Chas. C. Thomas, 1954.

White, J. C.: Care of the Severely Injured Patient—Neurosurgical Injuries. J.A.M.A. 165:1924, 1957.

SPINAL COLUMN (CORD)

Injury to the spinal cord occurs in children usually as a result of indirect violence. The force is directed toward the vertebral column and spinal cord as the result of a fall or trauma directly to the head, buttocks, or legs. It is most often associated with a fracture or dislocation of the spine, which is of the closed type.

Fracture-Dislocation. The cervical spine is the region of greatest mobility and hence is predisposed to the forward dislocation of the upper cervical vertebrae on the lower, accompanied by fracture. This occurs especially in C5, C6, and C7, often in auto accidents, where the weight of the head pushes the upper vertebrae forward on the lower.

Compression Fracture. This occurs most often in T12 and LI because the other thoracic vertebrae receive greater support and the other lumbar vertebrae are of greater strength and size. It may be accompanied by acute angulations of the spinal column and cord which result in hemorrhage into the gray matter of the cord (hematomyelia).
Compression of the cord may also be caused by bone fragments from the vertebrae or very rarely by a spinal epidural hematoma with or without fracture of the vertebral column.

Concussion of the Cord. This may be due to edema with temporary dysfunction of the cord.
In most cases the spine is acutely flexed following injury but occasionally it may be hyperextended. This is important in management. Finally, the cord may be injured without any evidence of bone fracture or dislocation. It is postulated that in these cases hyperextension of the neck causes cervical cord damage. Compound fractures rarely occur in children.

CLINICAL PICTURE: Fracture or cord damage in the region of C5 and C6 may produce flaccid paralysis of all extremities, sensory loss below the level of trauma, loss of tendon reflexes, and bladder retention. With injury to the lumbar spine there are loss of power in the legs, bladder retention, and sensory loss below the level of injury. These are the common types. If damage is in the thoracic area, there may be good function of the arms, but spastic paraplegia of the lower extremities may be present. In all these instances sensori-motor loss may be partial or complete.

LABORATORY: X-rays should be taken of the entire spine. Lumbar puncture with jugular compression (Queckenstedt) may be performed when there is complete sensori-motor loss to determine the presence of spinal fluid block. This level can be outlined with myelography. If block is present, the question of laminectomy arises.

MANAGEMENT: Spinal injury is suspected when there is a history of an accident, blow, or fall. Movements such as sitting up or walking should be forbidden in order to avoid increasing any deformity which might intensify pressure on the cord. The child should be placed on a stretcher and left on his back, with a pillow or blanket under the shoulders, allowing the head to remain in a neutral position.

Examination may show a deformity or tender areas along the spine. It should be determined if other organs are injured. If in shock, the child should receive blood and other fluids.

The surgical treatment of the various types of fractures of the spine and the indications for laminectomy are to be found in the articles by Scarff, Tarlov, and Cooper. The references of Talbot and Covalt discuss care of the bladder and rehabilitation.

PROGNOSIS: This depends on the degree of cord involvement. If there is complete transection, there will be no return of useful function. In partial cord injury there are good prospects for rehabilitation.

Cooper, I. S.: Neurosurgical Aspects of Treatment for Patients with Spinal Cord Injuries. J.A.M.A. 162:1205, 1956.

Covalt, D. A.: Rehabilitation of the Paraplegic Patient. J.A.M.A. 162:1208, 1956.

Ingraham, F. D. and Matson, D. D.: Injuries to the Spinal Cord, Neurosurgery of Infancy and Childhood. Springfield, Ill., Chas. C. Thomas. 1954, p. 201.

Maxwell, G. M. and Puletti, F.: Chronic Spinal Epidermal Hematoma in a Child. Neurology 7:596, 1957.

Scarff, J. E.: Injuries of the Brain and Spinal Cord and Their Coverings. Baltimore, Williams and Wilkins, 1949, p. 510.

Talbot, H. S.: Primary Care of the Urinary Tract in Spinal Cord Injury. J.A.M.A. 162:1203, 1956.

Tarlov, I. M.: Spinal Cord Injuries—Early Treatment. Surg. Clin. N.A. Philadelphia, W. B. Saunders Co., 1955, p. 591.

PERIPHERAL NERVES

Injuries to the peripheral nerves occasionally occur in children. They are often caused by bone fractures. A number of cases involving the sciatic nerve have been reported following injections into the buttocks, especially in prematures. In a few cases improper casts have been the agent because of pressure on the nerve. In a report on supracondylar fractures of the humerus in children, Lipscomb and Burleson found that 24 of 108 cases had neurological and vascular complications.

The clinical picture will depend on the nerve involved, e.g., the radial in fractures of the humerus, the median in cuts of the wrist or dislocation of the shoulder, and the ulnar in fractures of the elbow. In each instance the particular nerve can be determined by noting the sensory and motor disturbance.

TREATMENT: The neurosurgeon must decide whether surgery is indicated, including neurolysis or suturing of nerve ends. In other instances splinting followed by rehabilitation measures is used.

Lipscomb, P. R. and Burleson, R. J.: Vascular and Neural Complications in Supracondylar Fractures of the Humerus in Children. J. Bone and Joint Surg. 37A:487, 1955.

TETANUS

ETIOLOGY: Tetanus is caused by Clostridium tetani, a gram-positive, anaerobic, spore-bearing organism, which is found primarily in the soil and in the intestinal tract of herbivorous animals. The organism produces a soluble exotoxin which causes spasm of the muscles. The portal of entry is usually a puncture wound of the skin, a compound fracture, or a wound from fireworks. In the past, contamination of the umbilicus of the newborn produced tetanus, but this is rare today. Smallpox vaccination wounds have at times also been secondarily contaminated with this organism; this is now also unusual.

PATHOGENESIS: There are two theories as to the mode of action of the toxin: one, that spread is by way of the lymphatics to the blood stream and thence to the nervous system; the second is that the toxin traverses the axis cylinders of the nerves to reach the spinal cord and brain stem. After the toxin is combined with the nerve tissue, it cannot be detached. Hence, antitoxin is successful only against free-circulating toxin.

PATHOLOGY: No specific changes in the central or peripheral nervous systems are seen.

CLINICAL PICTURE: The incubation period is usually eight to twelve days, but symptomatology may begin as early as one day or as late as three weeks or more. The onset is insidious with increasing stiffness of the jaw and neck. Ultimately, the jaw cannot be opened (lock-jaw). Rigidity is noted in other muscles so that there are difficulty in swallowing, spasm of the facial muscles producing a fixed expression (risus sardonicus), and spasm of the back muscles resulting in an opisthotonic position. There are general restlessness and irritability, and usually little or no fever. Clonic convulsions may occur; these may be easily precipitated by loud noises or handling of the child. A series of tonic spasms soon follows with intervening periods of relaxation. They consist of extreme bodily rigidity, tightened, fixed jaws (trismus), and clenched fists. When the respiratory and laryngeal muscles are affected, there are marked cyanosis and asphyxia. Consciousness is retained, and the child is obviously apprehensive. There is urinary retention. In time, the intervening periods of relaxation become shorter and less frequent, so that there is severe pain from the almost continuous spasm. In a number of children fractures of the spine occur.

In the newborn infected via the cut end of the cord, the onset of symptoms occurs about a week after birth. Convulsions are noted. The baby is seen to twitch and go into spasms with feeding or with any noise. The spasms are similar to those previously described, with rigidity, opisthotonos, and trismus.

LABORATORY: The cerebrospinal fluid and urine are normal. The blood shows a moderate leukocytosis.

DIAGNOSIS: The diagnosis is based on a history of injury resulting in a penetrating wound or compound fracture, the characteristic early onset of trismus, and the facial spasms and general muscle rigidity. Strychnine poisoning rarely involves the jaw muscles, and periods of complete relaxation are present between spasms. In tetanus there is never complete relaxation, and as the disease progresses the intervening periods between spasms diminish so that eventually there is continuous spasm. In the newborn, tetany is eliminated by the normal blood calcium. In birth trauma there is a history of difficult delivery, the clinical appearance of the baby is somewhat different, and convulsions are not initiated by loud noises, etc. Meningitis and encephalitis have their characteristic spinal fluid pictures. In rabies, there are the history of a bite, general mania, and no trismus.

PROGNOSIS: The mortality is about fifty per cent. The disease is almost always fatal in infancy. The outlook is best when the incubation period is longer than a week and there are no fever and few or no convulsions. Death usually occurs three or four days after the onset, with marked fever and respiratory failure. In those who recover there are no sequelae.

TREATMENT: (Following the recommendations of the Committee of the American Academy of Pediatrics on the Control of Infectious Diseases):

1. Heavy sedation should be given as soon as the diagnosis is made, to the point where the child is practically asleep continuously. The child should be in a quiet room, free of extraneous stimuli, and have good nursing care. Avertin® per rectum, 30 mg./kg. every two to six hours, or phenobarbital should be administered.

2. Skin test for horse sensitivity. If negative, give 40,000 to 60,000 units of tetanus antitoxin intramuscularly. If the intradermal test is positive, inject 1 ml. epinephrine chloride (1:1,000) intramuscularly 15 *minutes* before the administration of antitoxin. Also give an antihistamine drug.

3. Treat the wound surgically, if indicated, after the sedative effect has occurred.

4. 300,000 units of procaine penicillin and one-half gram of streptomycin should be injected intramuscularly, once daily.

5. The position should be alternated from side to face down to prevent pneumonia.

6. Gentle mechanical suction of mucus. Keep the child in the Trendelenberg position. If mucus accumulates, tracheotomy may be necessary.

7. Continuous i.v. drip of electrolytes, glucose, and amino acid solutions.

8. The spine is X-rayed in convalescence for fracture or compression.

9. Before discharge, active immunization against tetanus is begun.

PREVENTION: When a wound has occurred, it should be actively treated by proper cleaning, and the opening should be exposed. Penicillin should be administered.

If the child has had his complete active immunization with tetanus toxoid, he should get a recall booster dose immediately following the injury, 0.5 cc. fluid tetanus toxoid.

If he has not had active immunization with tetanus toxoid, he should immediately receive tetanus antitoxin, subcutaneously, 5000 units or less, depending upon age and weight, first testing for horse serum sensitivity. If the injury is older than twenty-four hours when the child is seen, give 5000 units.

American Academy of Pediatrics: Report of the Committee on the Control of Infectious Diseases: Tetanus, P. 62-64, 1957.

Turner, T. B., Velasco-Joven, E. A. and Prudovsky, S.: Studies on the Prophylaxis and Treatment of Tetanus: II Studies Pertaining to Treatment. Bull. Johns Hopkins Hosp. 102:71, 1958.

CHAPTER 16

LIPIDOSES

This group is characterized by accumulations of large, lipid-containing cells which are primarily of reticuloendothelial origin. In some the nervous system is affected. It includes:

1. Gaucher's disease—the lipid is kerasin, a cerebroside.
2. Niemann-Pick—the lipid is sphingomyelin, a diaminophosphatide.
3. Tay-Sachs—the lipid is a ganglioside.

GAUCHER'S DISEASE

Infantile Form:

CLINICAL PICTURE: This type is often familial, probably inherited as a recessive condition, and is almost unknown in Jews (Van Creveld). It occurs acutely and has many neurological features. The early weeks of the infant's life are uneventful. Then there is noted enlargement of the spleen and liver with swelling of the abdomen. At this time mental sluggishness develops, the child appearing apathetic and indifferent. The muscles show increased tone, gradually changing from hypertonia to severe spasticity with opisthotonos, and the deep tendon reflexes are increased. There is a convergent squint. The fundi are normal. In the later stages there are general wasting and mental retardation.

PATHOLOGY: There are great numbers of large, pale, lipid-containing cells (Gaucher cells) in all the organs, causing marked enlargement of the liver and spleen. The lipid is kerasin. Some of the ganglion cells of the brain are swollen, but most appear sclerosed, shrunken, and destroyed. Their granules are similar chemically to those of the Gaucher cells in other organs. There is some glial reaction.

ETIOLOGY: There is a familial incidence, with several members in a single generation being affected. Others in the family may have subclinical disease. Gaucher cells may be present in the bone marrow of parents of affected children.

DIAGNOSIS: This is suggested by the familial history, enlarged spleen and liver, and the neurological picture. It is established by bone marrow smears showing the typical Gaucher cells.

Gaucher's is differentiated from amaurotic idiocy by the absence of the cherry red spot in the macula.

Niemann-Pick disease is familial and the baby may also appear normal after birth. Later an enlarged liver and spleen and mental retardation are seen. The child dies within two years. The differential from infantile Gaucher's is easy if the cherry red spot in the macula is present. Niemann-Pick occurs in Hebrews, whereas Gaucher's does not in the infantile form. Neurological findings, if present in Niemann-Pick, are similar to those of Tay-Sachs. Foam cells are present in the bone marrow, spleen, lymph nodes, liver, and peripheral blood. (There are no abnormal cells in the peripheral blood in Gaucher's.)

PROGNOSIS: Death occurs several months after the onset.

TREATMENT: There is no specific therapy.

Chronic Gaucher's Disease: This form appears in older children and almost entirely in Jews. There are no clinical neurological changes.

Geddes, A. K. and Moore, S.: Acute (Infantile) Gaucher's Disease, Report of a Case, the Second in a Family. J. Pediat. 43:61, 1953.
Giampalmo, A.: Über die Pathologie der Gaucherschen Krankheit im Frühen Kindesalter (mit Besonderer-Berücksichtigung der Neurologischen Form). Acta Paediat. 37:6, 1949.
Van Creveld, S.: The Lipoidoses. Advances in Pediatrics. Chicago, Year Book Publishers, 6:190, 1953.

FAMILIAL AMAUROSES (CEREBROMACULAR DEGENERATIONS)

This group has been described in four different forms, each type named after the physician most closely allied with its description:
1. Infantile (Tay-Sachs)
2. Late Infantile (Bielchowsky)
3. Juvenile (Vogt)
4. Adult (Kufs)

Infantile (Tay-Sachs). The infantile or Tay-Sachs disease is the classic type and the form which the physician is most likely to see (1/250,000 population). It is a degenerative disease with racial and familial characteristics, in which there are idiocy, blindness, and progression to eventual death. It gets its name from Tay, who described the cherry red spot in the fundus (1881), and Sachs, who subsequently collected a series of cases and described the pathology and clinical findings and recognized its familial characteristics (1887).

ETIOLOGY: Almost all the patients are of Jewish extraction. The disease is familial, but all the children of a family may not have it. Some are born normal and remain so. The condition is transmitted as a genetic recessive, and may be due to an enzyme defect. Consanguinity is present in over fifteen per cent, and twenty-five per cent have parents who are first cousins. Since the occurrence is early in infancy there is no direct transmission.

CLINICAL PICTURE: For the first two or three months the infant seems to be developing satisfactorily, but then appears listless and shows a progressive loss of motor power, with weakness and lack of voluntary activity. The head now falls back when unsupported, and any previous ability to grasp objects is lost. The baby appears to have no sight and takes no interest in its surroundings. This loss of vision is often the earliest suggestion of trouble. The muscles at first appear flabby and hypotonic, but subsequently become extremely rigid and hypertonic and are associated with active tendon reflexes and a Babinski sign. Hyperacusis occurs in some; that is, they become unusually sensitive to sound and may be startled out of their apathy at some slight noise. Along with the developing picture of apathy and weakness, the failure of vision goes on to total blindness. Ophthalmoscopic examination reveals the characteristic cherry red spot in the macula lutea and optic atrophy. In the last stages, there are likely to be decerebrate rigidity, twitching, and myoclonic seizures. Feeding becomes difficult, and tube feeding must be resorted to. Marasmus is noted, with general wasting and finally inevitable death between two and three years of age.

LABORATORY: The total serum neuraminic acid is only slightly increased; however, the serum globulin neuraminic acid ratio (alpha-2 and beta globulins) is increased. The serum glutamic oxalacetic transaminase level is markedly elevated.

PATHOLOGY: Grossly, there appear to be no malformations or abnormalities of the brain. If death occurs before fourteen months, there is some atrophy; if later, the brain may show a marked increase in size due to gliosis and edema. The microscopic changes involve primarily the neurons. The cytoplasm is swollen and the cells take on various shapes. The dendrites are balloon-like in appearance and may gradually disappear. The Nissl substance is decreased in amount and finely granular, and the nucleus is displaced to the periphery of the cell. The neurofibrils are displaced, but the axis cylinder and myelin sheath may be only slightly involved. In other cases there is demyelinization. Changes similar to those of the brain also occur in the retina. The ganglionic cells contain prelipoid cytoplasmic inclusions. The brain pathology is associated with an increase in gangliosides. The neuraminic acid content of the cortex is markedly increased. Perhaps an enzyme deficiency allows accumulation of these substances.

DIAGNOSIS: Differential diagnosis from other forms of poor development in infancy rests on the facts that the infant is of Hebrew extraction and is well for several months after birth before beginning to deteriorate with failing vision. The cherry red spot on examination of the fundus is pathognomonic. In one family in which the first born had died of amaurotic idiocy, we checked the fundi immediately after the birth of another offspring. At this time they were negative. However, after successive examinations the cherry red spots were noted in the retinae at two months.

PROGNOSIS: The outcome is death in two to three years.

TREATMENT: There is no specific therapy.

What should the parents be told about the chances of recurrence with future offspring? They should be informed that there is a twenty-five per cent risk with every pregnancy. This may be greater if consanguinity is present. If more children are desired and they do not wish to take the risk, the possibility of adoption should be discussed.

There has been a good deal of literature on the relationship between Tay-Sachs disease and Niemann-Pick disease. The latter also occurs in the Hebrew race; its times of onset and death are similar; and there may also be changes in the retina. The histologic changes in the brain may likewise be similar in the two diseases. Sphingomyelin and lecithin are present in the foam cells in Nie-

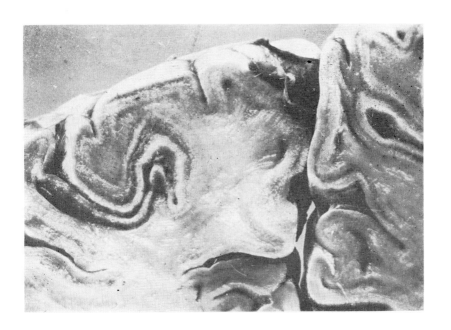

17. Tay-Sachs Disease. Linear degeneration of gray and white matter.

mann-Pick disease. In the peripheral blood, vacuolated monocytes and lymphocytes are present. There may be an increase in serum phospholipids in Niemann-Pick, but not in Tay-Sachs. The marked increase in the neuraminic acid content of the brain in Tay-Sachs is not present in Niemann-Pick or the other forms of amaurotic idiocy. Herdon feels that the genetic identity of the two diseases will not be settled until more extensive biochemical and genetic data are available. (Refer to the section on diagnosis in Gaucher's disease.)

Late Infantile (Bielchowsky). This type is rarely seen. Its onset is between three and five years. There is optic atrophy, but no cherry red spot in the macula lutea. It is not confined to Hebrews. The clinical course is much slower than Tay-Sachs. Seizures and especially cerebellar symptoms such as ataxia are prominent. The pathology is similar to Tay-Sachs but with greater emphasis on the location in the cerebellum. The outcome is death in a few years.

Juvenile (Spielmeyer-Vogt). This form was first described by Vogt in 1905. It differs from the infantile type clinically, though the pathology is similar. It is transmitted by a single recessive gene different from that causing Tay-Sachs. Fifteen per cent have first cousin parents.

CLINICAL PICTURE: The onset is at five to six years of age. The children develop normally up to this time. The first symptom is usually impaired vision. Examination of the fundi reveals a yellow-gray area at the macula with thin narrow vessels and no pigment; later examination shows small, black pigmented deposits in the macular area of degeneration and also around the periphery. This appearance has been called a "pepper and salt" picture. Later the pigment appears shaped in the form of "bone corpuscles." The patient gradually becomes blind because of optic atrophy. Following the onset of loss of vision, mental deterioration sets in. The child loses the ability to speak properly, memory fails, he absorbs nothing, and acts like an imbecile. He gradually develops a masked facies, tremors, rigidity, stooped posture, and a propulsive gait. Ataxia may set in, and convulsions also occur. As the years go on this picture of blindness, mental deterioration, constant seizures, general spasticity, and emotional changes of laughing and crying without reason ends with idiocy and complete helplessness. Death occurs by the twentieth year, secondary to infection.

SUMMARY: This type is not restricted to the Hebrew race; its age of onset is later; its clinical picture is different; and its course is slower than that of the infantile form. The pathology, however, is similar. The clinical picture consists of first, loss of vision, followed in the next two years by mental deterioration, epileptic seizures which are quite constant, extrapyramidal syndromes, cerebellar ataxia, and finally progressive dementia.

DIFFERENTIAL DIAGNOSIS: This form must be differentiated from Wilson's and Parkinson's diseases, which do not have the visual changes. Congenital syphilis with chorioretinitis must be considered; a positive serology occurs here. The unfolding clinical picture will separate this juvenile form from retinitis pigmentosa, in which the ophthalmoscopic picture may be identical. Some have questioned whether the two conditions might not be related. Retinitis pigmentosa is a primary degeneration of the neuroepithelium of the retina, usually transmitted as a Mendelian recessive. Mental deterioration and seizures do not usually occur. Retinitis pigmentosa is also present in the Laurence-Moon-Biedl syndrome and may secondarily follow measles, mumps, poliomyelitis, and smallpox vaccination.

Late Juvenile or Adult (Kufs). This form occurs in the late teens or in the twenties. There are mental deterioration and seizures, but no changes in the retina. The pathology is similar to the other forms of cerebromacular degeneration. Other members of the family may have retinal pigment changes.

Alfano, J. E. and Berger, J. P.: Retinitis Pigmentosa, Ophthalmoplegia and Spastic Quadriplegia. Am. J. Ophth. 43:231, 1957.
Aronson, S. M., Volk, B. W. and Epstein, N.: Morphologic Evolution of Amaurotic Family Idiocy. Am. J. Path. 31:609, 1955.
Aronson, S. M., Saifer, A., Kanof, A. and Volk, B. W.: Progression of Amaurotic Family Idiocy as Reflected by Serum and Cerebrospinal Fluid Changes. Am. J. Med. 24:390, 1958.
Bielchowsky, M.: Ueber Spätinfantile Familiare Amaurotishe Idiotie mit Kleinhirnsymptomen. Deutsche Ztschr. Nervenh. 50:7, 1914.
Elwyn, H.: Diseases of the Retina. 2nd ed. New York, Blakiston Co., 1953.
Globus, J. H.: Amaurotic Family Idiocy. J. Mt. Sinai Hosp. 9:451, 1942.
Hassin, G. B.: A Case of Amaurotic Family Idiocy, Late Infantile Type (Bielchowsky). Arch. Neurol. & Psychiat. 16:708, 1926.
Herndon, C. N.: Genetics of the Lipidoses. A. Res. Publ. Ass. Nerv. Ment. Dis. Proc. 33:239, 1954.

Kufs, H.: Über eine Spätform der Amaurotischen Idiotie une ihre Heredofamiliaren Grundlagen. Ztschr. f.d. ges. Neurol. u. Psychiat. 95:169, 1925.

Rothstein, J. L. and Welt, S.: Infantile Amaurotic Family Idiocy. Am. J. Dis. Child. 62:801, 1941.

Sachs, B.: On Arrested Cerebral Development, with Special Reference to its Cortical Pathology. J. Nerv. & Ment. Dis. 14:541, 1887.

Sjögren, T.: Die Juvenile Amaurotische Idiotie. Klinische und Erblichkeitsmedizinische Untersuchungen. Hereditos 14:197, 1931.

Symposium: Primary Chorioretinal Aberrations with Night Blindness. Tr. Am. Acad. Ophth. 54:607, 1950.

Tay, W.: Symmetrical Changes in the Region of the Yellow Spot in Each Eye of An Infant. Tr. Ophth. Soc. U. Kingdom, 1:55, 1881.

Thannhauser, S. J.: Diseases of the Nervous System Associated with Disturbances of Lipid Metabolism. A. Res. Publ. Nerv. & Ment. Dis. Proc. 32:238, 1953.

Volk, B. W., Aronson, S. M. and Soifer, A.: The Serum Neuraminic Acid Distribution. J. Lab. & Clin. Med. 50:26, 1957.

DISORDERS OF CONNECTIVE TISSUE

HURLER'S SYNDROME (GARGOYLISM)

This syndrome in its classical form consists of stunted growth (dwarfism), mental retardation, bone changes (kyphos), grotesque head, corneal clouding, and enlarged liver and spleen. However, incomplete forms or "formes frustes" are also present, in which one or more of the typical features may be absent. The disease was first described by Hunter in 1917. Hurler added the elements of mental deficiency and clouding of the cornea to the picture. Ellis added the word "gargoylism" or grotesque face.

CLINICAL PICTURE: The condition may be difficult to recognize during the first year. There may be evidence of mental retardation and some peculiarities of appearance, but nothing is distinctive. Then kyphos is noted, the liver and spleen become enlarged, and the skin grows thickened and inelastic. Cardiac murmurs are common. Gradually the clinical features unfold. Growth is stunted and the child appears grotesque and similar to a gargoyle, with a generally scaphocephalic skull shape. The nose is broad, the nasal bridge depressed, and the tongue thickened and protruding. The neck is short, the abdomen protuberant, and an umbilical hernia may be present. The hands and feet are broad, and extension of the fingers is limited. The eyes exhibit opacities of the cornea due to storage of lipid in the deeper layers. In the incomplete cases there may be no corneal clouding and no enlarged liver and spleen. However, osseous changes are usually present. The mental development varies.

LABORATORY: X-ray of the bones shows the abnormally shaped skull, with protrusions of the outer table near the coronal suture. The imperfect ossification of the lumbar vertebrae may be evident; also kyphos of the lumbodorsal spine. There is retarded development of the centers of ossification. According to Caffey there is an abnormal configuration of the shafts of the bones. The changes are most marked in the arms, and the central portions of the shafts of the upper extremities exhibit bizarre swellings which taper toward the ends. This appearance is very diagnostic. Blood studies show increased granularity of the white blood cells. The blood lipids and liver function are normal.

PATHOLOGY: The disease is a metabolic disorder involving various organs of the body, including the vascular system, connective tissues, and especially the liver and brain. Grumbach and Meyer suggest that the Hurler syndrome is a genetic disorder of connective tissue resulting in the abnormal storage and urinary excretion of acid mucopolysaccharides. Electrophoretic determinations show variations in the serum proteins. The defect may lie in the binding of mucopolysaccharides to proteins. According to some authors gargoylism is a lipoidal disorder similar to amaurotic idiocy.

ETIOLOGY: The disease runs in families. There is a ten per cent parental consanguinity. It is genetically transmitted and results from a single autosomal recessive gene. Herndon feels that there are two genetic types of gargoylism, the autosomal recessive which is characterized by a high incidence of corneal clouding and dwarfism, and the rarer sex-linked recessive, characterized by absence of corneal clouding, infrequent dwarfism, and frequent deafness.

DIAGNOSIS: This condition must be differentiated from Morquio's disease, in which a clouded cornea, large liver and spleen, peculiar facies, and mental retardation are not found. In the incomplete types of gargoylism there may be confusion with cretinism. In the latter the bone deformities are different, and the radioactive iodine uptake and serum BEI will establish the diagnosis. Mongolism may also require differentiation.

PROGNOSIS: The disease may go on for years at a slow rate. The majority of children die prior to adulthood, either from cardiac disease or intercurrent infection.

TREATMENT: There is no specific therapy.

Caffey, J.: Hurler's Syndrome. Pediatric X-Ray Diagnosis: Chicago, The Year Book Publishers, Inc., 1950.

Ellis, R. W., Sheldon, W. and Capon, N. B.: Gargoylism (Chondro-osteodystrophy, Corneal Opacities, Hepatosplenomegaly, and Mental Deficiency). Quart. J. Med. 5:119, 1936.

Gilbert, E. F. and Guin, G. H.: Gargoylism. A.M.A. J. Dis. Child. 95:69, 1958.

Grumbach, M. M. and Meyer, K: Urinary Excretion and Tissue Storage of Sulfated Mucopolysaccharides in Hurler's Syndrome. Soc. Pediat. Research. May 6-7, 1958.

Herndon, C. N.: Genetics of the Lipidoses. A. Res. Publ. Ass. Nerv. Ment. Dis. Proc. 33:239, 1954.

Hunter, C.: A Rare Disease in Two Brothers. Proc. Roy. Soc. Med. 9:104, 1917.

Hurler, G.: Über einen Typ. multipler Abartungen Vorwiegend am Skelettsystem. Zeitschr. f. Kinderh. 24:220, 1920.

Jervis, G. A.: Gargoylism (Lipochondrodystrophy). Arch. Neurol. & Psychiat. 63:681, 1950.

Lindsay, S.: The Cardiovascular System in Gargoylism. Brit. Heart. J. 12:17, 1950.

Uzman, L. L.: Chemical Nature of the Storage Substance in Gargoylism. A.M.A. Arch. Path. 60:308, 1955.

Van Creveld, S.: The Lipoidoses. Advances in Pediatrics. Chicago, Year Book Publishers, 6:190, 1953.

CHAPTER 17

VITAMIN DEFICIENCIES

Beriberi

Beriberi is a deficiency disease resulting from a lack of thiamine (B_1) in the diet. In the orient, where most cases are seen, it occurs most often within the first three months postpartum in breast-fed infants whose mothers are lacking this vitamin. It also develops in infants and children who are on inadequate or restricted diets.

CLINICAL PICTURE: Within one to four months after birth the breast-fed baby becomes whiny, restless, is lacking in desire to feed, and is constipated. If the onset is acute, there are vomiting, marked irritability, and edema, which may give a false appearance of weight gain. In some, the onset is sudden in an apparently healthy infant leading to a rapid cardiac death.

The clinical picture has been divided into four types: aphonic, polyneuritic, cerebral, and cardiac. Most often there is a combination of the polyneuritic and cardiac forms.

Aphonic. Slight hoarseness to complete loss of voice due to paralysis of the laryngeal branches of the vagus.

Polyneuritic. There are pain and weakness of the muscles with absent deep tendon reflexes, but not the distal selectivity of the adult type.

Cerebral. When the onset is acute, the symptoms of cerebral irritation include muscle spasms and convulsions, together with drowsiness and a comatose state; others show ptosis of the eyelids, ocular palsies, optic nerve atrophy, retrobulbar neuritis, and ataxia. Some of these are cases of Wernicke's syndrome (altered consciousness, ophthalmoplegia, and ataxia).

Cardiac. There are cyanosis, dyspnea, tachycardia, dilatation of the right heart, and changes in the ECG.

PATHOLOGY: The peripheral nerves show the usual changes of polyneuritis, with myelin sheath and axonal degeneration. The brain shows foci of congestion and hemorrhage in the gray matter of the brain stem and hypothalamus. In Wernicke's encephalopathy the lesions are mainly in the walls of the 3rd and 4th ventricles and periaqueductal gray matter of the midbrain. There are changes in the heart consisting of edema, dilatation, and fatty degeneration.

DIAGNOSIS: The clinical diagnosis is based on a history of nutritional deprivation together with gastrointestinal, polyneuritic, cerebral, and cardiac features. The neurological manifestations require differentiation from infantile spinal muscular atrophy, poliomyelitis, and diphtheritic disease, either the polyneuritic or laryngeal form.

LABORATORY TESTS:

1. Thamine level in the blood is decreased (below 3 mcg/100 ml.).
2. Thiamine assays of the urine:
   a. Oral—1 mg. of thiamine is given to the patient.
      Normal output is over 90 mcg. in the urine.
      In beriberi, the output is diminished.
   b. Intravenous—1 mg. Collect urine over the next four hours and measure the amount of thiamine.
      Normal output over 250 mcg.
      In beriberi output is decreased.
3. The blood pyruvic and lactic acid levels are increased.

PROGNOSIS: The average mortality in various large series has been about fifty per cent. When the patients have been untreated, this has risen to seventy-eight per cent. The most unfavorable outlook occurs when there is an acute onset. When the condition is more chronic and thiamine can be given, the prognosis is much better.

TREATMENT: Prophylactic: Women who are pregnant and those who are breast feeding should receive a nutritious diet and supplementary vitamins of all types, including thiamine, about 3 mg. per day. Infants and children should receive from 0.5 (for infants) to 1.5 mg. (for older children) of thiamine per day.

Therapeutic: The baby should be given 10 mg. of thiamine intramuscularly daily, for a week, and then put on a maintenance dose orally. There is a quick, dramatic improvement in the heart and the aphonia clears in about six weeks. However, the neuritis is more resistant, although the pain disappears. Mothers who are breast-feeding should get 50-100 mg. of thiamine intravenously and the same amount continued as a daily oral dose. Subsequently, the same therapy is used as in prophylaxis, namely, a good diet plus multiple vitamins, including B-complex.

Davis, R. A. and Wolf, A.: Infantile Beriberi Associated with Wernicke's Encephalopathy. Pediatrics 21:409, 1958.
Haridas, G.: Infantile Beriberi in Singapore During the Latter Part of the Japanese Occupation. Arch. Dis. Child. 22:23, 1947.
Spillane, J. D.: Nutritional Disorders of the Nervous System. Baltimore, Williams and Wilkins Co., 1947.
Van Gelder, D. W. and Darby, F. V.: Congenital and Infantile Beriberi. J. Pediat. 25:226, 1944.

PELLAGRA

Pellagra is a deficiency disease due primarily to a lack of niacin (nicotinic acid) in the diet.

CLINICAL PICTURE: While the term *pellagra* refers to skin lesions, there are also major gastrointestinal and neurological manifestations. The skin lesions appear early. There is erythema similar to a sunburn, which is intensified by exposure to light. It appears in symmetrical fashion over the extremities, including the backs of the hands and feet, wrists, ankles, and face; in other words, the exposed areas. When other parts of the body are uncovered, it is also noted over the neck and trunk.

⌐⌐ ⌐astrointestinal symptoms also appear early and include anorexia, diarrhea, abdominal pains, redness and fissuring of the tongue (Glossitis), excessive salivation, and stomatitis.

There may be psychic changes, including irritability, apathy, and depression. In the severe cases actual delirium and coma may occur.

Neurological manifestations occur mainly in adults, not in children. They may precede, accompany, or follow the skin and gastrointestinal features. They include polyneuritis, spinal cord lesions with spasticity and ataxia, extrapyramidal signs of tremor and rigidity, and cranial nerve involvement such as optic atrophy, retrobulbar neuritis, and occasionally nerve deafness.

LABORATORY: Anemia is present. The spinal fluid is normal, or there may be a slight increase in protein.

PATHOLOGY: There is edema of the brain. The Betz cells of the cortex and the Purkinje cells in the cerebellum show chromatolysis. There is myelin degeneration in the posterior columns of the cord, less so in the lateral columns and peripheral nerves. The last also show axonal degeneration. The skin and intestinal tract may also show changes.

DIAGNOSIS: In classical instances, especially in adults, the history of poor diet, plus the combination of skin, gastrointestinal, and neurological manifestations make recognition easy. In children, however, the condition is generally milder and the symptoms and signs more vague. A history of poor nutrition is important. If there are irritability, anorexia, gastrointestinal upsets, anemia, and perhaps skin lesions or mild mental changes, suspicion should be aroused. In school age children there are sleeplessness, soreness of the tongue, and burning pain in the abdomen.

PROGNOSIS: If treatment is not delayed too long, the outlook is good. The skin and gastrointestinal symptoms respond. However, mental impairment and neuritis may remain. The prospects are better in children than in adults.

TREATMENT: Prophylactic: This requires a nutritious diet plus the usual vitamins given to infants and children (A,B,C,D). When there is some question concerning the mother's health, 5 mg. per day of niacin should be added to the diet of infants who are nursing.

THERAPEUTIC: Nicotinamide, 100 mg., should be injected intravenously in urgent cases. Then 50 mg. to 300 mg. of niacin per day should be given orally in divided doses. A liberal diet, including B-complex, brewers' yeast (1½ ounces daily), and vitamins A,C,D, should be offered the child. Iron is added for the anemia. Children should be kept out of the sun to aid skin healing.

Spies, T. D., Walker, A. A. and Woods, A. W.: Pellagra in Infancy and Childhood. J.A.M.A. 113:1481, 1939.

PYRIDOXINE (B₆) DEFICIENCY

Convulsions have occurred in the newborn period from a deficiency of pyridoxine. This is discussed in the chapter on convulsions.

SCURVY

Scurvy, due to vitamin C deficiency, has only slight implications neurologically. It occurs primarily in the latter half of the first year and second year of childhood. The essential feature is hemorrhage, which occurs in the skin and subperiosteally. Occasionally hemorrhage into the orbit or a subdural hematoma occurs.

CLINICAL PICTURE: The clinical features include marked irritability and tenderness, especially in the lower extremities. The legs are held motionless because of pain, "frog-like." There may be swelling of the thigh due to subperiosteal hemorrhages. The gums are tender and swollen. Bleeding in the skin, bowel, or kidney may be noted. Fever may be present.

Neurologically, the major finding is subdural hemorrhage (discussed under this title). Rarely subarachnoid or intracerebral bleeding occurs. Orbital hemorrhage with exophthalmos may cause ocular palsies; this is also rare. Pain in the extremities along with diminished reflexes has been ascribed to involvement of the peripheral nerves, but this may all be due to a pseudoparalysis associated with the subperiosteal hemorrhages.

LABORATORY:

1. X-ray of the long bones is diagnostic. Changes include a subepiphyseal zone of rarefaction, calcification of the subperiosteal hemorrhage, and multiple spurs at the cartilage-shaft junctions.
2. The blood level of vitamin C is low.
3. The vitamin C saturation or blood loading test: Inject 400 mg. of vitamin C intramuscularly and collect urine for the next twelve hours. Normally 50% of the vitamin C appears in the urine in 8 hours. In vitamin C deficiency only a slight percentage appears.

DIFFERENTIAL DIAGNOSIS: A differential from poliomyelitis should be made by the spinal fluid findings in the latter. Suppurative arthritis and osteomyelitis may have positive cultures, and will have no bleeding manifestations and different X-ray findings. Congenital syphilis (pseudoparalysis) and blood dyscrasias should also be considered; these can be ruled out by appropriate blood studies.

PROGNOSIS: Symptoms disappear quickly with vitamin C therapy.

TREATMENT: Prophylactic: Every infant should receive two to four ounces of orange juice or 50 to 100 mg. of ascorbic acid daily.

THERAPEUTIC: 100-300 mg. of vitamin C per day should be given by injection, intramuscularly or intravenously. As soon as the baby takes food properly, vitamin C is given by mouth, either as ascorbic acid or orange juice, daily.

Caffey, J.: Scurvy: Pediatric X-ray Diagnosis, ed. 3. Chicago. The Year Book Publishers, Inc., 1956.

RICKETS AND INFANTILE TETANY

Tetany is a condition of hyperexcitability of the neuromuscular system, in which there are tonic spasms of the muscles along with convulsions. The major muscle groups involved are those of the hands and feet (carpopedal spasm) and larynx (laryngismus stridulus). Tetany of the newborn has been discussed under the subject of convulsions. The present discussion deals with the infantile tetany associated with rickets, both manifestations of a deficiency of vitamin D.

There are other factors aside from deficiency of vitamin D which may produce tetany or spasmophilia in childhood. These include hypoparathyroidism, and conditions like celiac disease in which there is lack of ability to absorb vitamin D. In vitamin D resistant rickets there is normal absorption but no response. In all of these types tetany is due to hypocalcemia. Gastric tetany, from vomiting secondary to pylorospasm, pyloric stenosis, or brain tumor, results from an alkalosis due to loss of chlorides. In hyperventilation, which can occur as a sequel of encephalitis, there is loss of CO_2 with the production of alkalosis and tetany. Irrespective of cause, the clinical picture is the same.

The onset of tetany due to vitamin D deficiency usually occurs in the late winter and early spring in infants from four months to two years of age. This seasonal incidence is due to the fact that with repeated respiratory infections and bouts of fever there is a tendency to restrict the diet and thus vitamin intake. Together with a lack of sunshine the conditions for expression of a vitamin D deficiency are ripe. The attack is often ushered in with an acute upper respiratory infection and fever.

The symptoms and signs depend on the fact that vitamin D is related to calcium and phosphorus metabolism. A lack of vitamin D causes rickets. While the calcium in the serum is usually normal, in a certain number of infants with rickets the calcium eventually becomes lowered below 7.5 mg. per 100 ml. (N 9-11 mg.). When this occurs, tetany results. Ionized calcium normally acts as a depressant on the neuromuscular junction. Release of this inhibitory action produces hyperexcitability of the nervous system. The serum phosphorus in rickets usually is lowered to 2-3 mg. per 100 ml. (N 4-6 mg.).

When active rickets is being treated, too rapid a flow of calcium from the blood to the bones may also cause tetany because of a sudden lowering of the blood calcium. In all these mechanisms the parathyroids and perhaps the kidneys may play a role. Why so few infants with rickets have a lowered calcium and tetany is unanswered, but it may be due to compensatory hyperactivity of the parathyroids.

Signs of Tetany (Manifest tetany). Carpal spasm is an early sign. It is bilateral and symmetrical. There is flexion of the wrist and metacarpalphalangeal joints and extension at the interphalangeal joints. The thumb is adducted. Pedal spasm usually follows. Here there is ventral flexion of the foot and flexion of the toes at the proximal joints with extension at the distal joints. The feet may be in a position of equinovarus. Any activity may increase the spasms. Carpopedal spasm is seen at all ages, but especially in childhood. Laryngospasm produces a contraction of the laryngeal muscles. There is a "crowing" sound with inspiration due to adduction of the vocal cords. Inspiratory stridor may occur. It is present in infants under two years of age. Convulsions, which are usually generalized, and loss of consciousness are especially prominent in the infantile period.

On examination there may be signs of latent tetany together with rickets. These are the Chvostek, Trousseau, Erb, and peroneal phenomena. Chvostek's sign is produced by tapping the cheek in front of the ear. This can be done with the finger or a percussion hammer. There is contraction of the facial muscles on the same side including those of the mouth, cheek, and eye, due to irritability of the branches of the facial nerve. It is especially valuable for diagnosis up to three years. Trousseau's sign is elicited by constriction of the arm above the elbow by means of a blood pressure cuff; this reduces the circulation and carpal spasm results. Erb's sign shows hyperirritability of the peripheral nerves: with the galvanic current less stimulation is required to obtain muscular contraction than in the normal infant. To elicit the peroneal sign, tap just below the head of the fibula (peroneal nerve). In tetany there is dorsiflexion and abduction of the foot. Signs of latent tetany are also present when convulsions indicative of active tetany have occurred.

DIAGNOSIS: Usually the first sign of tetany is a convulsive seizure. In such an infant blood should be drawn for a calcium level; if it is 7.5 mg. per 100 ml. or less the diagnosis is tetany. There will usually be clinical and X-ray evidence of rickets, an increased serum alkaline phosphatase, and some of the signs of tetany previously described.

PROGNOSIS: I have seen no deaths from tetany, although a three per cent mortality is quoted. Recovery is complete. There is no relation to epilepsy in later life.

TREATMENT: For the convulsions 10 cc. of a 10 per cent solution of calcium gluconate are given slowly intravenously. Do not give the calcium gluconate intramuscularly since calcification and subsequent necrosis of the muscle tissue may result. In one case, death from secondary infection with meningitis occurred. After the first injection, one more dose of calcium gluconate may occasionally be required, but usually there is a quick response. Calcium chloride may then be given orally in a five per cent solution. One teaspoon of the solution may be added to the milk formula four to six times a day, for two days. This should be followed by adding calcium lactate, gr. 10, to each bottle or glass of milk six times daily for several weeks. If the child does not take the calcium chloride because of the taste, begin with the lactate instead. After the first week, if rickets is present, vitamin D, 5000 units daily, is given. Thereafter, the usual prophylactic dose of 1000 units daily will suffice. Sodium phenobarbital, gr. 1, may also be given intramuscularly for the seizure.

Holt, Jr., L. E. and McIntosh, R.: Tetany, in Holt Pediatrics, ed. 12. New York, Appleton-Century-Crofts, 1953.

Lamm, S. S.: The Danger of Intramuscular Injection of Calcium Gluconate in Infancy. J.A.M.A. 129:347, 1945.

Nelson, W. E.: Tetany, in Textbook of Pediatrics, ed. 6. Philadelphia, W. B. Saunders Co., 1954.

CHAPTER 18

DISEASES OF MUSCLES

ELECTRODIAGNOSIS

Electrodiagnosis involves stimulation of a muscle by the introduction of a brief electric current. A contraction is produced which is followed by relaxation. The electrical current is applied through a small stimulating electrode to the motor point to be tested. The larger or dispersive electrode is near the examination area. Changes in electrical irritability are thus observed.

Reaction of Degeneration. A reaction of degeneration (RD) means that there is inability to stimulate the muscle to contract via the application of a tetanizing or faradic current. If there is a partial RD, some of the muscle may contract, but not to a normal degree. The presence of an RD indicates that there is lower motor neuron disease or injury. The RD may be used in prognosis. Since it takes about two weeks for the RD to develop, in peripheral nerve lesions such as Bell's palsy, if there is no RD at that time, a good outlook may be anticipated.

Myasthenic Reaction (Jolly reaction). In a normal muscle the application of a tetanizing current to the motor point causes the muscle to contract. If brief intervals of rest or relaxation are permitted, further stimulation of the muscle causes normal vigorous contraction for long periods. In myasthenia gravis such periodic stimulation after brief periods of rest will produce diminishing contractions, and finally none.

Myotonic Reaction. In this form, application of a galvanic or tetanizing current causes the usual muscle contraction, but following removal of the testing electrodes, the muscle contractions still continue for a few seconds followed by rest. This is seen in myotonia congenita (Thomsen's Disease) and myotonic dystrophy.

385

Chronaxy. The minimal intensity of current, measured in volts, required to produce muscle contraction is referred to as the rheobase. The minimal time required to stimulate contraction of the muscle, using a current twice the strength of the rheobase, is called the chronaxy. Alteration in chronaxy is helpful in the diagnosis of neuromuscular dysfunction since there are fixed values for specific muscles. When there are a normal nerve and muscle, the chronaxy is below one millisecond. In conditions like poliomyelitis or peripheral nerve degeneration, chronaxy values are increased.

ELECTROMYOGRAPHY

Electromyography records the electrical properties of muscle or muscle action potential. The needle electrodes are inserted into the muscle through the skin. They record primarily the activities of the motor unit, which includes the nerve cell, axon, end-plates, and muscle fibres. When the normal muscle is relaxed or at rest, no activity is recorded.

A most significant record is the fibrillation potential of denervation. This record is present in lower motor neuron degeneration and indicates individual muscle fibril denervation. It is noted in poliomyelitis, infantile muscular atrophy, and syringomyelia. Electromyography may be of aid in myasthenia gravis, where it may detect a defect in transmission at the neuromuscular junction. There is diminished amplitude of the action potential. In myotonias the action potential continues after the muscle relaxes; this is diagnostic. In the myopathies there are no spontaneous fibrillation potentials, and there is a low voltage potential.

The techniques of electromyography cannot be used to make a diagnosis of a particular clinical disease entity. They can be of help in distinguishing between primary myopathy and that secondary to a neurogenic cause. They may show reinnervation of the muscle before clinical evidence is present. In other instances, as in myasthenia gravis or myotonia, the findings may augment a clinical diagnosis.

Buchthal, F.: An Introduction to Electromyography. Scandinavian University Books. Oslo, J. W. Cappelen, 1957.

Licht, S.: Electrodiagnosis and Electromyography. New Haven, Conn. Publ. by Elizabeth Licht, 1956.

Mayo Clinic. Clinical Examinations in Neurology, Chap. XV, Philadelphia, W. B. Saunders Co., 1956.

Amyotonia Congenita

Amyotonia congenita is a term used to cover a syndrome of infancy in which there are hypotonia and generalized muscular weakness. The etiology is varied; hence, the clinical course, pathology, and prognosis are likewise variable.

Originally, amyotonia congenita was referred to as Oppenheim's disease. The onset is noted at birth or shortly thereafter. There is general hypotonicity so that the posture of the infant is altered and abnormal positions are noted. There are laxness and lengthening of the ligaments, permitting the back of the hand to touch the forearm and enabling the feet to be wrapped about the head. The infant's musculature may be small, weak, flaccid, and limp. The muscle can scarcely be felt within the surrounding mass of fatty tissue. The pathology is general, including the muscles of the extremities, back, and face. While the muscles are atonic, they are not paralyzed. The intercostals may be involved causing retraction of the thorax and interference with respiration; bronchitis and pneumonia may result. The diaphragm is usually spared. As a rule these infants do not support their heads or sit up. The muscles used in sucking and swallowing are usually not affected and any difficulty is due to the general weakness. The deep tendon reflexes are weak or absent. There is a diminution or loss of response of the muscles to electrical stimulation, but there is no reaction of degeneration. There are good sphincter control and no sensory disturbance. These children usually appear to be in good health and are normal mentally. There is no sex predilection. The spinal fluid is normal. There is a decrease in the creatinine output in the urine.

The diagnosis is based on the onset at birth, generalized atonia and weakness of the skeletal muscles, absent tendon reflexes, and absence of atrophic paralysis. The baby does not appear ill. There is normal mentality and at times a tendency toward improvement. The severe cases may die of intercurrent infection within the first year; in others there may be a remission followed by a period of slow improvement although never to the point of full recovery. The majority do not hold their heads up until two to four years and walk only at five years with a waddling type of gait. No specific therapy is available. Physiotherapy to avoid contractures is indicated.

With the passage of time it became obvious that amyotonia congenita (Oppenheim) was not a specific entity, but a clinical description of a syndrome which could be seen in varied forms. Walton

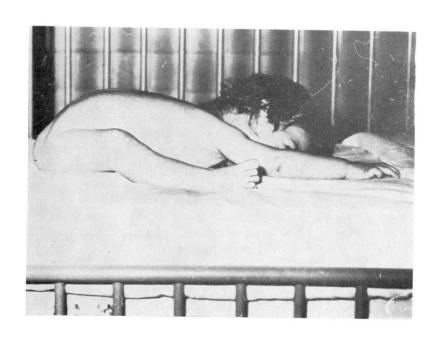

18. Hypotonia ("Limp child").

studied 109 cases of amyotonia congenita in which symptoms had existed from two to twenty-five years before the study. The diagnosis had usually been made in infancy. Of these, sixty-seven were cases of progressive infantile spinal muscular atrophy (Werdnig-Hoffman disease). Fifty-five of the sixty-seven died between five weeks and twelve years of age. Twelve remained disabled. In seventeen other cases, eight completely recovered and nine improved, still retaining weakness and hypoplasia of the muscles. This last group is now referred to as "Benign Congenital Hypotonia."

The clinical picture of benign congenital hypotonia probably also includes the benign, nonprogressive myopathy of Turner and the universal muscular hypoplasia of Krabbe. These patients exhibit a clinical picture similar to the one described above. The myopathies are nonprogressive. There are atonia, hypoplasia, and weakness of musculature. There are neither paralyses nor a reaction of degeneration. The patients recover completely or remain handicapped to some degree. In Turner's cases the muscle tissue showed atrophy similar to the changes of muscular dystrophy. In other cases similar to Krabbe's the muscle biopsy was normal. Shy and Magee, however, described a familial nonprogressive myopathy in five patients where there were specific alterations of the muscle fibres.

The section on infantile progressive muscular atrophy should be read in conjunction with the preceding discussion.

Burdick, W. F., Whipple, D. V. and Freeman, W.: Amyotonia Congenita (Oppenheim). Am. J. Dis. Child. 69:295, 1945.
Epstein, J. A.: Amyotonia Congenita. J. Mt. Sinai Hosp. 16:149, 1949.
Krabbe, K. H.: Kongenit Generaliseret Muskelaplasi. 338 meeting of the Danish Neurol. Soc. Feb. 27, 1946.
Schreier, K. und Huperz, R.: Über die Hypoplasia Musculorum Generalisata Congenita. Ann. Paediat. 186:241, 1956.
Shy, G. M. and Magee, K. R.: A New Congenital Non-Progressive Myopathy. Brain 79:610, 1956.
Turner, J. W. A.: On Amyotonia Congenita. Brain 72:25, 1949.
Walton, J. N.: Amyotonia Congenita. Follow-up Study. Lancet 1:1023, 1956.
Walton, J. N.: "The Limp Child." J. Neurol., Neurosurg., and Psychiat. 20:144, 1957.

INFANTILE PROGRESSIVE MUSCULAR ATROPHY
(WERDNIG-HOFFMAN)

This is a heredofamilial disease occurring in the first year of life, which involves the peripheral motor neuron and leads to progressive muscular atrophy.

CLINICAL PICTURE: The infant may appear well following birth, but at the fourth month or somewhat later during the first year, generalized hyptonia is seen. In about half the cases the onset is noted at birth or may even be suspected prenatally by the lack of fetal movements. There is a widespread muscle paresis with subsequent progressive wasting of the muscles. The infant is immobile, the head cannot be held up, the trunk and pelvic girdle are affected, and there is loss of ability to move the extremities. The intercostals may be involved. The deep tendon reflexes are diminished or absent. There is no sensory loss, and sphincter control is unaffected. The electrical reaction shows degeneration. Spinal fluid is normal. There is a diminished output of creatinine in the urine.

PATHOLOGY: The major changes are in the anterior horn cells, which are markedly reduced in number. Gliosis may be present. The histologic changes are noted in the motor nuclei of the cord primarily, and in the brain stem. The ventral roots are small and demyelinated. There is neurogenic atrophy of the muscles secondarily, with normal and atrophied fibres in juxtaposition. In one case there were lesions in the thalamus; in others, demyelination of the pyramindal pathways has been reported.

ETIOLOGY: The condition is rare. There is no difference in the sexes. The disease is strongly familial. The consanguinity rate is 5.8 per cent (Brandt), which is eight times greater than in a control group. Brandt regards the disease to be of recessive inheritance or incomplete dominance for some families.

PROGNOSIS: The outlook is poor. Eighty per cent die before four years of age, and almost all before twenty years of age. The remainder are severely disabled.

DIAGNOSIS: This is based on the familial occurrence, onset at birth or in early infancy, hypotonia, hypokinesia, absent reflexes, and muscular atrophy. The electrical reaction of degeneration is present and muscle biopsy shows atrophy. There are a number of diseases which must be differentiated:

Amyotonia Congenita

a) *Benign congenital hypotonia.* This includes Turner's infantile myopathy, Krabbe's universal muscular hypoplasia, and the congenital nonprogressive myopathy of Shy and Magee. This group is differentiated from progressive infantile muscular atrophy by the fact that the hypotonia is benign and usually nonprogressive. Muscle biopsy is practically normal and electrical reactions also normal. Electromyography may aid in establishing a primary myopathy or neuropathy.

b) *Progressive forms,* at present undifferentiated.

Arthrogryposis (amyoplasia). There are flexion contractures of joints with undeveloped local muscle groups and immobility of the limbs.

Ehlers-Danlos Syndrome. In this condition there are hyperelasticity of the skin, hyperextensibility of the joints, and fragile capillaries with a tendency to bleed.

Infantile Polyneuritis. If the onset is rapid and is later marked by improvement, polyneuritis is suggested. In polyneuritis there are early involvement of the trunk musculature, and increased protein in the spinal fluid. Electromyography shows compatible changes. Infantile polyneuritis has been proposed as a cause of amyotonia congenita. For a full discussion see the article by Brandt.

Congenital ataxia, mental deficiency, poliomyelitis, cretinism, mongolism, severe nutritional disturbance, rickets, scurvy, atonic diplegia, myasthenia gravis, and progressive muscular dystrophy may require differentiating.

Brandt, S.: Hereditary Factors in Infantile Progressive Muscular Atrophy. Am. J. Dis. Child. 78:226, 1949.

————: Werdnig-Hoffman's Infantile Progressive Muscular Atrophy. Copenhagen, Ejnar Munksgaard, 1950.

————: Course and Symptoms of Progressive Infantile Muscular Atrophy. Arch. Neurol. & Psychiat. 63:218, 1950.

Buchanan, D.: Some Disorders of the Motor Unit in Infancy & Childhood. Med. Clin. N.A. W. B. Saunders Co., 1950.

Chambers, R. and MacDermot, V.: Polyneuritis as a Cause of "Amytonia Congenita." Lancet 1:397, 1957.

Gruner, J. E. and Borgeton, E.: Thalamic Lesions in Myotonia of Infant. Rev. Neurol. 86:236, 1952.

Radermecker, J.: Infantile Spinal Amyotrophy (Werdnig-Hoffman) as Heredodegeneration. Rev. Neurol. 84:14, 1951.

ARTHROGRYPOSIS MULTIPLEX CONGENITA

Arthrogryposis multiplex congenita is a condition noted at birth in which there are multiple contractures with ankyloses of the joints. The latter appear curved (arthrogryposis). There is also a deficiency of muscle fibres or whole muscles (amyoplasia congenita).

CLINICAL FEATURES: The various joints are usually symmetrically affected, and may be fixed in flexion or extension. The extremities are rigid. The position most frequently noted is inward rotation of the arms with extension at the elbows, and flexion of the hands and fingers. The knees may be flexed or extended and the thighs rotated outward and flexed at the hips. There may be any number of positions, however.

The muscles are hypoplastic, and there are usually muscle weakness and hypotonia. Immobility of the joints occurs due to shortness of the muscles and ligaments rather than to involvement of the joints themselves, which are never completely ankylosed. Usually some amount of active and passive motion is possible. There is no reaction of degeneration, but a lessened response to electrical stimulation.

The skin is shiny, thick, and poorly nourished. The underlying tissues are soft, doughy, and flabby. The joints are swollen at the elbows and knees and appear cylindrical and large in contrast to the small limbs, but X-ray shows no abnormality except atrophy.

Various anomalies may be associated with this condition, including club foot, webbed fingers, hydrocephaly, polydactyly, absence of the sacrum, and defects in the spine. The general intellectual level is unaffected.

PATHOLOGY: The muscles may appear normal, atrophic, or absent. Histologically, the muscle fibres appear small. In the spinal cord the anterior born cells and the anterior root fibres are reduced in number.

ETIOLOGY: The cause of this condition is not known. There appears to be no hereditary or familial background. Adams and his associates feel that there are different types of amyoplasia congenita, including defective development of the spinal cord with failure of innervation of the skeletal muscles and developmental defects in the joints themsleves, which may produce contractures. They report a low mental level in some cases. Recently they reported two cases where there was primary myopathy.

The major problem is the explanation of the contractures. The presence of associated anomalies would tend to rule out intrauterine pressure by fixing the etiology early in the life of the developing embryo, before pressure could be a factor. On the other hand, defective development of the anterior horn cells of the spinal cord or their degeneration in fetal life with failure of muscle innervation does not explain them.

When myopathy is primary, there appears to be a greater probability of contractures.

DIAGNOSIS: The diagnosis is made on the basis of congenital immobility of the limbs and fixation in certain characteristic postures.

PROGNOSIS: The outlook is variable.

TREATMENT: Physiotherapy should be provided for the muscles and orthopedic correction for deformities due to contractures.

Adams, R. D., Denny-Brown, D. and Pearson, C. M.: Diseases of Muscle. New York, Paul B. Hoeber, 1953.

Banker, B. Q., Victor, M. and Adams, R. D.: Arthrogryposis Multiplex Due to Congenital Muscular Dystrophy. Brain 80:319, 1957.

Brandt, S.: A Case of Arthrogryposis Multiplex Congenita. Acta. Pediat. 34:365, 1947.

Sheldon, W.: Amyoplasia Congenita. Arch. Dis. Child. 7:117, 1932.

Stern, W. G.: Arthrogryposis Multiplex Congenita. J.A.M.A. 81:1507, 1923.

MUSCULAR DYSTROPHIES

The muscular dystrophies are characterized as heredofamilial disorders of motility with primary degeneration of the skeletal musculature leading to progressive, symmetrical weakness and dysfunction. Several types have been described in the literature by different authors, but often these cannot be clearly delineated in individual patients. In general the onset is in early childhood. There may be pseudohypertrophy or atrophy. No sensory loss is present. There is loss of deep tendon reflexes but no reaction of degeneration. Specific forms have been named in relation to the particular muscle groups involved and the age of onset. The nervous system is not involved.

PSEUDOHYPERTROPHIC

This is the most common form in childhood and is also referred to as the Duchenne type of progressive muscular dystrophy. The onset occurs before the fifth year, and the condition is rapidly progressive. It is transmitted by females as a sex-linked recessive condition and appears mainly in boys.

The onset may be insidious. Usually it is noted that the child is not walking so well as he did. He may climb stairs more slowly, drag his feet, or fall more readily. This is often the initial symptom. Soon he develops a waddling gait, his body swinging from side to side due to weakness of the gluteal muscles. A position of lordosis follows in which the pelvis is tilted forward, the abdomen is protuberant, and the shoulders are flung back due to weakness of the muscles of the lumbar spine. As the trunk muscles and those of the hips and knees become weaker, the child finds difficulty in rising from his seat or the floor. In arising from the floor he "climbs up on himself," that is, he turns on his side and uses his extended arms against the floor to support his trunk. The legs are brought forward and extended. He then places his hands against his legs, knees, and finally his thighs, thus getting his body in an erect position.

Other areas are also involved. In the shoulders the muscles which fix the scapula weaken, producing the "winged scapula" or flaring out of the vertebral margins. The weakness of the shoulder girdle can be brought out by placing the hands of the examiner under the armpits of the child and lifting him. The hands will slip up the child's arms because there is no resistance, and the child's shoulders will come up to his ears. Enlargement of the calf muscles is noted in most cases, occasionally the deltoid and glutei.

As indicated by the symptoms, first the muscles of the pelvic girdle and lumbosacral spine, and then later those of the shoulder girdle become atrophic with loss of power. These include the glutei, quadriceps femoris, sternal head of the pectoralis major, trapezius, and deltoid. The pseudohypertrophic muscles (mainly the gastrocnemius and triceps brachii) also show weakness, have a doughy feel, and seem to have no resistance or tone when palpated.

The involvement of the various muscles is symmetrical. It is the proximal muscles that are primarily involved; as a rule those of the hands and feet are unaffected. There is no sensory loss. The patellar tendon reflexes are present early, but are lost later because of the inability of the muscles to contract, whereas the ankle jerks persist longer. The cutaneous or superficial reflexes are intact. There are no fibrillations or fasciculations. While there is diminution of electrical excitation, there is no reaction of degeneration. There is no loss of sphincter control. The heart may show hypertrophy with disorders of rhythm and a rapid pulse. Occasionally there is con-

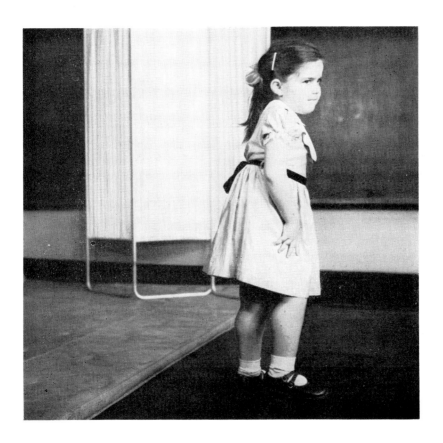

19. Muscular dystrophy. Pseudohypertrophy of calf muscles.

gestive heart failure. Ultimately, with confinement, flexion contractures of the knees, elbows, and hips may occur. The bones may show decalcification. Mental development is normal, but because of the physical difficulties the children may appear slow.

ATROPHIC FEMORAL DYSTROPHY OF LEYDEN AND MOEBIUS

This form is similar to the pseudohypertrophic except for absence of hypertrophy, occasional involvement of the face, and a somewhat slower course.

FACIO-SCAPULO-HUMERAL DYSTROPHY OF LANDOUZY AND DÉJERINE

This form occurs less often than the others but is not rare. It affects both males and females equally. The onset usually occurs in late childhood, at about ten years, and before the age of twenty. It may occur in several members of a family, or sporadically. In contrast to the childhood type, the face and shoulder girdle are initially involved. The eyes cannot be closed completely and there is failure to purse the lips with inability to whistle. The lips are loose and protruding, the face mask-like. Due to atrophy of the zygomaticus muscles there is inability to elevate the lip, resulting in a characteristic flat, transverse smile. Weakness of the shoulder girdle muscles, including the trapezius, pectoralis, serratus magnus, and latissimus dorsi, causes the loss of fixation of the scapula and the winging previously described. Later the biceps, triceps, and deltoid are involved, and finally, the pelvic girdle. This is in the reverse order of the childhood type.

The process is characteristically slow, continuing for years to middle life, and then often remaining stationary. Both dominant and recessive inheritance of the condition have been reported in the literature.

JUVENILE MUSCULAR DYSTROPHY OF ERB

This form has its onset in late childhood. In some instances its occurrence has been noted in late adult life. It is inherited as an autosomal recessive characteristic. Along with involvement of the shoulder girdle and upper arms, the proximal leg muscles are affected, but not the face. It has features similar to the Landouzy form as to longevity and slow course, but differs in the lack of facial involvement.

PATHOLOGY: In muscular dystrophy the color of the muscle, instead of being the normal brown-red, appears yellow or pinkish-

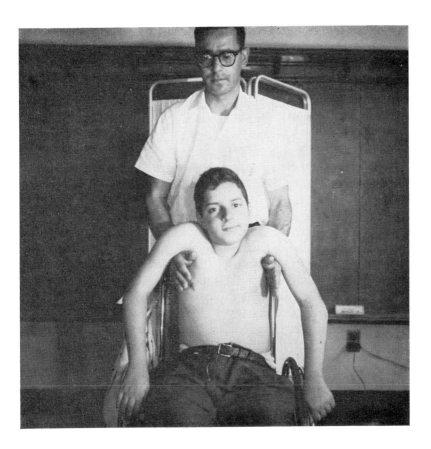

20. Muscular dystrophy. Weakness of shoulder girdle muscle.

gray due to replacement of muscle with fat and fibrous tissue. Microscopically, there is loss of many of the muscle fibres. Large and small muscle fibres are seen with many fat cells, much connective tissue and vacuolar degeneration. Swelling of the muscle fibres appears to precede atrophy. There is an increase in the sarcolemmal nuclei. The nervous system is essentially normal.

LABORATORY: X-ray of the long bones shows narrowing of the shafts and overtubulation of the metaphyses. Bone age may be retarded, and there may be demineralization. The spinal fluid is normal. The creatine in the blood serum (fasting level) is increased in muscular dystrophy and there is marked creatinuria. The creatinine in the blood serum is decreased, which leads to a low urinary creatinine. The phosphorus and calcium in the serum may be increased, chloride and cholesterol decreased. Tests for endocrine dysfunction are normal. Hypoglycemia may be present.

Of these findings, the most significant and constant is the decrease in output of creatinine in the urine. This decreased excretion becomes more marked as muscle wasting progresses. The other important finding is the creatinuria. Neither of these determinations is specific for muscular dystrophy; they are of particular value if other conditions where either of these changes may occur are ruled out. Diminished creatinine output may occur in other causes of muscular wasting such as myotonica atrophica, amyotonia congenita, muscular atrophy secondary to diseases of the central nervous system, and dermatomyositis. Creatinuria may occur in poliomyelitis, familial periodic paralysis, progressive muscular atrophy, and hyperthyroidism, where there is no muscular wasting.

The creatinine coefficient (mg. of creatinine eliminated daily per kg. body weight) of normal boys (six to eleven years) is 17 to 21. In muscular dystrophy the creatinine coefficient is diminished. Normal creatinuria averages about 10 mg. per kg. of body weight per day in boys six to eleven years. In muscular dystrophy there is an excessive output (20 mg.).

There may be an increased serum transaminase level. The normal range is 17 to 55 units, average 35. If cardiac and liver disease can be excluded, the presence of a high serum transaminase level suggests a primary myopathy and probably eliminates a neural etiology. A normal level of transaminase does not rule out muscular dystrophy, but might indicate that the process, if present, is not active. The serum aldolase is also elevated and this is of value diagnostically. The mean normal is 0.4 units. In muscular dystrophy the level averages 3.3 units. The rise has no relation to the degree of muscular involvement or prognosis.

DIAGNOSIS: Muscular dystrophy can usually be differentiated quite satisfactorily by keeping in mind the characteristic features: onset in early childhood but not, as a rule, in infancy; symmetrical, slow, progressive wasting of the muscles; pseudohypertrophy, or atrophy alone without preceding hyperthrophy; absence of sensory changes; heredofamilial background; involvement of proximal muscles rather than distal; method of rising from the floor; and involvement of particular muscle groups such as pelvic and shoulder girdle. Chemically, a diminished creatinine coefficient and marked creatinuria are helpful. Elevated serum aldolase and transaminase levels strongly suggest the diagnosis. Electromyography and muscle biopsy are also useful. Electromyography shows absent fibrillations and low voltage potential. In actual practice variations do occur and a differential diagnosis must be made:

Amyotonia congenita is evident in early infancy.

a) Benign congenital hypotonia. The atonia is unaccompanied by paralysis or atrophy, and is generalized. Muscle biopsy may show some atrophy. The course is not progressive.
b) Progressive forms of amyotonia of unknown etiology.

Werdnig-Hoffman disease is familial. There is marked wasting of the muscles and a reaction of degeneration. The course is progressive and usually fatal.

Polyneuritis. In this condition there may be a history of lead ingestion, infection such as diphtheria, or injection of serum. The etiology may be unknown (Guillain-Barré). The peripheral nerves are involved with paralysis, sensory changes, and marked pain and tenderness in the extremities. The protein in the spinal fluid may be elevated. The infantile form may be a cause of amyotonia congenita.

Poliomyelitis in the later stages is recognized by the history of acute onset and localized type of paralysis.

Neural muscular atrophy can be differentiated by the involvement of the distal muscles of the hands and feet.

Myasthenia gravis shows no muscle atrophy. The response to neostigmine is definite.

Dermatomyositis or polymyositis usually exhibit skin changes, and muscle biopsy shows an inflammatory reaction.

PROGNOSIS: The least favorable outlook is in the common childhood pseudohypertrophic form. Death usually occurs from infection in a debilitated child. These children rarely survive more than ten years after the disease is noted or beyond the age of twenty-one. Other forms progress more slowly and may go on for much longer periods.

TREATMENT: Specific therapy for permanent cure, thus far, has been of no avail, either in the form of vitamin E, glycine, or hormones. Klingman has reported some preliminary encouraging results from the use of adenylic acid (adenosine triphosphate, necessary for muscle contraction, is deficient in muscular dystrophy), thiamine, methionine, choline, and magnesium gluconate.

Adams, R. D., Denny-Brown, D. and Pearson, C. M.: Diseases of Muscle. New York, Paul B. Hoeber, 1953.

Danowski, T. S., Gillespie, H. K., Egan, T. S., Mateer, F. M. and Leinsberger, M. H.: Muscular Dystrophy. A.M.A. J. Dis. Child. 91:429, 1956.

Duchenne, G.: Note sur l'anatomie pathologigne de la pseudohypertrophique dans cinq nouveaux case, Gaz. d. hop Paris, 45:634, 1872.

Erb, W. H.: Ueber die "juvenile form" der progressiven Muskelatrophie ihre Beziehungen Zur sogenannten Pseudohypertrophie der Muskeln. Arch. Klin. Med. 34:467, 1884.

Fetterman, G. H., Wratney, M. J., Donaldson, J. S. and Danowski, T. S.: Muscular Dystrophy. A.M.A. J. Dis. Child. 91:346, 1956.

Klingman, W. O.: Treatment of Heredodegenerative Disorders. Neurology 8:633, 1958.

Landouzy, L. and Dejerine, J.: De la myopathie atrophique progressive; myopathie héréditaire, sans neuropathie, débutant d'ordinaire dans l'enfance, par la face. Rév. de Méd. 5:81-117, 253-366, 1885.

Milhorat, A. T.: Creatine and Creatinine Metabolism and Diseases of the Neuro-Muscular System. A. Res. Publ. Ass. Nerv. Ment. Dis. Proc. 32:400, 1953.

Moebius, P.: Progressive Muskelatrophie mit ungewöhnlichen Beginne, Memorabilien; Helibronn, 1:212, 1881.

Pearson, C. M.: Serum Enzymes in Muscular Dystrophy and Certain Other Muscular and Neuromuscular Diseases. I. Serum Glutamic Oxalacetic Transaminases. New England J. Med. 256:1069, 1957.

Perkoff, G. T. and Tyler, F. H.: The Differential Diagnosis of Progressive Muscular Dystrophy. Med. Clin. North America, W. B. Saunders Co., 1953, p. 545.

Rowland, L. P. and Ross, G.: Serum Aldolase in Muscular Dystrophies, Neuromuscular Disorders, and Wasting of Skeletal Muscle. A.M.A. Arch. Neurol. & Psychiat. 80:157, 1958.

Schapira, G. Dreyfus, J., Schapira, F. and Kruh, J.: Glycogenolytic En-
zymes in Human Progressive Muscular Dystrophy. Proceedings of the
Third Medical Conference of Muscular Dystrophy Association of Amer-
ica, Incorporated, New York. Edited by H. D. Bauman, 324 pp. Balti-
more, William & Wilkins, 1955. (pp. 313-319).
Symposium of Inquiry—What We Need to Know About Muscle: Bennett,
H. S., Szent-Gyorgyi, A., Denny-Brown, D., Adams, R. D.—Moderator:
Rose, A. S. Neurology 8:65, 1958.
Zatuchni, J., Aegerter, E. E., Malthan, L. and Shuman, C. R.: The Heart
in Progressive Muscular Dystrophy. Circulation 3:846, 1951.

CHRONIC PROGRESSIVE EXTERNAL OPHTHALMOPLEGIA
(OCULAR MYOPATHY)

This is a rare disease with an insidious onset which usually begins
in infancy or childhood. It is progressive and involves the ocular
muscles of both eyes. There is a familial history of ptosis or
ophthalmoplegia in half the cases. Ptosis appears early. A complete
external and rarely, an internal ophthalmoplegia follows. Occasionally ophthalmoplegia precedes the onset of ptosis. According to
Kiloh and Nevin, other muscles are involved in twenty-five per cent
of cases. The orbiculares oculi and the muscles of mastication are
especially affected. In ten per cent, the muscles supplied by the
spinal segments become dystrophic.

The course goes on for years with no other complications and a
normal span of life. At any point the progress of the disease may
halt temporarily or completely.

Neurogenic and myogenic causes for ophthalmoplegia have been
postulated. All the authors referred to in the references agree that
chronic progressive external ophthalmoplegia is a form of progressive muscular dystrophy.

Beckett, R. S. and Netsky, M. G.: Familial Ocular Myopathy and External
Ophthalmoplegia. Arch. Neurol. & Psychiat. 69:64, 1953.
Kiloh, L. G. and Nevin, S.: Progressive Dystrophy of the External Ocular
Muscles. (Ocular Myopathy). Brain 74:115, 1951.
Schwarz, G. A. and Liu, Chan-Nao: Chronic Progressive External Oph-
thalmoplegia. Trans. Am. Neurol. Ass. 78:143, 1953.

MYOTONIA ATROPHICA OR MYOTONIC DYSTROPHY

This disease combines myotonia and muscular atrophy. It has
been observed to occur in families and is more common in males.

Along with the myotonia and muscle atrophy, which has a fairly characteristic distribution about the face and neck, there are usually testicular atrophy, baldness, and cataracts.

CLINICAL PICTURE: The onset is usually in adult life, but occasionally cases have been reported which began in childhood. The first manifestation is usually myotonia. This is characterized by failure of relaxation (or persistent state of contraction) immediately following muscle contraction after active motion or mechanical stimulation. The phenomenon is noted following voluntary closing of the fist and shaking hands; there is a delay in opening the hand due to failure of the flexors to relax. The myotonia involves the muscles of mastication, the orbicularis oris, tongue muscles, sternomastoid, and muscles of the trunk and limbs. Percussion will bring out the prolonged and visible contraction of the muscles, especially by striking the thumb, deltoid, or tongue, using a tongue depressor under the latter. As atrophy develops and becomes more extensive, the myotonia begins to disappear.

The other component of the disease is atrophy. This involves the face and neck. The muscles affected include the zygomaticus, levator palpebrae, temporalis, and sternomastoid. There are severe ptosis, blepharoconjunctivitis, and a "myopathic facies." The distal muscles of the extremities become involved, including the hands, extensors of the forearms, and anterior tibial group.

Other features include cataract, which is present early and may be the only abnormality for a time. Also observed are baldness over the frontal region of the scalp, testicular atrophy in the male, early menopause in the female without ovarian involvement, and occasional endocrine dysfunction, such as hypothyroidism. There is no explanation for the paradox of baldness and hypogonadism. There are no sensory or sphincter disturbances. Cutaneous reflexes are intact. The deep tendon reflexes are variable and depend on the degree of muscle wasting. The mental level may be impaired.

LABORATORY: Blood, urine, and spinal fluid are normal. Creatinuria is variable. Radioactive iodine uptake is normal. Electromyography shows a slow relaxation phase.

PATHOLOGY: There is enlargement of the muscle fibres, which are rounded rather than polygonal. There is proliferation of the sarcolemmal nuclei, which are centrally placed in long rows or series. Subsequently, connective tissue and fat cells are evident.

The nervous system is normal. There may be changes in the thyroid and adrenals and atrophy of the androgenic cells of the testes.

ETIOLOGY: The cause is unknown. The condition is inherited, usually as a dominant, but variations occur so that transmission also appears to be recessive. Ancestors in preceding generations will often show one of the defects of the condition, most frequently cataract. Because of the testicular atrophy transmission of the disease by way of the male patient does not usually occur.

DIFFERENTIAL DIAGNOSIS: The features of myotonia and muscular atrophy of a characteristic type, together with cataract, testicular atrophy, and baldness differentiate this condition from progressive muscular dystrophy. The onset at birth and the lack of wasting of the muscles set myotonia congenita (Thomsen's disease) apart.

PROGNOSIS: The course is slowly progressive. In some, at old age, wasting produces a bedridden patient.

TREATMENT: Quinine, two grams a day, given in three divided doses, will relax the myotonia in adults. For children, less drug is used. Some value from cortisone has been reported where myotonia was the predominant symptom; the myotonia was reduced or abolished. Cataracts are treated in the usual surgical manner. Endocrine therapy may be tried.

Adie, W. J. and Greenfield, J. G.: Dystrophia (Myotonia Atrophica). Brain 46:73, 1923.
Caughey, J. E. and Brown, J.: Dystrophia Myotonia: An Endocrine Study. Quart. J. of Med. 19:303, 1950.
Liversedge, L. A. and Newman, M. J. D.: The Treatment of Myotonia. Brain 79:395, 1956.
Wohlfart, G. J.: Dystrophia Myotonia and Myotonia Congenita: Histopathologic Studies with Special Reference to Changes in the Muscles. J. Neuropath. and Exp. Neurol. 10:109, 1951.

MYOTONIA CONGENITA (THOMSEN'S DISEASE)

This disease was described in 1876 by Thomsen, who himself suffered from it. It is a heredofamilial condition found in many members of families through various generations, transmitted primarily as a Mendelian dominant. Occasional recessive, sporadic cases may appear.

CLINICAL PICTURE: The essential feature of Thomsen's disease is myotonia, which appears either in infancy or early childhood. It occurs equally in both sexes and may be transmitted by either. The rare cases in infancy may have difficulty in nursing, or there may be delay in the onset of walking. Most cases are observed in late childhood and during adolescence.

All the skeletal muscles are involved. In the hands there is the same lack of relaxation after a shake as noted in myotonia dystrophica. There is difficulty in beginning to walk after a rest, which often results in stumbling or falling. Continued repetition of the movement, however, does result in relaxation. The upper limbs, facial muscles, and extraocular muscles are also included in the spasms. As mentioned in myotonia dystrophica, percussion of any muscle will set up the spasm, showing the prolonged contraction with failure of relaxation.

The muscles are enlarged and may be hypertrophied. There is never any atrophy. Nor is there any loss of muscle power once the myotonia has been overcome by repeated movement. The tendon reflexes are normal. No contractions occur.

There is no creatinuria, and creatinine output in the urine is normal. Electromyography shows a delay in the onset of relaxation after the initial phase of prolonged contraction.

PATHOLOGY: There is hypertrophy of the muscle fibres. There are no degenerative changes or atrophic fibres. The central nervous system is not involved.

PROGNOSIS: There is no cure, but patients may go on for years with their limitation.

TREATMENT: Quinine is given, two grams per day for adults, in three individual doses. For children, dosage is proportionately reduced.

There is a question whether Thomsen's disease (myotonia congenita) should be considered as a monosymptomatic form of myotonia dystrophica. Those who feel that Thomsen's is a separate entity point out that the usual age of onset is earlier, the muscle distribution is more widespread, and that there are neither muscle atrophy nor associated features such as cataract, testicular atrophy, or baldness.

Those who favor inclusion of Thomsen's disease under myotonia dystrophica state that the classical differentials are only textbook descriptions and that the individual patient has features of both. Most cases beginning as Thomsen's end up as dystrophica. The remainder may be considered variants with only one form of the major disease of myotonic dystrophy.

Paramyotonia, a name given to those cases of myotonia developing with exposure of the muscle to cold, probably does not exist as a separate classification, but is seen in Thomsen's and myotonia dystrophica. However, Drager and his associates have recently reported a pedigree with paramyotonia as a separate clinical entity.

Drager, G. A., Hammill, J. F., Shy, G. M.: Paramyotonia Congenita. A.M.A. Arch. Neurol. and Psychiat. 80:1, 1958.

Maas, O and Paterson, A. S.: Myotonia Congenita, Dystrophia Myotonica and Paramyotonia. Brain, 73:318, 1950.

Thomasen, E.: Myotonia, Thomsen's Disease, Paramyotonia and Dystrophia Myotonica. A Clinical and Heredobiologic Investigation. Denmark, Aarhus, Universitets Forlaget i, 1:257, 1948.

CHAPTER 19

VASCULAR DISORDERS

Intracranial Aneurysms

The effects of congenital and other types of aneurysms are noted most often in the older age periods, only rarely in infancy and childhood. However, instances have been reported as early as one and one-half and two years of age. McDonald and Korb in their series of 1,125 cases of intracranial aneurysms reported only eleven per cent under twenty years of age. Hamby has grouped a number of reports on intracranial aneurysms which indicate that eighty-three per cent occur in the anterior or carotid segment of the Circle of Willis, and that seventeen per cent are in the posterior or vertebral segment. About fifteen per cent of aneurysms are multiple.

PATHOLOGY: Miliary aneurysms are due to atheromas of the media. Mycotic aneurysms are related to septic emboli, secondary to endocarditis. Trauma and syphilis are rare causes. Arteriosclerosis is a contributing factor. Congenital (saccular or berry) aneurysms are the result of congenital weakness of the vessel wall. The media is improperly developed and the defect occurs at a bifurcation in the Circle of Willis. The elastic membrane may be intact or absent. Intracranial aneurysms may be associated with other congenital anomalies such as coarctation of the aorta or polycystic kidney.

CLINICAL PICTURE: There are many aneurysms so small that they give no symptoms or trouble. When they do produce clinical disturbance, it is due to the effects of pressure by the aneurysm directly on nerve structures or brain tissue (local effects) and/or to the rupture or leakage of blood from the aneurysm into the subarachnoid space (subarachnoid hemorrhage). Finally, depending on the pathology, there may be the features of the original disease process which resulted in the aneurysm.

The most common focal signs occur with involvement of the third nerve, including pain in the eye, ptosis, dilatation of the pupil, and external strabismus, associated with aneurysm of the internal carotid artery in the carotid canal and the intracranial portion before it branches. Next in frequency to the third nerve is involvement of the sixth. Exophthalmos may occur when there is an aneurysm in the cavernous sinus. There are also visual disturbances consisting mainly of blindness due to compression of the optic nerve. Compression in the region of the optic chiasm by the intracranial carotid artery may produce contralateral or bitemporal hemianopia plus reduction in visual acuity. Compression of the hypothalamus may produce symptoms of diabetes insipidus. Aneurysms of the posterior segment of the Circle of Willis are much less common. They may give signs of compression when they involve the basilar and vertebral arteries. There may be convulsions, hemiplegia, and cranial nerve palsies, including bulbar palsy. Involvement of the middle cerebral artery in the Sylvian fissure may also produce convulsions, and rarely hemiplegia.

Rupture or leakage of blood into the subarachnoid space, "spontaneous subarachnoid hemorrhage," produces a sudden onset of symptoms. There is headache, a throbbing sensation, or pain in the back of the head. As a result of the subarachnoid hemorrhage, intracranial pressure is raised. The blood also acts as an irritant to produce signs of meningeal irritation. These include pain and stiffness of the neck, Kernig's sign, convulsions, loss of consciousness, and elevated blood pressure. The temperature is raised. Retinal "sub-hyaloid" hemorrhages may be noted. Cranial nerve palsies, especially third and fifth, may occur in the presence of hemorrhage. With involvement of the cortex there may be local signs of hemiplegia, variable reflexes and a Babinski sign.

LABORATORY: The spinal fluid is bloody when the rupture of the aneurysm has just occurred. As the days go by the deep red appearance is replaced by xanthochromia; finally, the fluid is completely clear. The pressure is elevated, and there may be an increase in mononuclear cells due to meningeal irritation, elevated protein, and a positive Pandy.

Following the initial rupture of the aneurysm the clinical course may be of several types. Some die in coma, which usually means a large vessel is involved. Others recover from the initial attack of coma, react temporarily showing confusion, and then relapse into coma and death a few days later, probably due to a second rupture. Still others regain consciousness, have some mental disorientation, low grade fever, headache, and local signs such as loss of visual acuity and paralysis of the third nerve. The general signs clear up rapidly, and after a few months the local signs clear as well.

When other disease processes are operating, as in a mycotic aneurysm secondary to endocarditis or in the case of coarctation of the aorta, there will be associated symptoms and signs.

DIAGNOSIS: A lumbar puncture with evidence of hemorrhage into the spinal fluid should eliminate meningitis and the encephalitides. Brain tumor may produce hemorrhage into the subarachnoid space, but there is usually a preceding history of severe headache, vomiting, and papilledema prior to the sudden onset of hemorrhage. With aneurysm the child is well until the sudden advent of the catastrophe. Trauma to the head is usually recognized by the history, signs of injury, and X-ray evidence of fracture. A history of endocarditis should suggest the possibility of a mycotic aneurysm secondary to septic emboli. In this case there may be fever, a positive blood culture, and carditis. The onset of the clinical picture is likely to be sudden, with hemiplegia. Coarctation of the aorta may be associated with the rupture of a cerebral aneurysm. In coarctation the blood pressure is elevated in the upper extremities and low in the legs (reverse of normal). The child may have had previous complaints of headache, epistaxis, a systolic murmur over the back, and absent femoral or dorsalis pedis pulsations. X-ray may show an enlarged heart, and notched ribs due to the increased pressure in the intercostal arteries. The electrocardiogram shows left axis deviation. Aortograms show narrowing at the isthmus. Because of the resultant increased pressure in the carotids and circle of Willis, a congenital aneurysm may rupture. Carotid angiography will demonstrate the aneurysm. Where necessary, ventriculography should be done to rule out tumor.

PROGNOSIS: The mortality following the first attack, as reported in different series, is about thirty per cent. In the three weeks following the initial onset, the mortality rises to about fifty-seven per cent due to recurrences of leakage. Of the remainder, the prognosis becomes increasingly good if recurrences do not occur within five years; most of these may carry on free of trouble, if there is no underlying disease process.

TREATMENT:

1. Absolute rest in bed for about eight weeks. Constipation and straining should be avoided (saline enemas). Use passive exercise.

2. Lumbar puncture on admission. It may be repeated to keep the patient comfortable and to reduce gradually the intracranial pressure, especially when severe headache and restlessness are present. This routine is controversial.
3. Angiography within two weeks to localize the aneurysm.
4. Surgical approach is extracranial ligation of the common or internal carotid or direct attack on the aneurysmal sac by "clipping the neck" or trapping the aneurysm with clips applied to the parent trunk on either side. The latter is used for an anterior cerebral aneurysm. Recently operations have been done under hypothermia, which permits prompter and more direct surgery. This should result in lower mortality rates.

A Classification and Outline of Cerebrovascular Diseases. Neurology 8:395, 1958.

Baumann, C. H. H. and Bucy, P. C.: Aneurysms on the Anterior Cerebral Artery. Evaluation of Surgical and "Conservative" Treatment. J.A.M.A. 163:1448, 1957.

Botterell, E. H., Lougheed, W. M., Morley, T. P. and Vanderwater, S. L.: Hypothermia in the Surgical Treatment of Ruptured Intracranial Aneurysms. J. Neurosurg. 15:4, 1958.

DeKaban, A. and McEachern, D.: Subarachnoid Hemorrhage, Intracerebral Hemorrhage and Intracranial Aneurysms. Arch. Neurol. & Psychiat. 67:641, 1952.

Ecker, A. and Riemenschneider, P. A.: Angiographic Localization of Intracranial Masses. Springfield, Ill., Chas. C. Thomas, 1955.

Forster, F. M. and Alpers, B. J.: Anatomical Defects and Pathological Changes in Congenital Cerebral Aneurysms. J. Neuropath. and Exper. Neurol. 4:146, 1945.

Graf, C. J.: The Modern Treatment of Ruptured Nonfistulous Intracranial Aneurysm. New York State J. Med. 56:3132, 1956.

Hamby, W. B.: Intracranial Aneurysms. Springfield, Ill., Chas. C. Thomas, 1952.

McDonald, C. A. and Korb, M.: Intracranial Aneurysms. Arch. Neurol. & Psychiat. 42:298, 1939.

Walker, A. E.: Clinical Localization of Intracranial Aneurysms and Vascular Anomalies. Neurology 6:79, 1956.

ARTERIOVENOUS ANEURYSMS

The essential feature of the arteriovenous aneurysm or fistula is that arterial blood enters the venous system without passing through a capillary bed.

PATHOLOGY: Arteriovenous fistulae involve the vessels of the brain itself, in contrast to the saccular aneurysms, which involve arteries outside the brain. These anomalies affect the surface of the brain and also penetrate into the tissue. They are made up of coils of blood, arterial and venous, the latter containing arterial blood, without intervening capillaries. The large artery supplying the mass of coils is usually of greater than normal size. It enters a mass of loops, usually below the surface of the brain, made up of arterial-venous channels which finally connect with other loops of veins. The shape of the mass from the surface downward is that of a cone. The veins receiving the arterial blood are likely to be engorged and dilated. Evidence of hemorrhage is often found; thrombosis is rare. There are strands of brain tissue (glia) between the loops. These aneurysms are most often situated in the region of the middle cerebral artery.

CLINICAL PICTURE: A number of reports have indicated that clinical onsets are not infrequent within the first decade of life. One of the most common early symptoms is a focal seizure. This may spread to other parts of the body (Jacksonian type). There is often associated transient paralysis of the extremity involved in the convulsion. A sudden hemiplegia with increased reflexes may occur due to cerebral hemorrhage. In some, the onset is associated with symptoms and signs of subarachnoid hemorrhage, including sudden headache, vomiting, neck stiffness with pain, seizure, and loss of consciousness. Unilateral exophthalmos may be found in conjunction with a fistula over the mastoid region; it appears on the same side and may be accompanied by a thrill and bruit. Bruits are often heard during systole in cases of arteriovenous fistula and are accentuated with the heart beat. There may be symptoms suggestive of brain tumor, such as headache and vomiting combined with papilledema. Hydrocephalus is present in some, due to obstruction of the aqueduct by pressure. Arteriovenous fistulae may be noted in the retina associated with proptosis of the eye, bruit, and nevi over the face. There may be fistulae involving the midbrain and cerebellum. These are associated with facial nevi, mental changes including lowering of the mental level, and psychic disturbances.

LABORATORY: There may be evidence in the X-ray of increased vascular markings in the skull and calcification. Encephalography and ventriculography show distortion of the ventricles and brain atrophy. Angiography of the internal carotid artery is valuable because it outlines the situation for surgery.

DIAGNOSIS: The major diagnostic points are the presence of recurring seizures, especially of a focal or Jacksonian type, and

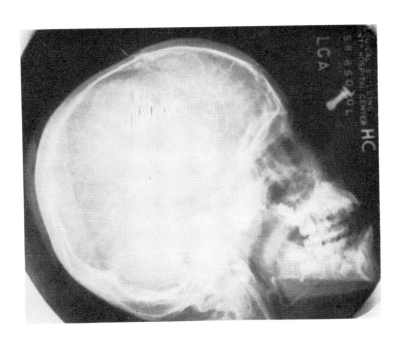

21. Arteriovenous malformation. Early filling of large veins in the arterial phase of injection.

the sudden onset of hemiplegia. There may be localizing signs with intracerebral hemorrhage. In others, the picture is one of spontaneous subarachnoid hemorrhage. When present, bruit, other vascular anomalies of the face and scalp, and calcium deposits in the skull are helpful. Arteriography will demonstrate the arteriovenous aneurysm. It should be performed as quickly as possible.

TREATMENT: Surgical excision of the mass is the best procedure and should be attempted when there are frequent seizures resulting in brain destruction. Generally the results are unsatisfactory.

Anderson, F. M. and Korbin, M. A.: Arteriovenous Anomalies of the Brain. Neurology 8:89, 1958.

Cushing, H. and Bailey, P.: Tumors Arising from the Blood Vessels of the Brain. Springfield, Ill., Chas. C. Thomas, 1928.

Dandy, W. E.: Arteriovenous Aneurysm of Brain. Arch. Surg. 17:190, 1928.

Hamby, W. B.: Intracranial Aneurysms. Springfield, Ill., Chas. C. Thomas, 1952.

Olivecrona, H. and Riives, J.: Arteriovenous Aneurysms of the Brain, Their Diagnosis and Treatment. Arch. Neurol. & Psychiat. 59:567, 1948.

Silverman, B. K., Breckx, T., Craig, J. and Nadas, A. S.: Congestive Failure in the Newborn Caused by Cerebral A-V Fistula. Clinical and Pathological Report of Two Cases. A.M.A. J. Dis. Child. 89:539, 1955.

Ward, C. E. and Horton, B. T.: Congenital Arteriovenous Fistulas in Children. J. Pediat. 16:746, 1940.

Wyburn-Mason, R.: Arteriovenous Aneurysm of Midbrain and Retina, Facial Naevi and Mental Changes. Brain 66:12, 1943.

VENOUS ANGIOMAS

These congenital malformations involve the venous blood vessels of the brain and carry venous blood. They may lie superficially or penetrate deep into the cortex. They may be single or multiple. They have been described as simple varices, serpentine, racemose, or plexiform. Others are cavernous in type, with numerous vascular venous channels occupying large areas of the cortex. These channels are thin walled, nonpulsating, and markedly dilated.

The clinical picture includes recurrent seizures, usually focal in character and occurring early in life, hemiplegia, and hemianopia. As with arteriovenous fistulae, there may be hemorrhage into the cerebral substance or subarachnoid space with the clinical features previously described, due to increased intracranial pressure and meningeal irritation. Thrombosis of the channels may occur. There are no bruits. There may be associated port wine stains or nevi on the face.

LABORATORY: X-ray may show calcification of the vessels.

DIAGNOSIS: Convulsions and hemiplegia in the absence of any obvious cause should bring up a consideration of venous angioma. Angiography should be performed.

PROGNOSIS: If convulsions are recurrent, there may be mental deterioration. If no surgery can be done, the seizures should be treated as recommended under epilepsy.

TREATMENT: Removal, if possible, is the procedure of choice.

TELANGIECTASES

These are vascular angiomatous malformations arising from the blood vessels of the brain, similar in many respects to the venous angioma, but consisting of a collection of dilated capillaries. They may be present in any part of the brain or spinal cord, especially in the upper part of the pons. The vessels are usually of small calibre with a thin-walled endothelial lining, but may at times have a cavernous appearance. There may be associated angiomas in the face, eyes, liver, bones, kidneys, and adrenals.

CLINICAL PICTURE: The essential features are recurrent focal seizures, contralateral hemiplegia, and mental impairment. A special type (Sturge-Weber syndrome) has been described. The calcification of the skull is characteristic in this condition (X-ray).

DIAGNOSIS: A combination of the above features should suggest the diagnosis.

PROGNOSIS: The outlook is poor.

TREATMENT: Remove the angioma if possible.

VASCULAR MALFORMATIONS OF THE SPINAL CORD

Vascular anomalies of the spinal cord are rarely seen in children. As in the vascular malformations of the brain, there may be congenital venous angiomas, arteriovenous fistulae, telangiectases, and arterial aneurysms. Males are mostly affected. The racemose angioma is the most common vascular anomaly of the spinal cord.

PATHOLOGY: The vascular anomaly, usually thoracic or lumbar, may produce pressure on the spinal cord with subsequent softening and necrosis. In some, rupture of the vessel occurs. As bleeding increases, cord compression develops.

CLINICAL PICTURE: With rupture the onset is sudden, with pain in the abdomen radiating down the legs. There are usually short attacks of recurrent pain and weakness in the legs preceding the major attack. Spastic paraplegia follows. With the passage of time, flaccid paralysis, atrophy of the muscles, loss of tendon reflexes, and sphincter disturbances develop. There is sensory dissociation with loss of pain and temperature and preservation of touch.

LABORATORY: The spinal fluid is xanthochromic and has a high protein content, with few or no cells. A spinal fluid block may be present. Rarely the fluid may contain frank blood. In hematomyelia secondary to an intramedullary angioma, the spinal fluid may be clear, but protein is elevated and there is a block. Myelography will indicate the level of the vascular anomaly.

DIAGNOSIS: A history of a sudden catastrophe of the type described above and the characteristic spinal fluid should suggest a vascular malformation of the spinal cord. Myelography will confirm the diagnosis. This abnormality must be differentiated from intramedullary tumor of the spinal cord, acute myelitis, spinal arachnoiditis, and Pott's disease. The arterial anomalies may be associated with coarctation of the aorta, patent ductus, or aneurysm of the cerebral arteries. Telangiectasias in the cord may be associated with others in the pons and cortex. The presence of skin nevi, especially in the same dermatome as the level of the spinal cord lesion, aids in the diagnosis.

PROGNOSIS: The outlook is poor for recovery.

TREATMENT: It is not possible to correct the anomaly surgically.

Brion, S., Netsky, M. G. and Zimmerman, H. M.: Vascular Malformations of the Spinal Cord. Arch. Neurol. and Psychiat. 68:339, 1952.
Buchanan, D. N. and Walker, E. A.: Vascular Anomalies of the Spinal Cord in Children. Am. J. Dis. Child. 61:928, 1941.
Odom, G. L., Woodhall, B. and Margolis, G.: Spontaneous Hematomyelia and Angiomas of the Spinal Cord. J. Neurosurg. 14:192, 1957.
Wyburn-Mason, R.: The Vascular Abnormalities and Tumors of the Spinal Cord and Its Membranes, London, Henry Kimpton, 1943.

CEREBRAL EMBOLISM AND THROMBOSIS

Embolism and thrombosis of the cerebral vessels in childhood occur in certain conditions which have been referred to elsewhere, e.g., hemorrhagic encephalitis, periarteritis nodosa, lupus erythematosus, and acute infantile hemiplegia (Strümpell). In the adult, arteriosclerosis is the major factor in thrombosis. This is, however, of little importance in childhood.

Thrombosis and embolism of the cerebral vessels occur in children most frequently in relation to infection and congenital heart disease. Rarely, trauma plays a role in introducing fat embolism following a bone fracture, or air embolism following cardiac catheterization or lung puncture.

In infancy, infections such as meningitis and septicemia, birth trauma, and hemorrhagic disease in the newborn will produce vascular occlusion, cerebral hemorrhage, and encephalomalacia. Acute endocarditis is a rare cause. This may be present with or without congenital or rheumatic heart disease. The common organisms are the streptococcus and pneumococcus. Another rare factor is subacute bacterial endocarditis due to streptococcus viridans, which attacks either congenital or acquired heart lesions.

The smaller cerebral vessels are involved with septic emboli and thrombosis. In addition, infection of the wall of the vessel with the development of a mycotic aneurysm may occur.

Congenital heart disease, especially the cyanotic type, can be associated with thrombosis and embolism of the cerebral vessels. Thrombosis results from the polycythemia and increased viscosity and from stagnation of the blood stream. Cerebral infarction follows. A picture of transverse myelopathy due to occlusion of the anterior spinal artery may occasionally be seen.

PATHOLOGY: In conjunction with the development of thrombosis or embolism of the cerebral vessels, the surrounding brain tissue undergoes varying degrees of necrosis due to ischemia. Emboli may be sterile or septic, the latter resulting in brain abscess.

CLINICAL PICTURE: The symptoms and signs are in part those of the underlying disease process. In congenital heart disease they will depend on the type of abnormality, e.g., patent ductus, coarctation of the aorta, tetralogy of Fallot, etc. There is a high incidence of aneurysm of the Circle of Willis with coarctation. If there is endocarditis, fever, chills, anemia, petechiae, and cardiac signs may be present.

There are also manifestations of the cerebral accident. These may begin with a convulsion, paralysis, and loss of speech. Depending on the areas involved there are evidences of hemiplegia, cranial nerve palsies, visual difficulties, and hemianopia. Extension of the pathology is indicated by signs of brain abscess, meningitis, or subarachnoid hemorrhage.

LABORATORY: The spinal fluid is normal unless embolism or thrombosis is complicated by meningeal infection or subarachnoid hemorrhage.

DIAGNOSIS: In children, cerebral vascular disturbance is to be considered when there is congenital heart disease, rheumatic carditis, or endocarditis, associated with symptoms and signs of a cerebral accident.

The location of the vascular accident will determine the clinical picture. It seems pointless to describe the syndromes associated with the specific involvement of each cerebral artery. It has been pointed out that children do not follow textbook pictures in their clinical behavior. Arteriograms will aid in localization.

THERAPY AND PROGNOSIS: The advances being made in cardiac surgery, and the use of chemotherapy and antibiotic drugs have all but eliminated the complications of embolism and thrombosis of the cerebral vessels. The prognosis when these complications do occur is poor if the underlying cardiac anomaly is not amenable to correction or is combined with anomalies of the cerebral vascular tree. If there is no contraindication, an anticoagulant (Dicumarol) and a vasodilator (nicotinic acid) may aid in recovery. Oxygen is also of value.

Berthrong, M. and Sabiston Jr., D. C.: Cerebral Lesions in Congenital Heart Disease. Bull. Johns Hopkins Hosp. 89:384, 1951.

Cabieses, F. and Saldias, C.: Thrombosis of the Internal Carotid in a Child. Neurology 6:677, 1956.

Gelfman, R. and Levine, S. A.: The Incidence of Acute and Subacute Bacterial Endocarditis in Congenital Heart Disease. Am. J. Med. Sc. 204:324, 1942.

Goldstein, S. L. and Burgess, J. P.: Spontaneous Thrombosis of the Internal Carotid Artery in a Seven-Year-Old Child. A.M.A. J. Dis. Child. 95:538, 1958.

Gross, R. E.: Arterial Embolism and Thrombosis in Infancy. Am. J. Dis. Child. 70:61, 1945.

Lindquist, B.: Syndrome of the Anterior Spinal Artery. Acta Paediat. 46:380, 1957.

Tyler, H. R. and Clark, D. B.: Incidence of Neurologic Complications in Congenital Heart Disease. A.M.A. Arch. Neurol. & Psychiat. 77:17, 1957.

HYPERTENSION

In childhood, hypertension, especially the malignant form, plays a great role in developing the clinical picture of vascular disease, with manifestations especially in the heart and kidney, but also in the brain, gastrointestinal tract, and adrenals. Hypertension in children may be associated with many factors:

a. Essential—no cause is found. This does not occur often in children.
b. Renal disease—This is most frequent in childhood. There may be glomerulonephritis, polycystic kidneys, tumors, and particularly congenital abnormalities of the genitourinary system including unilateral vascular aberrations.
c. Coarctation of the aorta or patent ductus.
d. Increased intracranial pressure.
e. Hyperthyroidism.
f. Pheochromocytoma.
g. Cushing's Disease
h. Periarteritis nodosa
i. Acrodynia and lead poisoning.

PATHOLOGY: The small arteries and arterioles show changes. The media is hypertrophied, the intima thickened; necrosis may occur in the arterioles resulting in expansion of the wall and closing of the lumen, causing ischemia. The brain shows evidence of ischemia in the form of softening, hemorrhage, and atrophy.

CLINICAL PICTURE: The onset may occur at any time in late childhood, but the average age is ten years. The major symptoms are severe headache and vomiting. The average blood pressure is 230/160. There is usually papilledema, and visual disturbances are frequent. Albuminuric retinitis with thickened retinal arteries and hemorrhages is noted. Convulsions occur, sometimes associated with hemiplegia. Aphasia may follow. Other organs are involved, resulting in hematuria and albuminuria, blood in the stool and vomitus, marked abdominal pain, and an enlarged heart.

LABORATORY: There are urinary changes and nitrogen retention. The spinal fluid is normal except for elevated pressure.

DIAGNOSIS: The cause of the hypertension must be determined. Each of the possibilities listed should be considered.

PROGNOSIS: Generally the outlook is poor. Death follows in a few years due to uremia, heart failure, or cerebral hemorrhage.

TREATMENT: Therapy depends on the etiological factor. Mild sedation is utilized. (Refer to the article of Haggerty and associates.)

Court, D.: Malignant Hypertension in Childhood. Arch. Dis. Child. 16:132, 1941.
Fisher, C. M.: Clinical Picture of Cerebral Arteriosclerosis, part of a Symposium on Arteriosclerosis by Minnesota Heart Assoc. and Univ. of Minn. (Edited by Ancel Keys), Reprinted from Minnesota Medicine, 38:731-808, and 829-935, 1955.
Haggerty, R. J., Maroney, M. W. and Nadas, A. S.: Essential Hypertension in Infancy and Childhood: Differential Diagnosis and Therapy. A.M.A. J. Dis. Child. 92:535, 1956.
Pickering, G. W.: The Pathogenesis of Malignant Hypertension. Circulation 6:599, 1952.

BLOOD DISORDERS

HEMOPHILIA

The central nervous system is rarely affected. Occasional signs of intracranial hemorrhage and bleeding into and around the spinal cord have been reported. In some instances the bleeding has occurred into the brain stem and ventricles. Peripheral nerve lesions are more common. They are caused by hemorrhages into the joints or muscles which involve nerves like the ulnar, peroneal, or femoral.

DIAGNOSIS: The diagnosis of hemophilia is based on the history of bleeding in a male, with delay in coagulation time and reduced prothrombin consumption. The neurological picture of a peripheral nerve lesion or intracranial hemorrhage is recognized as a complication.

TREATMENT: Blood or plasma is transfused to stop bleeding. Physical therapy is used to avoid contractures with joint involvement and peripheral nerve complications.

Davidson, C. S., Epstein, R. D., Miller, G. F., and Taylor, F. H. L.: Hemophilia. A Clinical Study of Forty Patients. Blood 4:97, 1949.
Schulman, I. and Currimbhoy, Z.: Hemorrhagic Disorders. Pediat. Clin. N. A. W. B. Saunders Co. p. 531, May 1957.

ANEMIA

In adults the major neurological disturbances occur in pernicious anemia. There is diffuse degeneration of the white matter of the spinal cord, brain, and peripheral nerves due to B_{12} deficiency. In children, this form of anemia is exceptional. The most common type is associated with infection. In addition, there are forms secondary to dietary insufficiency and prematurity, hereditary forms such as sickle cell anemia, and those due to blood loss.

Of all the anemias, sickle cell disease is most likely to have neurological complications because of the common occurrence of vascular thromboses due to the high viscosity of the sickled erythrocytes. Clinically, the onset is acute, and there may be convulsive seizures with hemiplegia. Rowland reported that in 92 cases of sickle cell anemia, 27, or 29 per cent, had neurological complications. In five instances, signs of meningeal irritation were the only manifestation of a sickle crisis. Three others had a spastic hemiplegia. The diagnosis depends on the presence of signs of an acute cerebral vascular disorder in a negro child with evidence of sickling in the blood smear. Since these attacks occur during a crisis, the treatment is transfusion.

Rowland, L. P.: Neurological Manifestations in Sickle Cell Disease. J. Nerv. & Ment. Dis. 115:456, 1952.

PURPURA

Hemorrhage in the brain occurs occasionally, and may be brought on by mild trauma. It takes the form of large masses of blood in the cortex or in the subarachnoid and subdural spaces. Petechial hemorrhages are also present.

As a result of the hemorrhage, the child may develop seizures, loss of consciousness, and paralyses. In other instances hemorrhages in the brain stem may lead to decerebrate rigidity. Subarachnoid hemorrhage causes the sudden onset of headache, vomiting, papilledema, and signs of meningeal irritation.

LABORATORY: In the thrombocytopenic type there is a diminution in the number of platelets, coagulation time is normal, bleeding time is increased, clot retraction is poor, prothrombin consumption is decreased, and a positive tourniquet test is present.

DIAGNOSIS: The neurological picture is recognized as a complication of the purpura. A differential diagnosis must be made among the thrombocytopenic forms of purpura, including those secondary to specific diseases. Of the latter, the most important are leukemia, aplastic anemia, and diseases of the spleen. Other factors producing purpura should be considered. These include drugs, chemicals, toxins, anaphylactoid purpura, acute infections, scurvy, and hemophilia.

COURSE AND PROGNOSIS: The outlook is variable depending on the type of purpura and the cause. In the thrombotic thrombocytopenic form the course is fatal. In the idiopathic thrombocytopenic type the disease lasts several months and usually ends in recovery, especially in the two to eight year group.

TREATMENT:

1. Cortisone and ACTH provide remissions.
2. Transfusions.
3. Splenectomy in severe cases that do not respond to medical therapy.

Adams, R. D., Cammermeyer, J., and Fitzgerald, P. J.: The Neuropathological Aspects of Thrombocytic Acroangiothrombosis. J. Neurol. Neurosurg. and Psychiat. 11:27, 1948.
Clement, D. H. and Diamond, L. K.: Purpura in Infants and Children. Am. J. Dis. Child. 85:259, 1953.
Lewis, I. C. and Philpott, M. G.: Neurologic Complications in Schönlein-Henoch Syndrome. Arch. Dis. Child. 31:369, 1956.
Mills, S. D.: Purpura in Childhood. J. Pediat. 49:396, 1956.
O'Brien, J. L. and Sibley, W. A.: Neurologic Manifestations of Thrombotic Thrombocytopenic Purpura. Neurology 8:55, 1957.

LEUKEMIA

Leukemia may involve the central nervous system. In childhood it appears most often as an acute disease. Irrespective of type, the leukemic cells infiltrate the brain and cord. The leukemic foci probably arise locally in the brain and are not blood borne.

PATHOLOGY: The brain may show intracranial hemorrhage. There may be infiltration of the meninges, cranial nuclei, and cranial nerves with leukemic cells. In the spinal cord there may occur localized or diffuse leukocytic infiltrations. When the spinal meninges are infiltrated there is compression of the cord with resultant softening. Hemorrhages may also occur in the cord. The nerve roots and peripheral nerves may likewise become infiltrated.

CLINICAL PICTURE: The clinical manifestations may include sudden death, convulsions, or hemiplegia. In others there are cranial nerve paralyses, especially the sixth and seventh nerves, with external rectus and facial paralysis. There may be paralysis of the lower extremities and loss of deep tendon reflexes with cord involvement. The clinical signs and spinal fluid may resemble those of acute bacterial meningitis. Although intracranial pathology is common in leukemia, related neurological symptoms were not frequently reported in the past. With the use of adrenal steroid hormones and chemotherapy, Sullivan reported that about twenty-five per cent of the children followed in her hospital developed signs of increased intracranial pressure (headache, vomiting, papilledema, suture separation). The spinal fluid pressure was increased; there were elevated protein and normal or low sugar. The pathogenesis of this syndrome is unknown.

LABORATORY: If there is meningeal irritation, the spinal fluid shows increased numbers of cells, increased pressure, elevation of protein, and low sugar. X-ray may show destruction of bone in the skull or spine, with collapse of vertebral bodies.

DIAGNOSIS: This is based on involvement of the nervous system in the presence of known leukemia. Bacterial meningitis should be ruled out.

TREATMENT: The complications of increased intracranial pressure should be treated by X-ray therapy to the entire skull. Aminopterin intrathecally and adrenal steroid hormones orally may also be tried.

Boss, M. H.: Leukemia in Children, with Special Reference to Lesions in the Nervous System. Amer. J. Med. Sc. 162:647, 1921.
Critchley, M. and Greenfield, J. G.: Spinal Symptoms in Chloroma and Leukemia. Brain 53:11, 1930.
Gilbert, E. F. and Rice, E. C.: Neurologic Manifestations of Leukemia. Report of Three Cases in Children Simulating Acute Bacterial Meningitis. Pediat. 19:801, 1957.
Schwab, R., and Weiss, S.: The Neurologic Aspect of Leukemia. Am. J. Med. Sc. 189:766, 1935.
Sullivan, M. P.: Intracranial Complications of Leukemia in Children. Pediat. 20:757, 1957.

HODGKIN'S DISEASE

In Hodgkin's disease the spinal cord and brain are rarely invaded. However, the granulomatous lesions do invade the dura, so that pressure phenomena may be present. Jackson and Parker reported 174 cases associated with nervous system involvement. Of these, nine showed paralysis of the legs; seven flaccid, two spastic, due to spinal cord disturbance. In three of their cases the brain was invaded, including the cerebellum and brain stem. Various types of pathology may involve the spinal cord, e.g., pressure from epidural and subdural deposits, vertebral lesions, and pressure on the blood vessels and lymphatics due to tumors in adjacent lymph nodes. The peripheral nerves are frequently involved, producing abdominal pain or herpes zoster. The meninges may be invaded with symptoms and signs of meningitis and increase of cells in the spinal fluid.

The diagnosis is made in the presence of nervous system pathology associated with Hodgkin's disease.

The outlook is poor. X-ray therapy may be given.

Diamond, H. D.: Hodgkin's Disease: Neurologic Sequelae. Missouri Med. 54:945, 1957.
Hutchinson, E. C., Leonard, B. J., Maudsley, C., and Yates, P. O.: Neurological Complications of the Reticuloses. Brain 81:75, 1958.
Jackson Jr., H. and Parker Jr., F.: Hodgkins Disease: Involvement of Certain Other Organs. New England J. Med. 233:369, 1945.

CHAPTER 20

ENDOCRINE GLANDS

CONGENITAL HYPOTHYROIDISM

Congenital hypothyroidism or cretinism is usually due to absence of the thyroid gland. In some instances there may be a slight rudimentary gland present, which is non-functioning. The cause of the embryonic defect is unknown. This condition is referred to as sporadic athyrotic cretinism. Occasionally there are other types of congenital hypothyroidism. In one, also sporadic, the thyroid gland is present and capable of taking up iodine but is unable to produce thyroid hormone; goiter may be present. A third type is endemic cretinism, due to a prenatal, iodine nutritional deficiency. Since the thyroid hormone influences body development and mental level, its absence in these various forms of cretinism accounts for the clinical picture.

CLINICAL PICTURE: The sporadic cretin may be recognized at birth. More often a period of one or two months elapses before the characteristic features appear or are recognized. The early symptoms are difficulties in feeding, marked sluggishness, and lethargy. The skin is pale and dry, with cool, mottled extremities. The forehead is low, there is a broad nasal bridge, and the eyes are widely separated. Later there are puffiness of the face and thick lips, tongue, and hair. Intestinal inactivity with constipation and umbilical hernia are associated with the poor muscle tone, which also causes a protuberant abdomen. There are circulatory changes with subnormal temperatures and slow pulse. Closure of the fontanels is delayed. Signs of retardation in development occur. There is marked diminution in stature, with a large head and short extremities. Bone development, including dentition, is delayed. The voice is hoarse. Sexual maturation is retarded. There is marked mental deficiency, including slowness in the onset of speech and walking. Other

423

evidences of cerebral dysfunction may be present in cretins, including tremor, lack of coordination, spasticity, and hyperactive reflexes.

LABORATORY:

A. X-ray
  1. Delayed osseous development (disproportion between chronological age and bone age—retarded epiphyseal centers).
  2. Epiphyseal dysgenesis—multiple irregular islets of ossification in the cartilages of the epiphyses ("stippled epiphyses"—Wilkins).
B. Basal metabolic rate is decreased.
C. Cholesterol level of serum is usually elevated (N 125-250 mg./100 ml.) Rise after withdrawal of thyroid or fall with its administration is presumptive evidence of hypothyroidism.
D. Protein-bound iodine level of the serum (PBI) is decreased (N 4-8 mcg./100 ml.).
E. Butanol-extractible iodine (BEI) of the serum is decreased (N 4.5-7.3 mcg./100 ml.).
F. Radioactive iodine (I^{131}) uptake is diminished with absence of the gland (N uptake 10-40 per cent in 24 hours).
G. Plasma chromatograph analysis for thyroid hormone.

Of these tests, the X-ray and serum PBI or BEI are most valuable for early diagnosis. The I^{131} uptake is of value in detection of the athyrotic type. The plasma chromatographic analysis will reveal the defect of hormone synthesis in the goitrous type.

Comment on Types. Sporadic athyrotic cretinism is a congenital condition, cause unknown, but there is a suggestion that it is due to environmental factors acting on the fetus in utero, since four sets of monozygotic twins with discordance have been reported.

In familial goitrous hypothyroidism, probably caused by genetic factors and rare, there is an inability of the gland to convert iodide into an organically bound form and failure to form iodothyronine derivatives. These patients are able to take in iodine and live where there is no deficiency of iodine.

Endemic cretinism is extremely rare in the United States. It occurs where goiter is endemic, as in Switzerland. The gland usually is enlarged. These cretins also have additional malformations such as hydrocephalus, ocular defects, or urogenital anomalies. Associated neurological disturbances have also been reported, such as spastic diplegia or paraplegia. Deafness and speech defects have been noted. The mothers of these cretins have goiters. The cretinism and cerebral anomalies are considered to be of prenatal origin. Since the use of iodized salt has eliminated goiters in children in these endemic areas, the offspring of these goiter-free children should likewise be free from cretinism.

DIAGNOSIS: Congenital hypothyroidism or cretinism must be considered as one of the causes of poor physical development and mental deficiency. The history, physical examination, and laboratory tests will help in differential. It must be looked for early since a good prognosis is dependent on early treatment to avoid mental and neurological sequelae. The appearance may occasionally be diagnostic at birth. In the next month or two lethargy and pale, cool skin should create suspicion. Certainly, much before six months sufficient symptoms and signs are present so that tests for cretinism should be performed.

The major differential is from mongolism. The latter will show the characteristic appearance at birth. There are neither the bone nor the blood changes which are seen in cretinism. If there is doubt, thyroid hormone may be given; it will improve the cretin and have no effect on the mongol. Birth injury is distinguished by the history and neurological examination. In the atonic type of cerebral diplegia there are signs of pyramidal tract disturbance such as increased deep tendon reflexes. Gargoylism is distinguished by X-ray of the shafts of the upper extremities, which exhibit bizarre swellings of the central portions with tapering toward the ends; there are also an enlarged liver and spleen and clouding of the corneas. Other types of dwarfism including chondrodystrophy have normal mentality.

TREATMENT: Desiccated thyroid extract (U.S.P.) should be given by mouth to the limit of tolerance. An infant is started with gr. ¼ (15 mg.) once daily. This is increased by ¼ grain every one to two weeks, as needed. The optimum dose should be attained as rapidly as possible. Usually a dose of 1 grain to 1½ grains is reached for infants and young children, while older ones will take between 2 and 4 grains per day. The dose may be given once a day or divided into two or three portions. The child should be observed for toxic symptoms. There should be follow-up studies of the centers of ossification, the serum cholesterol level, PBI and BEI, weight, height, and IQ. Treatment with thyroid extract is continued throughout life.

PROGNOSIS: The outlook for physical improvement if therapy is begun early is good. Skeletal maturation proceeds satisfactorily, sexual development is good, and the level of cholesterol in the blood serum falls. The mental response is varied: in some it is satisfactory, in others there is no response. The primary determinant appears to be early diagnosis and initiation of adequate treatment. Smith, Blizzard, and Wilkins reported that twelve of twenty-nine patients of the severe type (athyrotic) treated before a year of age attained an IQ greater than 90. None of the fifty patients in whom treatment was begun after one year or who were inadequately treated attained such an IQ. In mild cretinism and especially in hypothyroidism acquired after two years the results were very good. Electroencephalographic studies have shown cerebral dysfunction in those who did not improve mentally as contrasted with normal electroencephalograms in cretins who did respond to therapy. The former also showed neurological sequelae such as spasticity, tremors, and hyperactive reflexes. The question arises in those who do not respond whether there is not some associated mental defect due to brain damage acquired in utero, concomitant with the hypothyroidism, or as a result of it.

Cooke, R. E. and Man, E. B.: Management of Hypothyroidism in Infancy and Childhood. Pediat. 17:617, 1956.
Kunstadter, R. H., Kohlenbrener, R. M., and Oliner, L.: Thyroid Dysfunction in Goitrous Children. A.M.A. J. Dis. Child. 94:682, 1957.
Lotmar, F.: Histopathologische Befunde in Gehirnen von Endemischen Kretinismus Thyreoaplasie und Kochexia Thyreopriva. Zeitschr. f. d. ges. Neurol. u. Psychiat. 146:1, 1933.
Pickering, D. E. and Koulischer, N.: Discordance of Cretinism in Monozyotic Twins. A.M.A. J. Dis. Child. 92:63, 1956.
———, Sheline, G. E., and Crane, J. T.: Sporadic Familial Goitrous Hypothyroidism. A.M.A. J. Dis. Child. 93:510, 1957.
Silverman S. H. and Wilkins, L.: Radioactive Uptake in the Study of Different Types of Hypothyroidism in Children. Pediat. 12:288, 1953.
Smith, D. W., Blizzard, R. M., and Wilkins, L.: The Mental Prognosis in Hypothyroidism of Infancy and Childhood. A Review of 128 Cases. Pediat. 19:1011, 1957.
Stanbury, J. B., and McGirr, E. M.: Sporadic or Non-Endemic Familial Cretinism with Goiter. Am. J. Med. 22:712, 1957.
Talbot, N. W., et al.: Functional Endocrinology. Commonwealth Fund, Harvard Univ. Press, 1952.

Topler, A.: Mental Achievement of Congenital Hypothyroid Children. Am. J. Dis. Child. 81:233, 1951.

Warkany, J., and Wilson, J. G.: Prenatal Effects of Nutrition on the Development of the Nervous System. A. Res. Publ. Ass. Nerv. Ment. Dis. Proc. 33:76, 1954.

Wilkins, L.: The Diagnosis and Treatment of Endocrine Disorders in Childhood and Adolescence. Springfield, Ill., Charles C. Thomas, 1957.

HYPERTHYROIDISM

Excessive secretion of hormone into the blood stream by the thyroid gland causes hyperthyroidism (Graves' disease, thyrotoxicosis). Though not common in childhood, it may appear at any age, and is especially noted in the preadolescent and adolescent periods. It occurs in females 7:1.

Diagnosis is based on the cardinal features, which are usually present. They are nervousness, goiter, tachycardia, loss of weight, exophthalmos, and tremor. The useful laboratory tests include the increased radioactive iodine uptake, the elevated serum protein-bound iodine, and the increased BMR. If needed, the patient's response to drug therapy may be utilized diagnostically.

The tremors and nervous movements must be separated from chorea. Rheumatic fever with carditis may be confusing in the presence of an enlarged heart with a murmur. Simple goiter without exophthalmos may cause difficulty if it occurs in a nervous child, but ordinarily there are no toxic symptoms. Hypertension due to pheochromocytoma must be ruled out by specific tests. In hyperthyroidism the eye grounds are not likely to show papilledema.

In reviewing the relationship of neuromuscular disease to the thyroid, Millikan and Haines discuss thyrotoxicosis and its association with myasthenia gravis, chronic thyrotoxic myopathy, familial periodic paralysis, and exophthalmic ophthalmoplegia. The problems occur almost entirely in adults. Myasthenia gravis and thyrotoxicosis occurred together in 5 per cent of their series. Thyrotoxic myopathy was present in nine cases. The outstanding feature was weakness of the pelvic girdle. These patients all had symptoms and signs of thyrotoxicosis in addition.

Familial periodic paralysis occasionally occurs in association with Graves' disease. Of 400 cases of the latter, thirty had familial paralysis. Control of the hyperthyroidism improves the periodic paralysis.

Exophthalmic ophthalmoplegia occurred with thyrotoxicosis in twenty-one cases. The superior rectus was most frequently involved with the exophthalmos, but there may be total ophthalmoplegia. There is no improvement in the ophthalmoplegia with treatment of the thyroid condition.

PROGNOSIS: The outlook in children is good with treatment. Spontaneous remissions are rare and the disease usually progresses and results in toxic crises.

TREATMENT: Antithyroid drugs are used. Methimazole (15-60 mg.) or propylthiouracil (150-450 mg.) is given daily in three divided doses every eight hours. As remission occurs, the daily dose of methimazole is reduced to 5-15 mg., and of propylthiouracil to 25-50 mg. Therapy is continued for at least two years. If there is no response, thyroidectomy is performed. Some prefer immediate surgery. (See article by Arnold.)

Arnold, M. B., Talbot, N. B., and Cope, O.: Concerning the Choice of Therapy for Childhood Hyperthyroidism. Pediat. 21:47, 1958.
Boas, N. F. and Ober, W. B.: Hereditary Exophthalmic Goiter—Report of Eleven Cases in One Family. J. Clin. Endocrinol. 6:575, 1946.
Brain, W. R.: Exophthalmic Ophthalmoplegia. Quart. J. Med. 7:293, 1938.
Kepner, R. J.: Periodic Paralysis Associated with Hyperthyroidism. J. Neuropath. and Clin. Neurol. 1:316, 1951.
Levy, G., Meadows, R. W., and Gunnar, R. M.: Association of Graves Disease with Myasthenia Gravis. Am. Int. Med. 35:134, 1951.
McConahey, W. M., Owen, Jr., C. A., Keating, Jr., F. R.: A Clinical Appraisal of Radioiodine Tests of Thyroid Function. J. Clin. Endocrinol. and Metab. 16:724, 1956.
McEachern, D., and Ross, W. D.: Chronic Thyrotoxic Myopathy. Brain 65:181, 1942.
Millikan, C. H., and Haines, S. F.: The Thyroid Gland in Relation to Neuromuscular Disease. Arch. Int. Med. 92:5, 1953.

PARATHYROID

The parathyroid gland regulates the levels of calcium and phosphorus in the blood plasma and extracellular fluid. Physiologically, the hormone exerts an effect on the kidney tubule by preventing reabsorption of phosphorus at the same time that calcium is reabsorbed. Bone metabolism is also influenced by parathormone, with an increase of calcium and phosphorus in the body fluids resulting from an increased rate of dissolution of bone.

CHRONIC IDIOPATHIC HYPOPARATHYROIDISM

CLINICAL PICTURE: The onset of symptoms may occur during childhood and is characterized by convulsions. This may take the form of tetany, including numbness, tingling, and cramps in the extremities, twitching, carpopedal spasm, and the presence of the Chvostek sign. However, quite often there are no discernible signs, but only convulsive seizures with loss of consciousness, differing in no way from the epileptiform types. Both major and petit mal forms have been described. There may also be evidence of increased intracranial pressure with papilledema.

Other features which may be present in hypoparathyroidism include blurred vision due to cataract, photophobia, and gastrointestinal symptoms of vomiting, intermittent diarrhea, and abdominal pain. The skin is dry and thick, and the hair may fall out causing areas of alopecia; the nails are short and thick, and the teeth show defects (pitting) or are hyperplastic. In some cases with recurrent seizures there has been a lowering of the mental level or personality aberrations.

LABORATORY: The blood serum calcium is decreased below 7 mg./100 ml. (N 9-11). Serum phosphorus is increased (N 4-6 mg./100 ml.). Serum alkaline phosphatase is normal or low (N 4-14 Bodansky units). Calcium is absent from the urine (Sulkowitch test), and the urine phosphorus is low in proportion to the serum phosphorus.

X-ray of the skull may demonstrate calcification in the basal ganglia, cerebellum, or cerebral cortex. The long bones show increased ossification. There may be calcification in the soft tissues. The electrocardiogram shows an increase in the Q-T interval. In the electroencephalogram the most important finding is the occurrence of 2-5 per second slow waves, singly or in short series.

ETIOLOGY: The cause of parathyroid hormone deficiency is unknown.

DIAGNOSIS: The presence of tetany requires consideration of hypoparathyroidism. In rickets X-ray of the bones shows demineralization in contrast to the increased density of hypoparathyroidism, and there is a history of poor nutrition and lack of vitamin D intake. With kidney pathology there may be variation in bone density, and there are in addition changes in NPN (elevated in nephritis, normal in hypoparathyroidism) or in total protein (may be decreased in nephritis and normal in hypoparathyroidism). In alkalosis the pH is elevated and the calcium normal.

To differentiate hypoparathyroidism from pseudohypoparathyroidism a renal phosphorus clearance test (Ellsworth-Howard) may be used. In hypoparathyroidism there is an increase in clearance showing response to parathormone stimulation.

The seizures of tetany must be differentiated from those of a brain tumor, especially when papilledema occurs in hypoparathyroidism, and those of idiopathic epilepsy and tetanus. Response to therapy for hypoparathyroidism may help in the differential.

PROGNOSIS: Under therapy, as outlined below, patients are kept under control but never recover. If, however, the parathyroid has been injured and the effect is transient, they do get well.

TREATMENT: The initial therapy is the same as previously described for other forms of hypocalcemic tetany, namely, injection of intravenous calcium gluconate (10 cc. of 10 per cent solution) slowly, and subsequently calcium chloride given orally, well diluted in juice.

For immediate therapy vitamin D (Calciferol 200,000 to 400,000 units daily, and AT 10 (dihydrotachysterol) 1.25 mg. t.i.d. are given. After a few days, for maintenance the AT 10 is reduced to once a day and the vitamin D to 50,000 units. Further therapy is governed by blood calcium determinations and Sulkowitch tests for calciuria.

At the onset a diet low in phosphorus should be used (no milk, cheese, eggs). Aluminum gel aids phosphorus excretion via the intestines and is useful in maintaining a normal serum calcium. Parathormone is not used because of risk of toxic symptoms from too rapid and high an elevation of calcium and because refractoriness soon develops.

Bartter, F. C.: The Parathyroid Gland and its Relationship to Diseases of the Nervous System. A. Res. Publ. Ass. Nerv. Ment. Dis. Proc. 32:1, 1953.

Frame, R. and Carter, S.: Pseudohypoparathyroidism: Clinical Picture and Relation to Convulsive Seizures. Neurology 5:297, 1955.

Gotta, H. and Odoritz, J. B.: Electroencephalogram in Hypoparathyroidism with Tetany and Epilepsy. J. Clin. Endocrinol. 8:674, 1948.

Gribetz, D.: Hypocalcemic States in Infancy and Childhood. A.M.A. J. Dis. Child. 94:301, 1957.

Soper, R. T., Mason, E. E., and Buckwalter, J. A.: Hypoparathyroidism in Children and Adolescents. Pediat. 20:1097, 1957.

Steinberg, H., and Waldron, B. R.: Idiopathic Hypoparathyroidism: Analysis of 52 Cases, Including Report of a New Case. Medicine 31:133, 1952.

Talbot, N. B., Sobel, E. H., McArthur, J. W., and Crawford, J. D.: Functional Endocrinology from Birth Through Adolescence. Cambridge, Harvard Univ. Press, 1952.

HYPERPARATHYROIDISM

Hyperparathyroidism is characterized by excessive production of hormone by the parathyroid glands. It is associated with hypercalcemia and hypophosphatemia, and there are harmful effects on the nervous system, kidneys, and bones. It is termed primary when the pathology is essentially in the parathyroids. In the presence of severe kidney disease there may be secondary hyperparathyroidism.

PRIMARY HYPERPARATHYROIDISM

CLINICAL PICTURE: There are general manifestations of apathy, listlessness, and easy fatigability. The patients lose appetite and are constipated. There is reduction of muscle tone with diminished reflexes. Pain in the back and extremities may occur early. Walking becomes difficult. Gastrointestinal symptoms of nausea and vomiting with loss of weight may be present. Decalcification of bone produces deformities such as bowing of the legs, knock knees, and pathological fractures; shortening of stature occurs due to vertebral compression, kyphosis, or scoliosis. Bone cysts or tumors may occur. Rarely the spinal cord is compressed. There may be stones in any portion of the genitourinary system with renal colic. There may also be polyuria with low specific gravity and polydipsia. Ultimately nephritis, with infection and loss of function, sets in. There is an associated lowering of mentality.

ROENTGENOGRAPHY: Early there is marked decalcification of the bones and osteoporosis. Later there are fractures, deformities, bone cysts, and tumors. Renal calculi are visible. The skull has a granular appearance. Calcium deposits may be noted in the soft tissues.

LABORATORY: Serum calcium is usually elevated to 12-18 mg./100 ml. Serum phosphorus is low or normal if the kidney is functioning normally. Serum alkaline phosphatase is elevated when there is bone involvement. Urinary calcium is markedly increased.

PATHOLOGY: There is an adenoma in one of the four parathyroid glands or there may be general hyperplasia of the glands. Occasionally there are multiple adenomas. The bones show destruction and the marrow is replaced by fibrous tissue (osteitis fibrosa cystica). Cysts, fractures, and benign tumors of the bones are present. The kidney shows calcium stones and deposits, and evidence of infection.

ETIOLOGY: The cause of this condition is unknown.

DIAGNOSIS: The diagnosis of hyperparathyroidism is based on the presence of bone changes, renal stones and insufficiency, and general features attributable to hypercalcemia, many of which may be neuromuscular. Serum phosphorus is low. Other causes for hypercalcemia must be ruled out. In bone metastasis with malignancy, the phosphorus is usually normal or elevated; there are also other evidences of the primary disease. Polyostotic fibrous dysplasia may be confusing. The bones in fibrous dysplasia are likely to show both irregular areas of demineralization and normal spots, whereas in hyperparathyroidism there is generalized decalcification. The lesion in polyostotic fibrous dysplasia is often unilateral. Calcium and phosphorus are normal. Cutaneous pigmentation and precocious puberty in the female are also present. Hypervitaminosis D is ruled out by the lack of a history of excessive intake. Rickets in infancy is differentiated by the low or normal calcium. Osteogenesis imperfecta with multiple fractures can be differentiated by the normal serum calcium and phosphorus and clinically by the presence of blue sclerae. Secondary hyperparathyroidism is associated with primary renal disease; in these cases the serum calcium is low.

PROGNOSIS: This is good if the disease is recognized early and the parathyroid adenoma is removed. The patient improves in weight and well-being and the bones show healing. Deformities which do not spontaneously become corrected can be treated orthopedically. The status of the kidney is important; stones may disappear, but if too much damage has occurred, the outlook is more doubtful.

TREATMENT: Parathyroidectomy is indicated to remove the one or more adenomas. When the process is one of hyperplasia only, a portion of the glands should be removed so that function is preserved. Postoperatively there is a period during which tetany may develop. This is treated as previously described with calcium intravenously.

Albright, F. and Reifenstein, Jr., E. C.: The Parathyroid Glands and Metabolic Bone Disease. Baltimore, Williams & Wilkins Co., 1948.

Knuth, W. P. and Kisner, P.: Symmetrical Cerebral Calcification Associated with Parathyroid Adenoma. J.A.M.A. 162:462, 1956.

PITUITARY

The anterior pituitary contains three types of cells: basophilic, acidophilic, and chromophobic. The posterior portion contains cells and nerve fibres which are unmyelinated and originate from nuclei in the hypothalamus. Urine flow is regulated from the supraoptic nuclei of the hypothalamus. The anterior portion (adenohypophysis) elaborates such hormones as thyroid stimulating (TSH), gonadotropic, including follicle stimulating (FSH) and luteinizing (LH) or interstitial cell stimulating (ICSH), adrenocorticotropic (ACTH), and growth (PGH). The posterior portion (neurohypophysis) produces antidiuretic and oxytoxic substances.

The pituitary influences body tissues and other endocrine glands. However, it is in turn affected by these glands and is under nervous control of the hypothalamus. The hypothalamic centers appear to stimulate the release of a chemical substance, which in turn activates the production of ACTH and other hormones by the pituitary. Nerve transmission from the hypothalamus to the pituitary is by way of the tuber cinereum. The humoral agent is released from the eminence of the tuber cinereum and carried by the hypophyseal portal system to the anterior pituitary cells.

Pathological changes affecting the pituitary gland may exert their clinical effects either in the form of endocrine changes or through local effects on adjacent structures such as the sella turcica, hypothalamus, 3rd ventricle, optic chiasm, tracts, and nerves.

HYPOPITUITARISM

(SIMMONDS' DISEASE OR PAN-HYPOPITUITARISM)

This condition is very uncommon in children. All or almost all of the pituitary gland is destroyed. There are two clinical types. In one there are essentially manifestations of pituitary insufficiency. In the other there are signs of a tumor in the region of the sella turcica, and the clinical picture of an expanding lesion is outstanding; the symptoms of hypopituitarism are secondary.

In the first group, without tumor, the major feature in children is lack of normal growth and development. There are loss of weight, muscular weakness and atrophy, asthenia, and anorexia. There is evidence of hormonal deficiency from the thyroid, gonads, and adrenals. There are therefore in older children amenorrhea, lack of sexual development or regression, marked sensitivity to cold, low blood pressure, and dry skin. Fundus examination is normal.

LABORATORY: There are a low BMR, diminished excretion of 17-ketosteroids in the urine, and low I^{131} uptake and PBI. The serum sodium, chloride, and blood sugar are diminished; cholesterol is elevated. There is a normal eosinopenic response to ACTH. X-ray of the sella turcica is normal.

DIAGNOSIS: The differential diagnosis must be made from Addison's disease. In the latter there are skin pigmentation and a negative eosinopenic response to ACTH. In anorexia nervosa the epinephrine test (eosinopenic response) is normal as are the serum-bound-iodine and radioactive iodine uptake.

PROGNOSIS: The course is uncertain.

TREATMENT: ACTH is administered first, then thyroid, beginning with small amounts. In puberty, gonadal therapy is used. Most of the pituitary hormones are not as yet valuable or available.

In the second group, where tumor is present, there are signs and symptoms of increased pressure on the pituitary and neighboring structures. The symptoms secondary to hypopituitarism previously described are present, but may be overshadowed. The tumor may be derived from the chromophobe or chromophile cells. Primary optic atrophy, bitemporal hemianopia, and headache result.

LABORATORY: X-ray shows ballooning of the sella turcica.

PROGNOSIS: Poor.

TREATMENT: Extirpation of the tumor and X-ray therapy.

DWARFISM

We have already stressed lack of growth and development as the essential feature in hypopituitarism in children. This results in various degrees of dwarfism. The term includes lack of normal height, under 51 inches in the male and 48 inches in the female, and retention of childhood proportions, with the umbilicus in the mid-abdomen rather than nearer the symphysis. The children appear physically well. Mentality is usually normal.

The parents are usually well developed, and the birth history is uneventful. Development appears to proceed satisfactorily up to a point and then remains retarded. There is delay or absence of sexual maturation. Likewise there is delay in bone maturation and epiphyseal closure so that slow growth continues beyond the usual age. The appearance is that of a child, even in middle age, with a high-pitched voice, full, rounded, smooth face, and lack of pubic and axillary hair.

LABORATORY TESTS: These are similar to those described under panhypopituitarism. They show gonadal, adrenocortical, or thyroid hormone deficiency secondary to lack of pituitary stimulation.

DIAGNOSIS: A differential should be made from other causes of dwarfism or stunted growth. In primordial hereditary dwarfism there is a genetic transmission from the parents. These dwarfs are normal in all respects except for size and can transmit their dwarfism. They may also produce normal offspring.

The Laurence-Moon-Biedl syndrome is a hypothalamic disorder in which there may be dwarfism, marked obesity, mental retardation, and congenital defects like polydactylism, retinitis pigmentosa, and optic atrophy. Cretinism is recognized by the appearance, retarded mental development, and decreased PBI and radioactive iodine uptake. In ovarian agenesis there are a high urinary FSH and normal 17-ketosteroids showing no lack of pituitary function. There are associated anomalies such as webbed neck. The chrondodystrophies, osteogenesis imperfecta, rickets, and tuberculosis of the spine can be ruled out by X-ray. Other causes of dwarfism are hepatic, nutritional, renal, cardiac, and intestinal. Encephalitis may be followed by dwarfism. Brain tumors such as craniopharyngioma should be ruled out.

In progeria there is dwarfism of unknown origin associated with premature senility. The birth weight is below 2500 grams. Growth and development are slow in the first year. Other changes soon occur. There are loss of hair, small face, large head, beak-like facies, receding chin, and a high-pitched voice. The weight may reach only a three year level, and the height a five year level due to premature fusion of the epiphyses. Mentality is normal. Death results from arteriosclerosis of the coronary or cerebral vessels.

PROGNOSIS: If no growth has occurred by several years past adolescence, the outlook is poor.

TREATMENT: Testosterone may be tried in small amounts. Growth hormones are still experimental; however, their value has been demonstrated, and only the problem of production prevents their general use.

HYPERPITUITARISM

This condition is produced by adenomatous tumors of the adeno-hypophysis. The eosinophilic adenoma causes gigantism in children; after closure of the epiphyses, acromegaly results. The effects are due to an excess of growth hormone (PGH). Signs and symptoms of the tumor are also present. Basophilic adenoma is associated with Cushing's syndrome. The clinical picture is due to hyperadrenalism.

POSTERIOR PITUITARY GLAND

DIABETES INSIPIDUS

This is the major pathological condition due to diminished function of the posterior lobe of the pituitary. This portion of the pituitary, along with the associated nuclei (supraoptic and paraventricular) in the hypothalamus and the fibre pathways from the hypothalamus to the pituitary, is concerned with the production of the antidiuretic hormone. The pathogenesis of this condition depends on lesions which may involve the pituitary gland itself, the paraventricular and supraoptic nuclei of the hypothalamus, or the pituitary stalk.

ETIOLOGY: In a number of instances there is no demonstrable cause. Some instances are hereditary. Known causes in children include tumors such as craniopharyngioma, infections such as encephalitis, Schüller-Christian syndrome, and trauma.

CLINICAL PICTURE: The outstanding features are polyuria and polydipsia. The output of urine may reach ten liters per day. The children are constantly at the water faucet, drinking, and urinating. In addition to the symptoms of diabetes insipidus, there may be headache and visual disturbances associated with a pathological process in the brain, such as a tumor. In this case there may also be papilledema.

LABORATORY: The urine has a specific gravity below 1.005 and looks pale. Blood sugar and renal function tests are normal. X-rays of the skull (sella) may show a tumor or reticuloendotheliosis. The response to posterior pituitary extract is a concentrated urine. Restriction of water intake (6 hours) produces no increase in urine concentration.

DIAGNOSIS: The diagnosis depends on the symptoms of polyuria and polydipsia with a urine of low specific gravity, and normal blood sugar and kidney tests. A possible etiological factor should be sought, such as tumor, encephalitis, or reticuloendotheliosis.

Differential diagnosis can be made from: a) diabetes mellitus, where there are hyperglycemia, specific gravity of 1.015, and glycosuria; b) nephritis, in which the NPN is elevated and kidney function tests show pathology; c) nephrogenic diabetes insipidus, where there is failure of the kidney as an end organ to be influenced by the anti-diuretic hormone (therefore no response to an injection of pitressin); and d) psychogenic diabetes insipidus, in which restriction of water intake causes concentration of the urine.

PROGNOSIS: The outlook depends on the cause. In the so-called idiopathic types the patient continues normally, but requires constant therapy. Occasionally, if the cause is eliminated symptoms abate. In tumor the outlook depends on the outcome of the treatment of the tumor.

TREATMENT: Placing cotton saturated with a solution of pitressin into the nose for five minutes is a good method. The patient learns to repeat this several times a day as needed. Aqueous pitressin, 1 cc. t.i.d., or pitressin tannate in oil, 0.5 cc., b.i.d., may be injected intramuscularly; the latter is more slowly absorbed and lasts longer. As previously stressed, where there is an etiological factor such as tumor, therapy is directed at the underlying lesion with surgery and/or X-ray.

Cooke, J. V.: The Rate of Growth in Progeria—Report of 2 Cases. J. Pediat. 42:26, 1953.

Glaser, G. H.: The Pituitary Gland in Relation to Cerebral Metabolism and Metabolic Disorders of the Nervous System. A. Res. Publ. Ass. Nerv. Ment. Dis. Proc. 32:21, 1953.

Harris, G.: Pituitary—Hypothalamic Mechanisms. Arch. Neurol. and Psychiat. 73:124, 1955.

Munsen, P. D. and Briggs, F. N.: The Mechanism of Stimulation of ACTH Secretion. The Proceedings of the Laurentian Hormone Conference. New York, Academic Press, 11:83, 1955.

Pender, C. B. and Fraser, F. C.: Dominant Inheritance of Diabetes Insipidus; a Family Study. Pediat. 11:246, 1953.
Plotz, C. M., Knowlton, A. I., Ragan, C.: The Natural History of Cushing's Syndrome. Am. J. Med. 13:597, 1952.
Sheehan, H. L. and Summers, V. K.: The Syndrome of Hypopituitarism. Quart. J. Med. 18:319, 1949.
Talbot, N. B., Sobel, E. H., McArthur, J. W. and Crawford, J. D.: Functional Endocrinology from Birth Through Adolescence. Cambridge, Harvard Univ. Press, 1952.
Warkany, J. and Mitchell, A. G.: Diabetes Insipidus in Children. Am. J. Dis. Child. 57:603, 1939.
Williams, R. H. and Henry, C.: Nephrogenic Diabetes Insipidus, Transmitted by Females and Appearing During Infancy in Males. Ann. Int. Med. 27:84, 1947.

HYPOTHALAMUS

FRÖHLICH'S SYNDROME

Adiposogenital dystrophy or Fröhlich's Syndrome refers to a clinical condition in which there is obesity and delayed sexual development. Because the distribution of the adipose tissue is particularly noted in the breasts and pelvic region, boys appear to have a feminine appearance.

Fröhlich's syndrome may occur with suprasellar tumors or pathology involving the hypothalamus. In these cases there may be signs of increased intracranial pressure, blindness, diabetes insipidus, somnolence, and disturbances in growth. (Refer to tumors.) Encephalitis and trauma may also cause the preceding picture.

Most cases of adiposogenital dystrophy occur in children who are otherwise normal. In their preadolescent period they grow at a more rapid rate and develop obesity. Ultimately with the advent of adolescence these children mature satisfactorily both physically and mentally.

In making a diagnosis, one must differentiate between the normal preadolescent type of obesity and the adiposogenital syndrome which is due to tumor with hypothalamic involvement (Fröhlich's syndrome). The Laurence-Moon-Biedl syndrome should also be considered. Cases of true Fröhlich's syndrome are extremely rare. When they do occur, the outlook is poor.

Bruch, H.: Obesity in Childhood: Physical Growth and Development of Obese Children. Am. J. Dis. Child. 58:457, 1939.
————: The Fröhlich Syndrome: Report of the Original case. Am. J. Dis. Child. 58:1282, 1939.

PANCREAS

DIABETES MELLITUS

The neurological conditions associated with diabetes mellitus are polyneuritis, which has been discussed in the section on the latter, and the secondary effects on the nervous system of vascular disease and coma.

The etiology of diabetes mellitus is unknown. There appears to be an inherited factor of a recessive type. The onset and course of the clinical picture are usually rapid, within several weeks. In any child who is not gaining weight, irrespective of body build, diabetes must be ruled out. The major symptoms in childhood are thirst and polydipsia, polyuria, loss of weight in spite of a good appetite, enuresis, and fatigue.

Often in children the first manifestation of diabetes is coma. This is so when the initial symptoms of the disease have not been recognized. The attack may be ushered in by an acute infection. There may be vomiting and abdominal pain. Acidosis with resultant dehydration develops. This is marked by hyperpnoea, flushed face, red lips, odor of acetone to the breath, drowsiness, and finally complete stupor and coma. The skin is cold, the pulse weak, the blood pressure low, the abdomen often rigid, and breathing is labored.

LABORATORY: There are glycosuria, hyperglycemia, and ketonuria. A low CO_2 and low serum sodium and chloride are seen. The potassium is usually elevated.

DIAGNOSIS: This is based on the history and laboratory signs of hyperglycemia, glycosuria, and ketonuria. A glucose tolerance test may be done if needed. The diagnosis of diabetic coma is based on the history and laboratory data as previously given. Other causes to be considered when the patient is comatose are hypoglycemic shock due to insulin, lead encephalopathy, uremia, salicylate intoxication, and cerebral conditions such as tumor, meningitis, and encephalitis.

Hypoglycemic shock in children usually occurs with insulin therapy. It is quickly relieved by intravenous glucose (25 per cent). History, blood sugar, and acetone determination aid in differential.

With lead encephalopathy there are a history of lead ingestion, elevated blood lead level, and excess lead excretion in the urine.

Uremia is associated with chemical findings indicative of kidney disease.

Salicylates give a falsely positive test for diacetic acid in the urine. There is a history of taking aspirin or other tablets; there is no hyperglycemia.

Cerebral conditions give evidence of tumor, meningitis, or encephalitis by the history, neurological signs, papilledema, and spinal fluid findings.

PROGNOSIS: Recovery from diabetic coma is the rule. Since diabetes is diagnosed early in the present era, and antibiotics can control infections, the child progresses satisfactorily, and coma is now usually seen only when control of diabetes is irresponsible. However, adult life is complicated by the development of arteriosclerosis, hypertension, and neuropathies.

TREATMENT: This includes insulin, restoration of water and electrolyte balance, and antibiotics for any infection which may be present.

Bailey, A. A.: Neurologic Complications Associated with Diabetes. Diabetes 4:32, 1955.

Guild, H. G., Grubb, W., Chu, M. Y. F. and Sidbury, Jr., J. B.: Vascular Complications of Juvenile Diabetes. J. Pediat. 41:722, 1952.

White, P., Guest, G. M., Kennedy, W. B. and Harwood, R. The Young Diabetic-Panel Discussion. Diabetes 4:313, 1955.

HYPOGLYCEMIA

Hypoglycemia is considered to be present when the blood sugar falls below 50 mg. per cent and there are pathological consequences to the brain with resultant symptoms. The brain is the organ most vulnerable to a lack of carbohydrate; its oxygen consumption and metabolism depend on the utilization of sugar.

CLINICAL PICTURE: The early symptoms of hypoglycemia are likely to follow a period of fasting or strenuous exercise. They consist of weakness, a feeling of faintness, marked hunger, excessive irritability, sweating, pallor, and anxiety. If the condition is unrecognized and not relieved, a more serious picture develops. The child becomes irrational, confused, speech is incoherent, and convulsions and coma may occur. The neurological examination is normal except when seizure occurs, in which case there may be altered reflexes and a Babinski sign.

LABORATORY: Blood sugar is below 50 mg. per cent during the attack. The electroencephalogram shows abnormal patterns with slow waves.

ETIOLOGY:
a) Hyperinsulism associated with insulin therapy in diabetes is the most common cause in children.
b) Pancreatic islet adenomas.
c) Hyperplasia of the islets in the newborn, as in infants of diabetic mothers.
d) Liver—interference with storage of glycogen or delivery of glucose to the blood stream, as in infectious hepatitis, cirrhosis, or Von Gierke's disease.
e) Deficiency of the anterior pituitary and/or adrenal cortex (Addison's disease).
f) Functional or idiopathic—hypoglycemia without any obvious cause.
g) Starvation
h) Disorders of the central nervous system—encephalitis (hypothalamic).
i) Gastrointestinal disease with failure of absorption.
j) Protein administration (amino acids) in infancy.

PATHOLOGY: This depends on the cause of the hypoglycemia. There may be associated encephalopathy and myelopathy.

DIAGNOSIS: *Laboratory tests* (Talbot)
1. Fasting blood sugar level.
2. a. Epinephrine-glucose test.
   b. Epinephrine-eosinophil test.
3. Intravenous glucose tolerance test.
4. 24 hour fasting tolerance test.

The diagnosis will depend on the history and laboratory tests. When diabetes exists, an attack following insulin injection will make the cause obvious. In other instances there may be disease of the liver, pituitary, adrenal, or pancreas.

The laboratory tests will demonstrate a low blood sugar. The rise of blood sugar following epinephrine injection will show that the liver is performing its glycogenolytic function. The drop in eosinophiles following an epinephrine injection shows normal function of the pituitary-adrenal axis. If no diagnosis as to cause is made by these tests, exploration of the pancreas may be necessary. The condition may remain idiopathic.

PROGNOSIS: This is good in children when it is associated with insulin injection, as in diabetes. In other more rare types the outlook is poor as attacks grow worse with increasing damage to the brain.

TREATMENT: The child with diabetes is taught to take orange juice or a sweet as soon as he feels faint or hungry following an insulin injection. Epinephrine may be injected. Surgical exploration of the pancreas is performed for adenoma. For the idiopathic hypoglycemia of infancy, oral hydrocortisone may be given, using 1.5 mg./kg./day. As control is established, the maintenance dose may be reduced.

Cochrane, W. A., Payne, W. W., Simpkiss, M. J. and Woolf, L. I.: Familial Hypoglycemia Precipitated by Amino Acids. J. Clin. Invest. 35:411, 1956.
Hartmann, A. F. and Jaudon, J. C.: Hypoglycemia. J. Pediat. 11:1, 1937.
————: Hypoglycemia. J. Pediat. 43:1, 1953.
Himwich, H. E.: Hypoglycemia and Brain Metabolism A. Res. Publ. Nerv. Ment. Dis. Proc. 32:345, 1953.
McQuarrie, I.: Hypoglycemia in Infancy and Childhood: Differential Diagnosis and Therapy. Post. Grad. Med. 18:287, 1955.
Richardson, J. C. and Hill, F. M.: Neurologic Diagnosis of Pancreatic Islet Cell Adenoma with Hyperinsulism. Neurology 7:793, 1957.
Talbot, N. B., Sobel, E. A., McArthur, J. W., and Crawford, J. D.: Functional Endocrinology. Cambridge, Mass., Harvard Univ. Press. 1952.

ADRENAL

About thirty steroids have been isolated from the adrenal cortex. Some of these are concerned with maintenance of electrolyte balance and water metabolism, including control of sodium and potassium (mineralocorticoids). Others influence carbohydrate metabolism (glucocorticoids). Finally, other hormones are concerned with tissue growth and are androgenic.

The adrenal medulla produces epinephrine (adrenalin) and norepinephrine. Both increase mean arterial blood pressure.

INSUFFICIENCY OR HYPOFUNCTION OF THE ADRENAL CORTEX

Acute insufficiency occurs in children in the Waterhouse-Friderichsen syndrome, associated with acute infections, especially meningococcemia, septicemia, and diphtheria. It may also be present in the newborn associated with hemorrhage due to the trauma of delivery. The adrenal gland at autopsy may show hemorrhages and/or necrosis.

The symptom complex is one of shock, whether due to hemorrhage in the newborn or overwhelming toxemia. The skin is cold and clammy, the pulse is rapid and weak, fever is present, the blood pressure falls, and respiration is rapid and labored. In the newborn, masses may be palpable in the flanks (adrenal hemorrhage). Chemical studies are compatible with adrenal insufficiency: low sodium and sugar and high potassium.

PROGNOSIS: The outlook is serious, but since the advent of cortisone, it is much improved.

TREATMENT: This consists of electrolytes, blood plasma, cortisone, antibiotics, and norepinephrine. For a full discussion of the Waterhouse-Friderichsen syndrome refer to meningococcic meningitis.

Chronic insufficiency of the adrenal gland produces Addison's disease.

HYPERFUNCTION

PRIMARY ALDOSTERONISM

Primary aldosteronism, a clinical entity described by Conn in 1955, is due to excessive secretion of aldosterone by the adrenal cortex. This mineralocorticoid regulates the metabolism of sodium and potassium.

Clinically there is severe muscular weakness, which recurs periodically. During the attack the patient appears paralyzed (hypokalemia). There are also tetany, hypertension, polyuria, and polydipsia.

LABORATORY: Blood-Hypokalemia is outstanding. There is also at times hypernatremia and alkalosis (rise in pH and CO_2 combining power).

Urine—Excessive output of aldosterone (N less than 6.0 mcg. of aldosteronediacetate in 24 hours). 17-hydroxycorticoids are normal.

Electrocardiographic findings indicate hypokalemia with prolongation of the QT interval and inversion of T waves.

TREATMENT: Therapy consists of surgical removal of an adrenal cortical tumor. If there is no tumor, subtotal adrenalectomy is done.

PROGNOSIS: Of sixteen patients reported by Hewlett and his group, twelve have been cured, ten by removal of the tumor (adrenocortical adenoma), one by total and one by subtotal addrenalectomy. Three cases were proved at autopsy; one was an adrenal carcinoma.

Conn, J. W. and Louis, L. H.: Primary Aldosteronism: A New Clinical Entity. Tr. Ass. Amer. Phys. 68:215, 1955.
Hewlett, J. S., McCullagh, E. P., Farrell, G. L., Dustan, H. P., Pontasse, E. F. and Proudfit, W. L.: Aldosterone-Producing Tumors of the Adrenal Gland. Report of Three Cases. J.A.M.A. 164:719, 1957.

ADRENAL MEDULLA

Tumors arising from the medulla vary depending on the type of cell:

1. Sympathogonioma—arising from an early embryonic cell—malignant.
2. Sympathicoblastoma or Neuroblastoma—from an intermediate cell—malignant.
3. Ganglioneuroma—from ganglion cells—benign.
4. Pheochromocytoma—the only one which produces hormones —epinephrine and norepinephrine—from chromaffin cells.

Pheochromocytoma. This is a rare tumor of the chromaffin cells of the medulla. It occurs more often in male children, occasionally bilateral, and may occupy extra-adrenal sites. It produces symptoms because of the increased secretion of epinephrine and norepinephrine. There are headaches, hypertension, either constant or paroxysmal, palpitation, abdominal pains, excessive sweating, discomfort from heat, anxiety, vomiting, diarrhea, and rapid pulse.

Examination reveals marked increase in blood pressure. There may be an enlarged heart and papilledema.

LABORATORY: A pyelogram may show a displaced kidney.

1. In the paroxysmal types, when the blood pressure is not elevated at the time of testing, histamine injected intravenously causes a marked rise in blood pressure. This is a potentially dangerous test.
2. In the sustained type, Regitine® injected intravenously low-

ers the blood pressure temporarily (this drug is adrenolytic and antagonistic to pressor amines).

3. Antidiuretic response to (Benodaine®). In this test, administration intravenously causes a reduction in the output of urine in the presence of pheochromytoma; no effect or an increased output is found in hypertension due to other causes.

4. Quantitative determination of 24 hour urinary catechol amines. N 15-60 mcg. These are increased in pheochromocytoma.

DIAGNOSIS: This is based on the specific tests in any child with paroxysmal or persistent hypertension. To be ruled out are other types of adrenal tumor, familial dysautonomia, renal disease, coarctation of the aorta, and acrodynia.

PROGNOSIS: Smid and DuShane reported 31 cases in children, of whom 22 were treated surgically and 14 recovered.

TREATMENT: Surgical removal of the tumor should be performed.

Cone, Jr., T. E., Allen, M. S., Pearson, H. A.: Pheochromocytoma in Children. Report of Three Familial Cases in Two Unrelated Families. Pediat. 19:44, 1957.

Haggerty, R. J., Maroney, M. W., and Nadas, A. S.: Essential Hypertension in Infancy and Childhood. Differential Diagnosis and Therapy. A.M.A. J. Dis. Child. 92:535, 1956.

Jailer, J. W., Longson, D., and Christy, N. P.: Cushing's Syndrome—An Adrenal or Pituitary Disease. Clin. Endocrinol. and Metab. 16:1276, 1956.

Leiser, A. E. and Corcoran, A. C.: Antidiuretic Response to Piperoxan as a Diagnostic Test of Pheochromocytoma. J.A.M.A. 162:540, 1956.

Report of the Thirteenth M. & R. Pediatric Research Conference. Adrenal Function in Infants and Children. Columbus, Ohio, M. & R. Laboratories, 1955.

Robinson, H. J.: Adrenal Cortical Hormones and Infection. Pediat. 17:770, 1956.

Smid, A. C. and DuShane, J. W.: Pheochromocytoma in Children. Report of a Case. A.M.A. J. Dis. Child. 90:81, 1955.

Wilkins, L.: The Diagnosis and Treatment of Endocrine Disorders in Childhood and Adolescence. Springfield, Ill. Chas. C. Thomas, 1957.

CHAPTER 21

MISCELLANEOUS

Lead Poisoning

Unfortunately, lead poisoning is seen quite often in children. In the summer of 1955, during July and August there were seventeen admissions in one ward of the children's service at the Kings County Hospital (State University Division). Since in infants and children the effect of lead ingestion is manifested primarily as an encephalopathy, there are serious possibilities for permanent brain damage or death.

The chronic type of lead poisoning is almost always seen. It is due to the child's putting things into his mouth, irrespective of their utility or safety. In many instances a history of pica or perverted appetite is obtained, and it is learned that the child has been constantly chewing paint from window sills, woodwork, cribs, painted walls, or furniture. Most cases of lead ingestion occur between one and three years of age. Our experience is the same as reported by others, that the patients originate mostly from slum and poorer economic areas, often where buildings have been torn down to allow for a new housing development, leaving peelings, chipped paint, plaster, or putty around. In some instances wet paint is left around the house in open cans preparatory to painting and this is ingested. Licking of paint off toys is a lesser form of exposure. Infants occasionally are exposed to lead nipple shields. In rare instances lead fumes may be inhaled. Most cases are seen in the summer months, from May to September. There is no race or sex predilection.

Lead is absorbed into the body by way of the skin, lungs, and gastrointestinal tract. It has been observed that the greater the length of time during which lead has entered and remained in the body the more serious the effect. In children this form of low grade, chronic exposure is characteristic.

The lead enters the systemic circulation and is carried to the liver, brain, pancreas, and kidney, ultimately leaving the soft tissues to go in high concentrations to the bones. The lead in the bones is deposited as an insoluable tertiary phosphate and goes especially to the epiphyseal portions of the long bones. Excretion is by way of the kidney and bowel, the feces containing mainly unabsorbed lead.

Factors which influence the distribution of lead, which is normally carried by the red blood cell but appears in the blood plasma when in excess, include a diet high in calcium and phosphate which helps to deposit the lead in the bones. On the other hand, a low calcium, high phosphate intake causes deleading. Acids and parathyroid hormone also increase excretion of lead.

PATHOLOGY: The brain shows intense edema, and there is some degree of nerve cell and fibre injury with glial proliferation. The primary effect is in the cerebral cortex, which is distended in places by the marked serous exudate. The cerebellum is also involved. Peripheral neuritis with involvement of the axon and myelin sheath may be noted. The spinal cord is also affected together with the corresponding muscles. The liver, pancreas, and kidneys show intranuclear inclusion bodies.

CLINICAL PICTURE: The onset may be insidious with gradually developing lack of appetite, anemia, vomiting, persistent constipation, loss of weight, irritability, marked pallor, and colicky abdominal pain. Progression of symptoms depends on whether the child continues to ingest lead. If deprived of the source, the picture may abate. Renewal of the pica will again bring on the picture of lead poisoning. An infection may bring on acidosis, which increases the solubility of lead, so that the more acute picture of a cerebral lead encephalopathy may appear.

The younger the child, the greater the probability of a more acute onset. In any event, the characteristic and serious picture in children occurs with involvement of the brain, and is manifested by the onset of convulsions, both general and focal. The seizure may come on abruptly and precede any of the previous symptoms mentioned, or may accompany or follow them. Often there are coma and marked lethargy. Paralysis of various types such as hemiplegia occurs. Rarely cranial nerve palsies of the third, sixth, and seventh nerves are noted. There may be signs of cerebellar involvement with ataxia and muscular incoordination. Tremors, decerebrate rigidity, or papilledema may be present. There is evidence of elevated blood pressure and irregular pulse. In infancy the anterior fontanel may bulge and the cranial sutures be separated. The temperature is normal unless seizures continue, in which case hyperpyrexia may develop.

Peripheral neuritis occasionally occurs in older children, not in infancy. The adult type of foot or wrist-drop is unusual in children. There is more likely to be a general involvement including various muscle groups, more commonly of the lower extremities. The tendon reflexes are absent, the spinal fluid is normal in the presence of neuritis, and there is some tenderness. Sensory signs are not marked.

Aside from the nervous system, the other clinical feature is the lead line, a black line on the gum margins due to lead sulfide deposition. I have rarely seen it in children.

LABORATORY: The blood shows a hypochromic, microcytic anemia, and basophilic stippling of the red blood cells. The urine may contain albumin and sugar. There is an increase in urinary coproporphyrin, a valuable early sign. The spinal fluid is under increased pressure with elevation of protein and a positive Pandy. A slight cellular increase, 20-100 cells per cu. mm., mostly lymphocytes, is present in some cases. In a number of our recent cases at Kings County Hospital there was no cellular increase.

Urinary excretion of lead. This determination is very valuable in diagnosis. Normally a child will excrete less than 55 micrograms in 24 hours. Values between 55 and 80 micrograms suggest a lead contact and possible lead poisoning. Excretion above 80 micrograms in 24 hours indicates active lead poisoning. In severe lead poisoning with inadequate renal blood flow, excretion of lead may be impaired and normal values may be present. This exception to the general rule must be kept in mind if the remainder of the picture fits lead poisoning.

Blood lead is especially diagnostic. The normal level is up to 0.03 mg. to 0.06 mg. per 100 gms of whole blood. There is an increased lead level in the blood, over 0.1 mg. per 100 gms blood, in lead poisoning.

X-Ray. Increased density due to lead deposition, is noted at the ends of the shafts of the long bones. Spots due to lead may be seen in the intestines on roentgenography of the abdomen. In infants, skull films may show suture separation due to the intense cerebral edema and pressure.

DIAGNOSIS:

1. The major point in the diagnosis of lead poisoning is a history of ingestion of paint flakes or peelings containing lead. Rarely one of the other forms of exposure may occur.
2. Increased concentration of lead in the blood, in excess of 0.06 mg. per 100 gms.
3. Increased urinary excretion of lead, above 80 micrograms in 24 hours.
4. Basophilic stippling of the red blood cells; hypochromic, microcytic anemia.
5. Roentgenographic evidence of increased density in the ends of the shafts of the long bones, and lead spots in the abdomen.
6. Coproporphyrin increased in the urine.

In evaluating these findings, one must remember that lead remains in the bones for long periods. There may therefore be a zone of density on X-ray, but the acute episode for which the patient is admitted may be due to some other cause. On the other hand, roentgenographic evidence may be absent in a case of lead poisoning which has other positive evidence for a diagnosis. It is therefore necessary to use the diagnostic criteria as a group, particularly elevated blood lead and lead and coproporphyrin increase in the urine together with the clinical picture, to prove that there is active lead poisoning to account for the present symptomatology of the child.

DIFFERENTIAL: Convulsions are a frequent cause of admission to a children's ward. Since encephalopathy with seizures and coma is the characteristic clinical picture of lead poisoning in children, lead as a cause, must be considered in every case of convulsion.

Meningitis. In the purulent types the spinal fluid contains thousands of cells per cu. mm., polymorphonucleated mainly, organisms, and a low sugar. In lead poisoning the spinal fluid is clear, has few cells (lymphocytes), and a normal sugar. In tuberculous meningitis the spinal fluid contains organisms and there is a low sugar. A positive tuberculin test is present. The encephalitides have a spinal fluid similar to that in lead poisoning; the history will help rule out postinfectious encephalitis following measles, etc. The viral types will require serum antibody studies, two stage. With papilledema, brain tumor and abscess must be considered. The latter usually has a history of preceding infection in the ears,

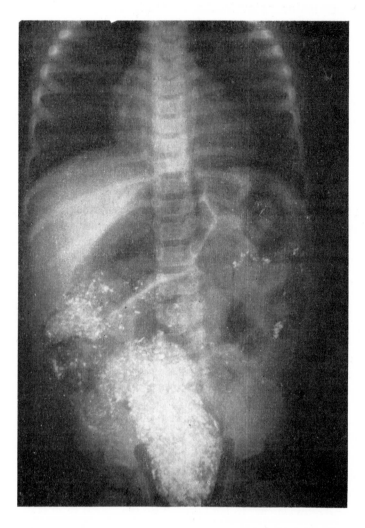

22. Lead encephalopathy. X-ray showing lead in the intestines.

sinuses, etc., and is less often seen today because of antibiotics. Tumors may be confusing. If there are no clear signs of lead pathology, exploration may be required. When polyneuritis occurs, causes in addition to lead must be considered. Poliomyelitis must also be ruled out in the summertime.

It is worthwhile repeating that lead must be proved the active cause of the clinical picture, for occasionally there may be another factor in addition to the lead. Lead encephalopathy may be engrafted on a retarded child with pica or brain tumor. Tuberculosis or purulent meningitis may occur in a child who has had lead exposure in the past.

PROGNOSIS: The outlook in children, once encephalopathy has set in, is poor. Mortality figures of 25 per cent persist in spite of present methods of therapy. In those surviving, mental retardation, residual paralysis, seizures, and emotional disturbances have occurred. Even in mild cases subsequent follow-up studies have revealed a failure of proper mental development. These children have language difficulty, short attention span, and marked distractability, which makes learning difficult (the characteristics of the brain-injured child).

However, since the advent of calcium disodium versenate the reports appear to be more encouraging with respect to sequelae. In older children and those with peripheral neuritis the outlook is much better.

TREATMENT: The first principle in therapy is prophylaxis. There must be a community drive, by means of posters, press, radio, and schools to acquaint parents, especially in the areas where houses are being torn down, of the seriousness of lead ingestion and how it may be avoided. Along with this, efforts should be made to control pica in children by greater attention to their emotional needs.

Stress should be laid on the importance of checking for lead in any child between one and five years who comes from slum areas with complaints of lack of appetite, pallor, apathy, severe persistent constipation, or vomiting. Suspicion of lead should be especially strong in the summer months.

Treatment of the acutely ill child with convulsions is, at present, best carried out by the use of calcium disodium versenate. This drug combines with certain metals forming non-ionized, water-soluble complexes (chelates), which are non-toxic and readily excreted in the urine. The calcium disodium salt is used since the versenate otherwise might combine with plasma calcium, which would cause hypocalcemic tetany. Metals such as lead and copper displace calcium from the complex. The dosage is 75 mg./kg. body weight/24 hours. The total daily dose is divided in two parts, and each half is administered intravenously in 250 cc. of 5 per cent glucose or normal saline over one or two hours. This procedure is carried out once on admission, and again later in the day. It is repeated twice a day for five days.

In addition to specific therapy the patient should be sedated for his seizures with i.m. sodium phenobarbital, gr. 1 for a child. Rectal paraldehyde or ether may be added. Surgical cerebral decompression should be used, if needed, to relieve increased intracranial pressure due to cerebral edema. McLaurin and Nichols, Jr. recommend that bilateral, massive, fronto-parieto-temporal decompressive craniectomy be performed when the seizures and elevated cerebrospinal fluid pressure are not responding to the EDTA. Lumbar puncture may first be tried every few hours, withdrawing only a few cc. at a time, for reduction of pressure above 300 mm. There is risk in this procedure for it may allow herniation of the brain through the tentorial incisura or foramen magnum.

Prevention of further exposure by the prophylactic measures previously outlined will permit the patient slowly to delead himself in about six months to one year. However, in the presence of acute infection or acidosis, a recurrence of lead encephalopathy may require repeat of the calcium disodium versenate regimen. Chisolm, Jr. and Harrison therefore suggest the use of quantitative coproporphyrin determinations as a guide. One might continue chelation until the coproporphyrin is present in the urine in near normal amounts, which would indicate that the lead in the soft tissues is at a non-toxic level.

At any rate, a period of about two weeks should be allowed after the first course of chelation before considering further therapy. Then if the output of coproporphyrin in the urine is in excess of 250 micrograms/24 hr., or if the blood lead is in excess of 0.1 mg./100 grams of whole blood and there is a positive qualitative test for coproporphyrin in the urine, of if serious neurologic manifestations persist, the course of versenate can be repeated.

Oral iron may be given for the anemia.

Blackman, Jr., S. S.: Intranuclear Inclusion Bodies in Kidney and Liver Caused by Lead Poisoning. Bull. Johns Hopkins Hosp. 58:384, 1936.
———: The Lesions of Lead Encephalitis in Children. Bull. Johns Hopkins Hosp. 61:1, 1937.

Byers, R. K., and Lord, E.: Late Effects of Lead Poisoning on Mental Development. Am. J. Dis. Child. 66: 471, 1943.
————, Maloof, C. A., and Cushman, M.: Urinary Excretion of Lead in Children. Am. J. Dis. Child. 87:548, 1954.
Chisolm, Jr. J. J., and Harrison, H. E.: The Exposure of Children to Lead. Pediat. 18:943, 1956.
———— and Harrison, H. E.: The Treatment of Acute Lead Encephalopathy in Children. Pediat. 19:2, 1957.
Deane, G. E., Heldrich, Jr., F. J. and Bradley, J. E.: Use of BAL in Treatment of Acute Lead Encephalopathy. J. Pediat. 42:409, 1953.
Goodman, L. S., and Gilman, A.: The Pharmocological Basis of Therapeutics. New York, Macmillan Co., 2 ed., 1955.
Markus, A. C. and Spencer, A. G.: Treatment of Chronic Lead Poisoning with Calcium Versonate. Brit. Med. J. 2:883, 1955.
McLaurin, R. L. and Nichols, Jr., J. B.: Extensive Cranial Decompression in the Treatment of Severe Lead Encephalopathy. Pediat. 20:653, 1957.
Mellins, R. B., and Jenkins, C. D.: Epidemiological and Psychological Study of Lead Poisoning in Children. J.A.M.A. 158:15, 1955.

ACRODYNIA (PINK DISEASE)

CLINICAL PICTURE: Acrodynia occurs primarily in infancy and early childhood. It is present in both sexes and in all races. The onset is insidious, frequent colds may be noted, and there are fretfulness and refusal of food with resultant loss of weight. The baby appears to shun the light (photophobia). The hands and feet are cold, moist, and have a pinkish appearance. Desquamation of the palms and soles occurs. The tip of the nose and cheeks are scarlet and pink. As the illness becomes more marked the classical features are present, including anorexia, profuse sweating, miliary rash, raw beefy hands and feet with shedding of skin, flabby musculature, marked hypotonia, and relaxation of the ligamentous structures. Pain appears to be intense. One observes scratching of the skin, loss of nails, and the fingers and toes may become gangrenous. The baby is without sleep, cannot rest, cries constantly, and lies face down in the pillow.

The neurological features include hypotonia and diminished to absent tendon reflexes. In some children there is inability to walk, in others there is a waddle similar to the gait in muscular dystrophy, probably due to the weak, atrophic musculature. Hyperaesthesia and pain along the nerve trunks may be noted. Tremors and convulsions may occur. Clinical pictures similar to polyneuritis, myelitis, and the Landry-Guillain-Barré syndrome are seen.

In older children the features previously described are present. There is marked inertia evidenced by the child's desire to sit in one area constantly. Fever usually is not present unless there is associated infection. There may be tachycardia and hypertension. Allergic phenomena such as wheezing and skin rashes are prominent. The children are wakeful at night. There may be loss of teeth, associated with inflammation of the gums and intense salivation. Delusions and hallucinations occasionally occur.

LABORATORY: No significant changes in blood count or spinal fluid are present. Mercury is present in the urine. Cheek has found a depletion of water and of sodium and chloride ions in the blood serum. There is loss of electrolyte with the excess sweat.

PATHOLOGY: There is no characteristic pathology in acrodynia. Changes in the peripheral nerves, cord, and brain have been described.

ETIOLOGY: Warkany and Hubbard have advanced data incriminating mercury as the cause of acrodynia. In twenty-eight patients they demonstrated the presence of mercury in the urine (100-400 mg. per liter) or obtained a history of exposure to mercury. It is true that mercury may occasionally be found in the urine of healthy children, so that there appears to be individual variation in the rate of excretion and reaction to mercury in those who ingest it. The greatest number of those demonstrating mercury in the urine were found in those areas where it was most often prescribed. Where teething powders are used, as in England and the southern United States, the greatest incidence is under one year, whereas in other areas, where mercury or calomel is given at a later age period, the greatest incidence is in the two to four year group. The response to BAL is also evidence in favor of mercury as the etiologic agent.

DIAGNOSIS: The classical picture of pink hands and feet, scarlet cheeks, hyperirritability, wakefulness, photophobia, abnormal sweating, hypotania, hypertension, peculiar position, and abject misery in a baby between a few months of age and four years is diagnostic. There may be a history of ingestion of mercury.

PROGNOSIS: The outlook is good. The mortality is about ten per cent. The disease lasts several months followed by slow recovery. Neurological sequelae may persist in some of the children.

TREATMENT: Prophylactic therapy consists of avoiding any form of treatment utilizing mercury. For the active disease Bivings uses BAL, 3 mg./kg. per day divided into injections q 4 h for 48 hours, then q 6 h for 24 hours, and finally q 12 h for 7 days. This is administered in 10% sol. of dimercaprol (BAL) in oil, intramuscularly, preceded by 0.5 ml. of 2% procaine. He noted rapid recovery in many cases. Others have not confirmed this. When the case is of long standing, rapid recovery is not so probable. If there is no response to BAL, EDTA may be tried (see under lead). For the pain and irritability phenobarbital may be used.

In addition to BAL, a high vitamin intake, sufficient calories, fluids, and electrolytes should be provided. Good nursing care is essential, especially skin cleanliness.

Bivings, L.: Acrodynia; A Summary of BAL Therapy Reports and a Case Report of Calomel Disease. J. Pediat. 34:322, 1949.
Cheek, D. B.: Pink Disease (Infantile Acrodynia). J. Pediat. 42:239, 1953.
Warkany, J., and Hubbard, D. M.: Adverse Mercurial Reactions in the Form of Acrodynia and Related Conditions. Am. J. Dis. Child. 81:335, 1951.
———— and Hubbard, D. M.: Acrodynia and Mercury. J. Pediat. 42:365, 1953.

HAND-SCHÜLLER-CHRISTIAN DISEASE

The three forms of reticuloendotheliosis, eosinophilic granuloma, Hand-Schüller-Christian disease, and Letterer-Siwe disease, are thought to be interrelated manifestations of a common disorder. Cholesterol accumulation is secondary to a primary disorder of the reticulo-endothelial system of unknown etiology. Only Hand-Schüller-Christian disease has significant neurological abnormalities.

CLINICAL PICTURE: This condition was originally described as a triad of defects in the membranous bones, mainly the skull, exophthalmos, and diabetes insipidus, due to xanthomatous deposits (foam cells containing cholesterol). This classical picture, however, is rarely seen.

The manifestations of the disease usually develop in early childhood. There is no familial tendency. Diabetes insipidus is usually the first symptom, but the disease may begin with swollen gums and loss of teeth, a bone lesion with impairment of gait, or with skin eruptions. Defects in the membranous bones of the skull may produce irregular swelling and may be palpable. Other skeletal bones are similarly involved. There are xanthomatous deposits in the region of the tuber cinereum, hypophysis, and mammillary bodies causing diabetes insipidus, obesity, dwarfism, or the adiposogenital syndrome. In other instances the deposits may produce an enlarged skull simulating hydrocephalus or signs of increased intracranial pressure with choked discs. Other neurological features may include mental retardation, severe headaches, and pains in the extremities (polyneuritis). Orbital deposits produce exophthalmos. There are cutaneous manifestations which include papular eruptions and seborrhea of the scalp. The lungs may show lesions. There may be discharge from the ear due to mastoid involvement.

LABORATORY: The blood shows anemia. Blood total lipids and cholesterol are normal. X-ray of the skull shows irregular defects in the bones and sometimes decalcification of the sella. Other bones, such as the pelvis, long bones, and spine show rarefaction. The spinal fluid is normal.

PATHOLOGY: The bone lesion is due to the accumulation of foam cells containing cholesterol, which produce defects especially in the skull and retro-orbital tissue. The defects also contain fibrous connective tissue. Deposits are present in the dura and base of the brain as well. Xanthomatous lesions are also produced in the skin, lungs, lymph nodes, and liver.

DIAGNOSIS: This is based on the combination of bone symptoms with other features of the disease as described. X-ray shows the bony defects in the skull and other areas. A biopsy of bone will reveal the characteristic granuloma. Other bone diseases like multiple myeloma, eosinophilic granuloma, tuberculosis, and lymphoma should be ruled out.

PROGNOSIS: The course is generally progressive and chronic. Remissions may occur. The younger the age of onset, the more severe the course.

TREATMENT: X-ray therapy should be offered for the bone lesions. Nasal pituitrin is used for the diabetes insipidus. The use of ACTH and cortisone is questionable.

Batson, R., Shapiro, J., Christie, A., and Riley Jr., H. D.: Acute Nonlipid Disseminated Reticuloendotheliosis. Am. J. Dis. Child. 90:323, 1955.

Davison, C.: Xanthomatosis and the Central Nervous System (Schüller-Christian Syndrome). Arch. Neurol. and Psychiat. 30:75, 1933.

Karlen, K. H.: A Case of Hand-Schüller-Christian Disease Treated with Cortisone. Acta Pediat. 41:282, 1952.

Knighten, R. S. and Fox, J. D. Diagnosis and treatment of Eosinophilic Granuloma of Skull. J.A.M.A. 162:1294, 1956.

Lichtenstein, L.: Histiocytosis X. A.M.A. Arch. Path. 56:84, 1953.

Rowland, R. S.: Xanthomatosis and the Reticulo-endothelial System: Correlation of an Unidentified Group of Cases Described as Defects in Membranous Bone, Exophthalmos and Diabetes Insipidus (Christian's Syndrome). Arch. Int. Med. 42:611, 1928.

Sosman, M. C.: Xanthomatosis (Schüller-Christian's Disease: Lipoid Histiocytosis). J.A.M.A. 98:110, 1932.

Van Creveld, S.: Hand-Schüller-Christian Disease. Advances in Pediatrics. Chicago, Year Book Pub. 6:209, 1953.

MYASTHENIA GRAVIS

Myasthenia gravis is characterized by abnormal fatigability and weakness of the striated musculature.

CLINICAL PICTURE: There are two types of myasthenia gravis in children. One is referred to as "neonatal" and includes babies born of mothers who have myasthenia gravis. The duration is short and with therapy to tide them over the babies in most instances recover in a period of a few days to several weeks and then continue normally without need of further medication. A few deaths, however, have occurred. The other clinical type is referred to as juvenile myasthenia gravis with symptoms beginning in the newborn period or in later childhood. The mothers of this second type do not have myasthenia gravis. Transmission is possibly recessive.

In babies there is muscle weakness, often symmetrical, and hypotonia. The Moro reflex is weak or absent. There are inability to suck or swallow, lethargy, poor cry, and general lack of movements. Ptosis, so classical at a later age, is uncommon in the infantile period. Strabismus is present. Prostigmine, 0.05 to 1 mg. parenterally or 1-5 mg. by mouth with each feeding, will relieve the symptoms and also confirm the diagnosis.

In the juvenile type there is fatigue, increasing with exercise and as the day goes on. One of the earliest signs is impaired function of the extraocular muscles. Ptosis of one or both eyelids may occur. Strabismus and diplopia may be present. The muscles supplied by the cranial nerves are involved so that there is difficulty in mastication, deglutition, and phonation. The trunk muscles and those of the neck are usually affected later, but occasionally may be the first areas to exhibit difficulty.

The child usually appears well in the morning, and the eyes are fully open. But as the day goes on the muscles become much weaker, and ptosis of the lids appears. The visceral musculature is spared. Occasionally the extremities may be involved. Characteristically, as the muscles are used they become weaker, but with rest they may improve. They do not ache nor are they tender.

There is no muscle atrophy except in a small proportion, mostly due to disuse. Deep tendon reflexes are normal. There are no sensory changes. Mentality is intact. With continued electrical excitation the muscles gradually do not react, but with rest reactivity is demonstrated.

In rare instances the onset in children is acute rather than insidious. Thus, in acute respiratory emergency of unknown etiology myasthenia gravis should be thought of. In these cases, tracheotomy and a respirator may be required until the effects of drug therapy can overcome the weakness of the respiratory and laryngeal muscles.

ETIOLOGY AND PATHOGENESIS: There are no morphologic abnormalities of muscle, central nervous system, or peripheral nerves. Tumor of the thymus or lymphoid follicle formation in the medulla of the thymus is found in some cases. There are also a small number of cases in which hyperthyroidism and myasthenia gravis are associated.

Attempts have been made to incriminate acetylcholine. The latter is liberated at the motor end plate and controlled by its antagonist, cholinesterase. Deficiency of the former or excess of the latter have been postulated but not substantiated. Bernsohn and his associates found a high true cholinesterase activity in the cerebrospinal fluid in seven cases. No hereditary trait has been proved, but there are a number of instances in the juvenile form where more than one sibling is affected.

LABORATORY: Blood, urine, and spinal fluid are normal. Electromyography shows diminution of the muscle action potential which can be converted to normal by neostigmine.

DIAGNOSIS: The major diagnostic considerations include the onset of weakness of the voluntary musculature, especially the ocular or bulbar muscles, without atrophy, and the response to neostig-mine. Bulbar palsies of any type, encephalitis, muscular dystrophy, hyperthyroidism, nuclear ophthalmoplegia, and poliomyelitis must be differentiated. The use of drugs which produce immediate im-provement in myasthenia gravis may aid in separating this condition from the others. Two mg. of Tensilon®, a cholinergic drug, injected intravenously produces a temporary increase in muscle strength within two minutes. In the normal individual there is no increase in strength and fasciculation develops.

PROGNOSIS: The child may go on to progressive death or may have remissions and exacerbations. Infections aggravate the myas-thenia. The mortality rate in children is reported as 4 per cent against 15-28 per cent in adults.

TREATMENT: There is no cure, but with neostigmine therapy the patient survives longer and is more comfortable. This drug re-duces the blocking effect of cholinesterase, thus permitting acetyl-choline to function more properly. One 15 mg. slow-release tablet of neostigmine bromide is given orally, three times a day. For the side effects of nausea, cramps, or diarrhea, atropine or Tinct. Bel-ladona may be used. Mestinon Bromide® slow-release tablets may also be used orally three times a day. One 60 mg. tablet is equivalent to a 15 mg. tablet of neostigmine. The slow-release tablets eliminate the need of medication during sleeping hours.

The reports of Eaton and his co-workers and of others suggest that thymectomy has some value. However, the indications for the procedure, except when there is pressure from a definite tumor, are still in doubt. ACTH and cortisone have been tried for their effect on shrinking the thymus. They may first produce an exacerbation of symptoms and therefore they may be dangerous.

Another approach has been the combined use of betaine and glycocyamine to correct creatine metabolism, urecholine, a choline ester which is a precurser of acetylcholine, and B_{12} which potenti-ates urecholine.

Adams, R. D., Denny-Brown, D., and Pearson, C. M.: Diseases of Muscle. New York. Paul Hoeber & Co. 1953.

Bastedo, D. L. A.: Acute Fulminating Myasthenia Gravis in Children. Canad. M.A.J. 63:388, 1950.

Bernsohn, J., Boshes, B., and Possley, L.: A Study of Cholinesterase and Ali-esterase in Various Neurologic Diseases. Neurology. 8:221, 1958.

Billig, Jr., H. E. and Morehouse, L. E.: Performance and Metabolic Alterations during Betaine Glycocyamine Feeding in Myasthenia Gravis. Arch. Phys. Med. 36:233, 1955.

Eaton, L. M., Clagett, O. T., and Bastron, J. A.: The Thymus and Its Relationship to Diseases of the Nervous System: Study of 374 Cases of Myasthenia Gravis and Comparison of 87 Patients Undergoing Thymectomy with 225 Controls. A Res. Publ. Nerv. Ment. Dis. Proc. 32:107, 1953.

Geddes, A. K., and Kidd, H. M.: Myasthenia Gravis of the Newborn. Canad. M.A.J. 64:152, 1951.

Kane, C. A., and Weed, L.: Myasthenia Gravis Associated with Adrenal Insufficiency. New England J. Med. 243:939, 1950.

Levin, P. M.: Congenital Myasthenia in Siblings. Arch. Neurol. and Psychiat. 62:745, 1949.

Mackay, R. I.: Congenital Myasthenia Gravis. Arch. Dis. Child. 26:289, 1951.

Osserman, K. E.: Studies in Myasthenia Gravis, Part I. Physiology, Pathology, Diagnosis and Treatment. New York States J. Med. 56:2512, 1956. Part II, Relationship of Thymus to Myasthenia Gravis. 56:2672, 1956.

Randt, C. T.: Myasthenia Gravis. Med. Clin. N. A. W. B. Saunders Co., 1953, pp. 535.

Schwab, R. S., Osserman, K. E. and Tether, J. E.: Treatment of Myasthenia Gravis. J.A.M.A. 165:671, 1957.

Schwarz, H.: Urecholine in Myasthenia Gravis. Canad. M.A.J. 72:346, 1955.

FAMILIAL PERIODIC PARALYSIS

This is a rare type of recurrent or periodic flaccid paralysis associated with strong familial incidence, loss of deep reflexes, and electrical excitability.

CLINICAL PICTURE: The onset is usually during childhood or adolescence. The attack may follow a period of rest, especially after a night of sleep. There may be no prodomata and the patient may have felt fine prior to going to sleep only to awaken with inability to get out of bed. In other instances the child may not feel well or may awaken with weakness, thirst, hunger, and tingling or pain in the extremities. An attack may follow ingestion of too much food, especially carbohydrates, exposure to cold, or prolonged exertion.

When the child tries to arise, he finds he cannot move his legs or back. Subsequently all the extremities and neck are affected. The paralysis is flaccid, involving the proximal muscles rather than those of the hands or feet. Generally the muscles of the face, eyes, and tongue are spared. There is usually no disability in speech, chewing, or respiration. Sphincter control is intact. There is no unconsciousness, and mentality remains clear. There are occasional cases reported, however, in which the cranial nerves are affected, with ptosis and dysphagia; in others there have been bladder retention, bradycardia, and intercostal paralysis with disturbed respiration. Along with the paralysis of the muscles, there are loss of deep tendon reflexes and lack of reaction to galvanic or faradic excitation. There may also be loss of superficial reflexes. There is no sensory disturbance.

With the end of the attack, which may last from several hours to two days, the reflexes and electrical reactions return to normal and there is recovery of muscular power. The attacks occur every week or less often and reach their peak of frequency in the first forty years, becoming less frequent and of shorter duration thereafter.

PATHOLOGY: A few autopsies and muscle biopsies have been performed. There is nothing distinctive for diagnostic purposes. However, when the patient is on a high salt intake, biopsy of the muscle shows vacuolar myopathy. With a low salt diet, the vacuolar myopathy disappears. There are no nervous system findings.

ETIOLOGY: The cause of familial periodic paralysis is unknown. Males are involved more frequently. In many of the patients there is a strong familial incidence. Hereditary transmission occurs through both male and female, essentially as a dominant condition with reduced penetrance, but also recessive.

PATHOGENESIS: It has been assumed that potassium plays a role in this disease because in most instances the blood serum level is decreased following an attack. Goss and his group induced attacks with large amounts of glucose. Attacks can also be precipitated by insulin injection, marked loss of extracellular fluid as in diarrhea, and ACTH or cortisone therapy with a low dietary potassium intake. Since urinary potassium is not increased before or after an attack, the drop in serum potassium must be due to an increase in the liver and muscles.

On the other hand, Tyler and his group could not correlate the attacks with serum potassium levels. An association with hyperthyroidism has been observed, but what effect, if any, the thyroid may have in producing an attack of periodic paralysis is unknown.

Recently Conn and his associates reported that a large increase in urinary aldosterone with an intense retention of sodium precedes the onset of a spontaneous attack of periodic paralysis. The retention of sodium is followed by potassium sequestration in the tissues and an abrupt fall of potassium in the blood serum and urine. With recovery, a large excretion of sodium occurs and subsequently relatively small amounts of potassium. Serum sodium and potassium then return to normal together. Aldosterone excretion also returns to its baseline in the urine. On a restricted sodium intake Conn and his group were unable to induce attacks of periodic paralysis or sequestration of potassium with glucose and insulin. Furthermore, if a sodium-retaining corticoid is given, an attack is induced only if there is a high sodium intake; it does not occur if sodium is unavailable for retention in the body. From their evidence they conclude that marked sodium retention within the muscle cell is in part the cause of muscle paralysis. Hypokalemia, when it occurs, may be a contributing factor. The stimulus for excessive aldosterone secretion is probably extra-adrenal.

PROGNOSIS: The course is favorable, since, as mentioned, the attacks become infrequent with middle age. Care should be taken during the attack since occasionally death may occur from respiratory or cardiac distress.

DIAGNOSIS: There is little difficulty in diagnosis if one keeps in mind the cardinal characteristics of a heredofamilial history, recurrent attacks of weakness, loss of reflexes and electrical excitability during the attack, and lowered potassium in the serum. The attack is best brought out by vigorous exercise followed by complete rest. In adynamia episodica hereditaria where the clinical picture is similar, serum potassium is elevated.

TREATMENT: For the attack itself four grams of potassium chloride are given orally. For prophylactic purposes a total of two to four grams of potassium chloride, made up in aqueous 25 per cent solution, are taken, either once before bedtime or in divided doses. The child should not eat large meals or too much carbohydrate.

Following the evidence of Conn and his associates, one should use a diet low in sodium to prevent attacks of periodic paralysis. As an initial step one might "desalt" the patient with mercurial diuretics or carbonic anhydrase inhibitors.

Adrenalectomy to remove the source of aldosterone is not advised since the attacks of paralysis ultimately disappear spontaneously.

Parents should be warned of future inheritance possibilities if their child marries.

Conn, J. W., Louis, L. H., Fajans, S. S., Streeten, D. H. P. and Johnson, R. D.: Intermittent Aldosteronism in Periodic Paralysis, Dependence of Attacks on Retention of Sodium, and Failure to Induce Attacks by Restriction of Dietary Sodium. Lancet, pp. 802-805, April 20, 1957.

Gamstorp, I., Hauge, M., Helwig-Larsen, H. F. and others: Adynamia Episodica Hereditaria: A Disease Clinically Resembling Familial Periodic Paralysis but Characterized by Increasing Serum Potassium During the Paralytic Attack. Am. J. Med. 23:385, 1957.

Goss, H., Cherhashy, M. and Savitsky, M.: Potassium and Periodic Paralysis: A Metabolic Study and Physiological Considerations. Medicine 27:105, 1948.

Hosotte, A., Ferrand, M., Philippori, J., Widlocher, D. and Soulayrol, R.: Two Cases of Periodic Familial Paralysis. Rev. Neurol. 91:347, 1954.

Typler, F. H., Stephens, F. E., Gunn, F. D., and Perkoff, G. T.: Studies in Disorders of Muscle: VII Clinical Manifestations and Inheritance of a Type of Periodic Paralysis Without Hypopotassemia. J. Clin. Invest. 30: 492, 1951.

IDIOPATHIC HYPERCALCEMIA OF INFANCY

This clinical entity was described in 1952 by Fanconi, et al. It consists of anorexia, vomiting, constipation, and loss of weight, and begins at about two to three months of age. As the months pass by, these children show a characteristic peculiar facies and dwarfism. There may be a small skull, recessive mandible, epicanthal folds, wide mouth, and a depressed nasal bridge. There are mental and motor retardation and hypotonia, but hyperactive reflexes are present. Marked irritability is noted. Hypertension and a heart murmur were present in many of the infants. There is also impaired kidney function.

LABORATORY: Serum calcium is increased to 15 mg./100 ml. The BUN is elevated. X-ray shows osteosclerosis and premature craniosynostosis.

ETIOLOGY: The cause is unknown. However, it has been suggested that this disease may be due to hypersensitivity to vitamin D with excessive calcium absorption. Others have postulated a defect in the metabolism of vitamin D.

PROGNOSIS: The disease occurs in mild and severe forms. The latter is fatal.

TREATMENT: The infant should be placed on a calcium-free diet with restricted intake of vitamin D. Cortisone may be used.

Daeschner, G. L. and Daeschner, C. W.: Severe Idiopathic Hypercalcemia of Infancy. Pediat. 19:362, 1957.

Fanconi, G., Giradet, P., Schlesinger, B., Butler, N., and Black, J.: Chronische Hypercalcamie; Kombiniert mit Osteosklerose, Hyperazotamie, Minderwuchs und Kongenitalen Missbildungen. Helvet, Paediat. Acta. 7:314, 1952.

Schlesinger, B. E., Butler, N. R., and Block. J. A.: Severe Type of Infantile Hypercalcemia. Brit. M. J. 1:127, 1956.

Fellers, F. X. and Schwartz, R.: "Vitamin D Activity" in Idiopathic Hypercalcemia. Soc. Pediat. Research. May 6-7, 1958.

DISSEMINATED LUPUS ERYTHEMATOSUS

This condition is an acute or chronic systemic disease affecting tissues of mesenchymal origin and resulting in prolonged fever and a variety of clinical features. Involvement of the blood vessels of various organs is prominent.

CLINICAL PICTURE: There is an acute febrile course, which becomes protracted with intermittent remissions. Joint pains are prominent. The skin shows a "butterfly erythema" over the bridge of the nose, neck, and chest. The serous membranes may give evidence of involvement in the form of pleurisy or pericarditis. There is enlargement of the liver and spleen, and glomerulitis may occur.

The central nervous system findings include generalized and focal seizures, transient cranial nerve palsies, hemiplegia, delirium, and aphasia. There may be a peripheral neuritis or cerebrovascular accident.

LABORATORY: There are anemia, leukopenia, and occasionally thrombocytopenia.

The urine is positive for albumin and red blood cells, and the blood may show an elevated NPN and urea. Lupus erythematosus cells (LE phenomenon) may be demonstrated. The sedimentation rate is increased, and the serum gamma globulin is elevated. There may be a false positive test for syphilis.

PATHOLOGY: The essential lesion is a "fibrinoid" degeneration of the connective tissue, particularly in the smaller arteries and arterioles. In the brain, as elsewhere, there is an endarteritis resulting in encephalomalacia. There may be gross or petechial hemorrhages in the cortex. The gray matter is especially involved.

ETIOLOGY: This is unknown, although the evidence would seem to incriminate an immunological mechanism. The disease occurs mostly in females in the second and third decades. However, children are also affected.

DIAGNOSIS: The major features are protracted fever, the rash on the face, pericarditis and pleuritis, joint, cardiac, and kidney involvement. The blood studies, especially the presence of the LE phenomenon, are significant. Since the manifestations are so varied and may not be typical, there may be great difficulty in diagnosis. At times, rheumatic fever, nephritis, thrombocytopenic purpura, erythema nodosum, dermatomyositis, and periarteritis nodosa must be ruled out.

PROGNOSIS: The outlook is poor.

TREATMENT: Cortisone or ACTH does not cure, but ameliorates the symptomatology and produces a good response. In some instances, however, while seizures have been reduced, other untoward cerebral effects such as hemorrhage have been brought on.

Glaser, G. H.: Lesions of the Central Nervous System in Disseminated Lupus Erythematosus: Arch. Neurol. and Psychiat. 67:745, 1952.
Ogryzlo, M. A. and Smythe, H. A.: Systemic Lupus Erythematosus and Syndromes Possibly Related. Pediat. 19:1109, 1957.

PERIARTERITIS NODOSA

Periarteritis involves the medium and smaller sized arteries.

CLINICAL PICTURE: The disease has protean manifestations. There are fever, pains in the mucles of the extremities, joints, and abdomen, weakness, and loss of weight. Skin eruptions may occur, either urticarial or macular. There is some degree of hypertension. The clinical picture may simulate an acute infectious disease of the brain or tumor, with bulbar and cerebral symptoms. There may be hemorrhages into the brain or subarachnoid space from rupture of the arteries. The neurological features include convulsions and paralyses. Peripheral neuritis, especially of the nerves of the upper and lower extremities, may occur. This is due to occlusion of the nutrient arteries in the nerve trunks with subsequent infarction of the nerve bundles. There are pain and tenderness along the nerve trunks, paresthesias, muscle weakness with loss of function, and loss of tendon reflexes.

LABORATORY: The blood shows a leucocytosis with eosinophilia and anemia. Culture is sterile. The sedimentation rate is elevated. The blood NPN may be elevated. The spinal fluid is normal, unless hemorrhage has occurred; it is then xanthochromic. The urine may be positive for albumin, red blood cells, and casts.

PATHOLOGY: There is an inflammatory reaction involving all parts of the artery. The process appears to begin in the media resulting in a hyaline-like necrosis; there is proliferation of the intima followed by infiltration of the adventitia. Thrombosis and occlusion of the vessels occur. Periarterial nodules may be felt along the arterial walls. The arteries of the heart, kidney, adrenals, liver, gastrointestinal tract, skin, and brain are involved.

ETIOLOGY: The cause of periarteritis nodosa is unknown, but it may possibly be due to hypersensitivity. Drugs such as sulfonamides have been incriminated.

DIAGNOSIS: The clinical picture is so varied that many diseases must be considered in differential, especially rheumatic fever, lupus erythematosus, dermatomyositis, and nephritis. When the neurological picture develops, it may appear similar to meningitis, tumor, or peripheral neuritis. The etiological factor may be obscure. When peripheral neuritis is present, its association with renal or gastrointestinal symptoms or hypertension may make the diagnosis. Muscle biopsy showing the vascular lesions is very helpful.

PROGNOSIS: The prospects are bleak in this condition.

TREATMENT: Cortisone may bring temporary remission, but usually there is not a good response and the ultimate downhill course is unaffected.

Griffith, G. E., and Vural, I. L.: Polyarteritis Nodosa. Circulation 3:481, 1951.
Lovshin, L. L. and Kerhohan, J. W.: Peripheral Neuritis in Periarteritis Nodosa. A Clinicopathologic Study. Proceedings Staff Meeting Mayo Clinic, 24:48, 1949.
Parker, H. L., and Kernohan, J. W.: The Central Nervous System in Periarteritis Nodosa. Proceedings Staff Meetings Mayo Clinic, 24:43, 1949.

Physical Expression (In Terms of the Nervous System) of Psychogenic Disturbances in Children

Physicians have from time to time encountered children who refer their complaints to some part of the body for which there seems to be no adequate organic explanation. A few examples follow.

J. F., a girl of fourteen, had not been attending school for the past five years because of recurrent chorea (Sydenham's). The first attack occurred within a month of the time the maternal grandmother had come to live with the family. The child, after a period of hospitalization, was sent to a convalescent home. Shortly after she returned to her home, her father died. This precipitated a second attack. Her condition was diagnosed as a conversion hysteria of the hyperkinetic type. In this instance, the subacute type of chorea appears to have involved both organic and psychological factors, making for slow and uncertain progress.

F. L., a thirteen year old boy, was admitted to the hospital because of tremors of the arms and fingers. Two weeks earlier he had had severe palpitation of the heart and had awakened from his sleep saying he was going to die. Study of the case revealed marital discord in the home. The mother was having an affair with another man, and the boy had witnessed frequent quarrels. Emotional insecurity, fear, and anxiety provided the basis for the clinical picture.

A girl of eleven was referred because she cleared her throat so frequently that it was annoying to those around her. Physical examination, including laryngoscopy, was negative. Questioning revealed that a great deal of financial difficulty existed in her home. The movement on the part of the child to clear her throat was unconscious and compulsive.

Tics may be a means of alleviating emotional tension. Encephalitis and chorea must be differentiated. As a rule these children are normal physically. There is no history of encephalitis or rheumatic fever. The treatment is directed at eliminating the causes of the emotional disturbances. No direct attempt is made to affect the motor movements, and parents and teachers are told not to urge the child to stop the movements. Analysis of the day's routine should be made to avoid excessive fatigue and stimulation. (See Chorea).

Hysterical manifestations may involve paralysis of any or all extremities. With careful testing it can be shown that while use of the extremity appears to be impaired, the muscles themselves are functioning. Hoover's sign brings this out. Normally, when the child is placed on his back, a request to raise one leg automatically causes the heel of the other leg to press down. If the examiner places his hand under the heel he can feel this downward pressure. If there is true paralysis of a limb, an attempt to raise it creates a marked pressure on the hand of the examiner from the automatic downward movement of the normal limb. If there is hysterical paralysis, a request to raise the "paralyzed limb" results in no increase in the downward pressure of the normal limb, for no real effort to use the muscle is made. The tendon reflexes and electrical reactions are normal. Another form of motor impairment is astasia abasia, in which the child cannot walk or stand. If placed in bed, however, he has full use of his limbs, which indicates that there is no organic paralysis. It may be a symptom of an underlying neurosis.

G. F. was admitted for headaches and decreasing vision of two months duration. Examination revealed diplopia and concentric contraction of the visual field. The fundi were normal. General neurological examination was negative. On the third day of hospitalization the patient's visual defects cleared suddenly and completely and the headache also disappeared. In this case, the child had a friend who had similarly lost her vision. While the background for the hysterical manifestation was a maternal conflict, the form was suggested by the friend's failure of vision. This patient had a hysterical amblyopia, not a brain tumor for which she was admitted. Wolff and Lackman reported two cases in which emotional conflicts were engendered through loss of affection and resulted in hysterical blindness. Various tests may be used to detect hysterical amblyopia. The fundi are normal and the pupils react to light. The patient can walk in a room without running into furniture. There is concentric contraction of the visual fields. Furthermore, the field does not change with variation in distance or size of objects (tubular field).

Other types of somatic manifestations include sensory symptoms, such as pains of all types in the head, abdomen, and lower limbs, and anaesthesia, often of the glove and stocking type, in the extremity. Another characteristic of the anaesthesia is that it stops at the exact midline of the head or body, contrary to the anatomical nerve supply of the area and the course of any nerve.

Hysterical seizures may occasionally occur. This has been discussed under epilepsy. There may also be anaesthesia of the pharynx and loss of the pharyngeal reflex. Anorexia nervosa may also occur, in adolescent females especially. The failure of appetite and resultant undernutrition are due to a hysterical disturbance resulting from underlying tension or worry.

DIAGNOSIS: The diagnosis of the psychogenic cause for a somatic manifestation rests upon a careful history, which may furnish evidence of a neurotic personality, parental discord, or other environmental factors producing fear, insecurity, etc. The physical examination is normal, suggesting that the complaints are not on a neuroanatomic basis. The onset in hysteria is likely to be sudden, and often recovery takes place by suggestion, persuasion, change of environment, or re-education. Differential must be made from organic disease. It should be kept in mind that brain tumor, encephalitis, etc., may occur in hysterical individuals. If there are neurological signs such as the Babinski, papilledema, etc., it is certain that organic disease exists.

TREATMENT: The basic treatment is a thorough study of the child and his surroundings. The explanation is to be sought in some environmental factor in the home, school, or neighborhood which is acting upon the hereditary make-up of the child. The psychogenic disorder may arise through a sense of insecurity or anxiety because of parental conflict. Fears and frustrations because of intellectual inadequacy may play a role. Detailed attention must be given to the every day experiences of the child.

For the immediate and temporary cure of symptoms, techniques such as pretended surgery, electrical stimulation, sham X-radiation, or hypnotism have been used. It is obvious that these measures are only of short term value, and there is a question as to their desirability. Primarily, one should deal with the psychological aspect of the problem so as to get to the underlying causes of the trouble. The outlook is generally good in children if early therapy is instituted. In special instances psychiatric help may be required.

Hinman, A.: Conversion Hysteria in Childhood. A.M.A. J. Dis. Child. 95:43, 1958.
Lamm, S. S.: Physical Expression of Psychogenic Disturbance in Children. J. Pediat. 20:237, 1942.
Walsh, F. B.: Clinical Neuro-ophthalmology. Baltimore, Williams and Wilkins Co., 1947.
Wolff, E. and Lachman, G. S.: Hysterical Blindness in Children. Report of Two Cases. Am. J. Dis. Child. 55:743, 1938.

BRAIN-INJURED CHILDREN

Strauss restricts the use of the term "brain-injured child" to children with minimal brain damage and normal family constellation. The cerebral damage is caused by environmental factors acting either pre, para, or postnatally. He calls these factors exogenous. Examination reveals some slight neurological signs even if there is no conspicuous motor retardation. In general the growth of these children is satisfactory and their mental level is within or near the normal range. Bender has added developmental deviations including heredodegenerations. These are referred to as endogenous and are based on inheritance. Others have included children with gross neurological damage, as in the cerebral palsied.

Whether the brain damage is minimal or gross, obscure or obvious, of exogenous or endogenous origin, the children in this brain-injured group are characterized by poor quality of school work, behavior disturbances, and poor physical performance. Even with a normal mental level these children show perceptual difficulties, disturbed spatial relationships, and impaired ability to think abstractly. Their psychological patterns include restlessness, short attention span, distractibility, tendency to impulsiveness, and unpredictable behavior. There may be noted a regression in motor pattern, disturbances in muscle tone, and generally poor functioning reflexes. In some, hyperactivity is outstanding.

It should be made clear that not all children who have had brain injury due to trauma or infection have these behavior disorders. Some recover completely. In others there may be motor disturbances such as hemiplegia, seizures, or impaired mental level. However, in many brain-injured children this disturbance of behavior leading to disruption and disorganization of the personality is the outstanding feature. The child is doing poorly in school, has personality problems, is unpredictable, or is awkward.

ETIOLOGY: There is usually a history of congenital or acquired pathology. In the latter group infections, e.g., encephalitis, especially within the first five years of life, are significant. The congenital pathology is due to prenatal or natal factors.

CLINICAL PICTURE: There may be cranial nerve palsies, alteration of reflexes, disturbance in coordination, changes in muscle tone, poor gait, and poor speech. Electroencephalography may show a focus of excitation if seizures are present, or an abnormal pattern.

Psychological. The intelligence level may be normal, but peculiarities show up in tests for reasoning, thinking, and concept formation. The child who is brain-injured exhibits a disturbance in spatial relationships and is easily distracted by background. He shows perseveration or stereotypy. There is also visual-motor incoordination. All of this makes it difficult to learn. Body image or the child's conception of himself is disturbed so that the world around him is distorted. Visual and auditory perception are affected. As a result, speech and reading disabilities develop.

Behavior and Personality. There may be marked aggressiveness, unpredictability of behavior, and feelings of inadequacy. The work in school suffers. These children have a short attention span and are easily distractible, going from one thing to another. As a reaction to their inadequacies they act selfishly, and show a generally immature reaction pattern.

DIAGNOSIS: The criteria for recognition of the brain-injured child consist of a history of brain injury in a generally normal family with minimal or gross neuromuscular effects in terms of motor weakness, incoordination, or changes in muscle tone. There are intellectual and personality disturbances with inability to adjust in school. In a condition in which the major complaints on the part of the parents are of intellectual and personality difficulties, there must be a distinction made from childhood schizophrenia. This may be difficult. The childhood schizophrenic is characterized by generalized withdrawal of interest from the environment and seclusiveness. The other differential is from acute encephalitis where specific sequelae of a more antisocial type may occur such as stealing, lying, rape, and arson.

TREATMENT: As in other handicapped areas treatment is a team approach. It requires parental education as to the nature of the problem. Special educational methods are required to overcome the perceptual difficulties. Specific psychiatric therapy may be used in conjunction with the team approach. (Refer to cerebral palsy).

Drugs may be of some value in helping the child meet his school problems and in aiding social adjustment. Amphetamine each morning or a tranquilizing drug such as chlorpromazine 15 mg., may be used t.i.d. Sedatives such as phenobarbital seem to act adversely in these children and should not be given. Favorable results have also been reported with Benadryl ®, Tolserol ®, and Suvren®.

PROGNOSIS: The outlook is variable depending on the factors previously discussed. The behavior patterns are favorably influenced by a sound therapeutic regimen, which includes aid to the child and parents. The hyperkinetic behavior syndrome disappears in early adult life (Laufer).

Bender, L.: Psychopathology of Children with Organic Brain Disorders. Springfield, Ill. Chas. C. Thomas, 1956.

Bradley, C.: The Behavior of Children Receiving Benzedrine. Am. J. Psychiat. 94:577, 1937.

————: Schizophrenia in Childhood. New York, Macmillan Co., 1941.

————: Characteristics and Management of Children with Behavior Problems Associated with Organic Brain Damage. Pediatric Clinics N. A. Philadelphia, W. B. Saunders Co. p. 1049, 1957.

Gesell, A., and Amatruda, C. S.: Developmental Diagnosis. New York, Paul B. Hoeber, 1947.

Ingram, T. T. S.: Characteristic Form of Overactive Behavior in Brain Damaged Children. J. Ment. Sc. 102:550, 1956.

Laufer, M. W. and Denhoff, E.: Hyperkinetic Behavior Syndrome in Children. J. Pediat. 50:463, 1957.

Milman, D. H.: Organic Behavior Disorder. A.M.A. J. Dis. Child. 91:521, 1956.

Potter, H. W.: Schizophrenia in Children, Am. J. Psychiat. 89:1253, 1933.

Silver, A. A.: Postural and Righting Reflexes in Children. J. Pediat. 41:493, 1952.

Strauss, A. A., and Lehtinen, L. E.: Psychopathology and Education of the Brain-Injured Child. New York, Grune and Stratton, 1947.

———— and Kephart, N. C.: Psychopathology and Education of the Brain-Injured Child. Vol. II. New York, Grune and Stratton, 1955.

APHASIA

The term aphasia is applied to a defect in symbolic language due to cerebral pathology. It is realized that in the infant or young child who has never learned to speak or is only just beginning there is technically no aphasia in the sense that there is no loss of a skill previously acquired; however, for purposes of discussion the term is retained so that we can differentiate cerebral from other causes of language disorders. One might use the term "aphasoid."

The visual and auditory senses are normal, as is speech, and testing shows adequate mental development. Nevertheless, the child cannot comprehend or use language properly or may not speak at all. The term congenital aphasia is applied to the failure of speech development which occurs in young children. It is based on faulty development of the cerebral cortex or injury to those areas or their association pathways concerned with the reception, interpretation, or production of language. Aphasia may also result from infections, such as meningitis and encephalitis, trauma with hemorrhage, or brain tumor. A particular type of receptive aphasia acquired in association with manifestations of a convulsive disorder has been reported in some children.

In the older child the aphasic syndrome may approach the adult type. In young children under five years of age there are some differences. Whereas in the adult a left hemisphere lesion with right hemiplegia is associated with speech disturbance, in the very young child with a similar clinical picture, speech may not be affected. Speech disturbance in the child appears to require a more diffuse pathology.

There are various areas devoted to speech:

a. Broca's in the 2nd and 3rd left frontal convolution at the foot of the motor area.
b. Other areas in the parietal (above the Sylvian fissure), temporal, and superior frontal lobes just anterior to the Rolandic foot region.

The primary area for auditory reception is in the transverse temporal gyrus of Heschl. Other areas of interest include the superior temporal gyrus of Wernicke where auditory interpretation occurs, the visual area in the occipital lobe, and the visual word area in the angular gyrus.

The previous discussion suggests that multiple lesions may be needed to produce aphasia in children. Some feel that each form of aphasia requires involvement of the specific area controlling the particular function. Others, however, consider that all parts of the brain are involved in language aphasia. It may be that local and non-local factors operate together.

PATHOLOGY: There may be defective development of part of the cortex. In others, encephalitis, meningitis, occlusion of the middle cerebral artery, or thrombosis of the veins may be present. There may also be evidence of cerebral anoxia.

TYPES OF SPEECH APHASIAS

1. *Receptive or Sensory,* also known as congenital word deafness, auditory aphasia, or Wernicke type. The child is unable to comprehend language although his hearing is normal. The result is unintelligible speech or no speech at all. Words, if used, are indiscriminately chosen. When the same word is repeated it is not

used in relation to the original idea. Speech is unaccompanied by gestures. It is a jargon. The child is brought for study because of failure of speech development or inadequate use.

The physical and neurological examination usually reveal no abnormalities. The muscles of the tongue, jaw, larynx, and respiration are normal. Hearing is adequate. Vision is good. Mentality is normal.

2. *Motor or Expressive.* The child comprehends but cannot use language to express himself. This is less common than receptive aphasia. He cannot express himself by the use of words (no speech) or makes only primitive sounds. However, he does respond to sound. Physical, neurological, and special sensory examinations are usually normal.

3. *Sensory-Motor (Receptive-Expressive).* This consists of inability to comprehend and express oneself and is probably the most common type in children and adults. It may be associated with speech disturbances similar to the receptive type.

4. *Global or Central Aphasia.* The child cannot use symbols or language for any purpose. All processes are interfered with.

VISUAL APHASIA

Congenital Word Blindness (developmental alexia). In this type of aphasia there is inability to comprehend the written or printed word and as a result the child reads poorly. In some there is poor writing as well (agraphia). These children have a normal visual apparatus and mentality. However, they tend to develop mirror reading or mirror writing, i.e., there is a reversal in their visualization of words—"was" becomes "saw," "god" becomes "dog," or "on" becomes "no." These mistakes are made when reading or writing. Letters similar in appearance are confused, such as p and q, b and d.

The name of strephosymbolia or twisted symbols was given by Orton to these reversals. These children can do arithmetic well, speak fluently, and read musical notes correctly, but their reading ability is several years below their mental level.

The etiology of this condition has been ascribed to failure of unilateral cerebral dominance by Orton. Other authors have indicated as factors emotional tensions, unstable personality, disturbances in visual-motor pattern organization, and abnormal conditions associated with birth. Drew regards dyslexia or primary-reading retardation as a defect in Gestalt function and states that not only reading, but also writing, spatial orientation, and auditory-visual integration are involved, perhaps due to a failure of maturation of the parietal lobes. The reversals, mirror writing, mixed hand-eye preference, spatial disorientation, and phonetic disintegration which are basic in congenital dyslexia are thus looked upon as due to a fundamental defect in correct figure-background recognition. This holds for both familial and nonfamilial congenital dyslexia. The familial form of congenital dyslexia has an autosomal dominant mode of inheritance.

DIAGNOSIS: Aphasia in children is rare and difficult to diagnose. Obviously defects in vision or hearing or a low IQ indicate that one is not dealing primarily with aphasia. If the mentality is normal and special sensory tests are normal, there may be a personality disturbance with emotional immaturity.

Special tests should be carried out to determine handedness (see how the ball is thrown, preferred hand in writing) and eyedness (sighting with microscope or through a hole in a cardboard). Mental testing should include the general level of intelligence, educational achievement tests, and personality tests as needed (Rorschach, Bender, Visual-Gestalt, Drawing of a Figure).

In general, these children are found to be normal intellectually and physically; yet they fail to develop speech. In the reading disability type there is normal performance elsewhere in school work. All of these disabilities occur mainly in boys.

TREATMENT: There are various points which should be considered in therapy. Educationally, visual and tactile methods as well as speech training should be utilized for the speech aphasias. For the visual type of aphasia with reading difficulties remedial reading methods under trained personnel should be employed. In all forms of aphasia early recognition will aid in preventing the personality and behavior problems which develop along with and probably because of aphasia. Psychiatric help may be needed. Early diagnosis by the physician, full discussion of the problems with the parents, and proper specialty assistance are the requirements for good therapy. Obviously, in acquired aphasia the problem is one of prevention by treating the meningitis, etc., early and actively.

Drew, A. L.: A Neurological Appraisal of Familial Congenital Word-Blindness. Brain 79:440, 1956.

Kanner, Leo: Child Psychiatry. Springfield, Ill. Chas. C. Thomas, 2nd ed. 1948.

Karlin, I. W.: Aphasias in Children. Am. J. Dis. Child, 87:752, 1954.

Kawi, A. A. and Pasamanick, B.: Association of Factors of Pregnancy with Reading Disorders in Childhood. J.A.M.A. 166:1420, 1958.

Krynauw, R. A.: Infantile Hemiplegia Treated by Removing One Cerebral Hemisphere. J. Neurol. Neurosurg. & Psychiat. 13:243, 1950.

Landau, W. M. and Kleffner, F. R.: Syndrome of Acquired Aphasia with Convulsive Disorder in Children. Neurology 7:523, 1957.

Laub, G. R.: Aphasia after Meningitis. Am. J. Dis. Child. 72:728, 1946.

Myklebust, H. R.: Auditory Disorders in Children. New York, Grune & Stratton, 1954.

Nance, L. S.: Differential Diagnosis of Aphasia in Children, Speech Disorders, 11:219, 1946.

Orton, S. T.: Reading, Writing and Speech Problems of Children: A Presentation of Certain Types of Disorders in the Development of the Language Faculty. New York, W. W. Norton & Company, 1937.

Penfield, W., and Rasmussen, T.: The Cerebral Cortex of Man: A Clinical Study of Localization of Function. New York, The Macmillan Co. 1950.

——— and Jasper, H.: Epilepsy and the Functional Anatomy of the Human Brain. Boston, Little, Brown & Co. 1954.

Schuell, H.: A Short Examination for Aphasia. Neurology 7:625, 1957.

Van Gelder, D. W., Kennedy, L., and Laguaite, J.: Congenital and Infantile Aphasia. New Orleans, Med. and Surg. J. 104:241, 1951.

STUTTERING

In stuttering there is a break or interruption in the rhythmic progress of speech, with repetition of words, syllables, or sounds due to tonic and clonic spasms of the muscles involved in speech. Stuttering and stammering are used interchangeably.

CLINICAL PICTURE: The onset of stuttering usually occurs from two to five years of age. It is normal during this early period for occasional moments of hesitation to occur as the child speaks; he will grope for a word or repeat one. It is a period when new ideas and experiences are constantly crowding in. Most children go on to develop fluency. Some, however, become more tense, begin to repeat more frequently, and develop muscle spasms, including those of the tongue, larynx, and muscles of respiration. Parental anxiety becomes marked and may become evident to the child. He now senses that something is wrong with the way he speaks, even though he may not have been too aware of this before. Thus, anxiety and subjective tension begin to develop. This is referred to as primary stuttering. In older children and young adolescents associated personality distortions may develop (secondary stuttering) and facial grimaces appear. Anxiety, fear of stuttering, and psychological disturbances are added to the primary stuttering picture. Physical examination, including neurological, is generally normal. The organs involved in speech show no neuromuscular abnormalities and the electroencephalogram shows no significant pattern.

ETIOLOGY: Next to the disorders of articulation, stuttering is the most frequent cause of speech disturbance in children. It occurs about four times more often in boys and is often noted in more than one member of a family. A number of theories have been offered to explain stuttering.

Heredity. This theory postulates a relationship between stuttering and heredity. The objection to this idea is that in the stutterer there are no physical or neurological characteristics which are specific or different from the normal. The condition is found in children with a high degree of intelligence as well as in those mentally retarded. There is, however, a definite familial tendency, with a greater percentage of stutterers in families of stutterers (33 per cent) against a control of 9 per cent (Johnson).

Karlin has proposed that delayed myelinization of the cortical association areas associated with speech is the basic cause of stuttering. Earlier myelinization in the female might be correlated with less stuttering. He concedes the importance of psychologic and environmental factors.

Handedness. This theory was expounded by Orton and Travis. They believe that there is a dominance of one cortical hemisphere. In most individuals this consists of left cortical dominance with selective use of the right side (dextral). This control is expressed in handedness, eyedness, speech, and footedness. When there is no cortical dominance and hence no preferred laterality, or when, as in a sinistral (right cortical dominance with use of the left side), there is an attempt to effect conversion to the right hand which is incomplete, so that again there is lack of dominance, confusion results, with speech disturbances such as stuttering. No difference in the two hemispheres anatomically or psysiologically is postulated. It is purely one of function.

Psychological. Many hold stuttering to be psychological due to emotional difficulties, fear states, psychoneurosis, or disturbed parent-child relationships. Van Ryper gives a list of causes and states that because of the "stress felt by most children, if driven by their parents, they try too swiftly to master the art of talking in phrases and sentences." This last is probably the most common cause.

TREATMENT: The child's stuttering should be managed by treating the parents. First, the latter should be given reassurance that complete study has revealed no abnormalities of vision, hearing, or neuromuscular function of the organs of speech. Then the parents should be told of the importance of good family relationships and of avoiding emotional outbursts and quarreling in front of the youngster. The child should not be corrected or interrupted in his speech by parents or teachers. He should not be advised to speak slowly, etc., as these criticisms draw his attention to the stuttering and make him fearful. The subjects or words which produce the child's block should be avoided. Whatever value derives from the theory of laterality should be taken advantage of by encouraging one-sided dominance.

In the later age period of childhood and adolescence with the onset of secondary stuttering, the psychological and personality problems come into play. There is now marked anxiety and fear of stuttering. Therefore, irrespective of the cause, therapy should be directed toward lessening the child's fear and tension. Tranquilizing drugs may be tried as an adjunct. In some children psychotherapy may be required.

PROGNOSIS: Most stuttering disappears in adult life, especially if early treatment is instituted. In some the outlook is poorer as emotional and environmental factors produce a disordered personality.

Blau, A.: The Master Hand. Research Monographs—No. 5. American Orthopsychiatric Ass. New York, 1946.

Bloomer, H. H.: Speech and Language Disorders—A Summary of a Round Table. Pediat. 20:738, 1957.

Barbara, D. A.: Stuttering. A. Psychodynamic Approach to Its Understanding and Treatment. New York, The Julian Press, 1954.

Johnson, W.: Speech Handicapped School Children. New York, Harper & Bros., 1948.

Karlin, I. W.: Stuttering—Evaluation and Treatment. New York State J. Med. 56:3719, 1956.
———: Speech- and Language-Handicapped Children. A.M.A. J. Dis. Child. 95:370, 1958.
Travis, L. E.: Speech Pathology. New York, D. Appleton-Century Co., 1931.
Van Riper, C. V.: Speech Correction—Principles and Method. Ed. 3. New Jersey, Prentice-Hall, 1954.
Lillywhite, H.: Doctor's Manual of Speech Disorders. J.A.M.A. 167:850, 1958.

DISORDERS OF HEARING

The loss of hearing in an infant or child is reflected in the failure to develop speech which may be utilized for normal communication. The incidence of deafmutism is 1/3000. About 5% of children of school age are said to have a hearing loss based on a pathological condition. When an infant or child has not developed speech (deaf-mute), there are four major considerations as to the etiology. First, there may be involvement of the end organ for hearing, either congenital or acquired. Other causes include aphasia, emotional and psychological factors, and mental deficiency. Myklebust studied 228 children between the ages of six months and eight years who were referred during one year for lack of speech development. In 45 per cent of the children the difficulties in speech were due to hearing deficiency.

Deafness may be congenital or acquired. In most all instances the deafness is not total, and the hearing loss is largely in the high frequencies. The loss of hearing is due to involvement of the middle ear, labyrinth, cochlear branch of the eighth nerve, or its end organ of Corti. In congenital deafness, which comprises about 50 per cent of all cases, there is in most instances failure of development or malformation of the saccule and membranous cochlea. These are heredofamilial cases. Genetic transmission is usually recessive, sometimes dominant. Kinney reported that of 186 cases of bilateral congenital deafness, 59 or 32 per cent were of the true Mendelian type.

Other factors in congenital deafness include malformation of the external or middle ear, viral infections, maternal syphilis, and drug intoxications such as quinine or salicylates. Occasionally birth injury may play a role. Erythroblastosis might be included as a prenatal factor. When kernicterus occurs, deafness, either central (cranial nuclei) or peripheral, may develop. In the Rh group there may be combined deafness and aphasia (refer to references for complete discussion).

In the acquired type, meningitis, encephalitis, acoustic neuritis (viral), and reaction to inoculation may affect the nerve pathways to produce difficulties in perception of sound with ultimate effect on speech. Conduction deafness in older children may originate from obstruction of the Eustachian tube by lymphoid tissue and recurrent middle ear infections.

CLINICAL PICTURE: In early infancy the parents may note that the baby does not respond to the closing of a door or other sounds or does not vocalize much, but usually no real significance is attached to the infant's behavior until the end of the first year, when it is evident that the baby fails to comprehend or is not speaking with understandable words. The tone of the voice is not varied and is harsh. Tests may be tried at this age, especially when the parents are deaf-mute, for they wish to know as early as possible if the baby can hear. One of these tests consists of striking a tuning fork or making a loud noise and observing if the eye lids blink. This is a reflex reaction and is not too exact. Psychogalvanic skin resistance audiometry (PGSR) may be utilized, if available. Another technique makes use of the conditioned reflex. A variety of other tests involving the use of sound instruments, toys, or whispered voice may be tried.

DIAGNOSIS: Deafness should be suspected in any child who has not developed normal speech by two years of age. Its presence should be established by various methods of testing hearing, including audiometry in the older child. A careful history should be obtained, including any familial loss of hearing, the type of pregnancy, especially as to maternal infections, the labor, and any post natal infections. The examination should include a complete neurological survey and also tests for vision and vestibular function as well as hearing. Finally, a complete psychological study should be performed, not only for the intellectual level but also for personality and emotional development. A mentally deficient child will also show delay in speech. Distinguishing between deafness and mental retardation is an important differential. The child with deafness and normal I.Q. is likely to show up normally in mental testing. He is active, uses gestures, watches lip movements, and makes use of visual and tactile stimuli. The retarded child will earn a low I.Q. on mental tests, and his behavior in speech and understanding will be compatible with his intellectual level. Another differential must be made from children with normal I.Q. and normal hearing who have psychological difficulties. The severe cases may show the autistic behavior characteristic of the childhood schizophrenic or the hyperactivity and poor attention span of the brain-injured child. In others there is fear of speech caused by too much parental concern or criticism or no speech because all needs are anticipated. Finally, aphasia must be differentiated. In aphasia the intelligence and hearing are normal, but the child cannot understand the spoken word or express himself through speech (receptive or expressive aphasia). Refer to the section on aphasia for the discussion of this subject.

TREATMENT: The problem must be completely discussed with the parents. Trained specialists should be utilized for speech therapy. Hardy and Paul state that children whose hearing is impaired down to 75 db. below normal can make use primarily of audition for language comprehension, and secondarily of vision. They state that the child can learn to hear by amplification and constant use of speech in the home and can then be given training in language skill. If below 75 db. he should learn mainly by vision and attend a school for the deaf.

Management of the psychological types of hearing loss will require advice by the physician as to the proper handling of the child. The speech problem is only a part of the total maladjustment, and with improvement in the parent-child relationship the speech retardation will be rectified. In the case of the emotionally immature child for whom everything is being done by the parents so that the child does not require speech to fulfill his needs, the therapeutic procedure is obvious. In the severe psychological disorders psychiatry may be needed. Aphasics must have specific therapy. The lack of speech in the retarded is part of the entire problem of mental deficiency.

PROGNOSIS: If deafness is recognized early, before school age, 75 per cent have a good outlook. They can be habilitated. In older children rehabilitation must be carried out. These children need special education as soon as deafness is discovered. The parents must be educated to accept it. A hearing aid should be used even in an infant as soon as deafness is discovered, and auditory training should be given. Speech training (lip reading) must be added to auditory training of sounds.

Dix, M. R. and Hallpike, C. S.: The Peep Show: A New Technique for Pure-Tone Audiometry in Young Children. Brit. Med. J. 2:719, 1947.

Hardy, W. G. and Bordley, J. E.: Special Techniques in Testing the Hearing of Children. J. Speech Disorders, 16:123, 1951.

——— and Pauls, M. D.: The Test Situation in PGSR Audiometry. J. Speech and Hearing Disorders, 17:13, 1952.

——— and Pauls, M. D.: Hearing Disorders—Symposium on Hearing, Speech and Reading Difficulties in Children. Pediat. 12:81, 1953.

Herman, G.: Hearing Problems. A Summary of a Round Table. Pediat. 20:739, 1957.

Kinney, C. E.: The Pathology of Hereditary Deafness. Ann. Otology, Rhinology and Laryngology. 59:1117, 1950.

Lurie, M. H.: The Membranous Labyrinth in the Congenitally Deaf Collie and Dalmation Dog. Laryngoscope 58:279, 1948.

Myklebust, H. R.: Auditory Disorders in Children. New York, Grune & Stratton, 1954.

Stephens, F. E. and Dolowitz, D. A.: Hereditary Nerve Deafness. Am. J. Human Genet. 1:37, 1949.

Rh Child: Deaf or 'Aphasic.'

Cohen, P.: 'Aphasia' in Kernicterus. J. Speech & Hearing Disorders, 21:411, 1956.

Goodhill, V.: Clinical Pathologic Aspects of Kernicteric Nuclear 'Deafness.' J. Speech & Hearing Disorders, 21:407, 1956.

Hannigan, H.: Language and Behavior Problems of the Rh 'Aphasic' Child. J. Speech & Hearing Disorders, 21:413, 1956.

Myklebust, H. R.: Some Psychological Considerations of the Rh Child. J. Speech & Hearing Disorders, 21:423, 1956.

Rosen, J.: Variations in the Auditory Disorders of the Rh Child. J. Speech & Hearing Disorders, 21:418, 1956.

INDEX

INDEX